Imaging of the Reproductive Age Female

Editor

LIINA PÕDER

RADIOLOGIC CLINICS OF NORTH AMERICA

www.radiologic.theclinics.com

Consulting Editor
FRANK H. MILLER

March 2020 • Volume 58 • Number 2

ELSEVIER

1600 John F. Kennedy Boulevard ● Suite 1800 ● Philadelphia, Pennsylvania, 19103-2899

http://www.theclinics.com

RADIOLOGIC CLINICS OF NORTH AMERICA Volume 58, Number 2
March 2020 ISSN 0033-8389, ISBN 13: 978-0-323-68195-7

Editor: John Vassallo (j.vassallo@elsevier.com)
Developmental Editor: Donald Mumford

Radiologic Clinics of North America (ISSN 0033-8389) is published bimonthly by Elsevier Inc., 360 Park Avenue South, New York, NY 10010-1710. Months of issue are January, March, May, July, September, and November. Periodicals postage paid at New York, NY and additional mailing offices. Subscription prices are USD 513 per year for US individuals, USD 980 per year for US institutions, USD 100 per year for US students and residents, USD 594 per year for Canadian individuals, USD 1253 per year for Canadian institutions, USD 703 per year for international individuals, USD 1253 per year for international institutions, USD 100 per year for Canadian students/residents, and USD 315 per year for international students/residents. To receive student and resident rate, orders must be accompanied by name of affiliated institution, date of term and the signature of program/residency coordinatior on institution letterhead. Orders will be billed at individual rate until proof of status is received. Foreign air speed delivery is included in all *Clinics* subscription prices. All prices are subject to change without notice. **POSTMASTER:** Send address changes to *Radiologic Clinics of North America*, Elsevier Health Sciences Division, Subscription Customer Service, 3251 Riverport Lane, Maryland Heights, MO63043. **Customer Service: Telephone: 1-800-654-2452** (U.S. and Canada); **1-314-447-8871** (outside U.S. and Canada). **Fax: 1-314-447-8029. E-mail: journalscustomerservice-usa@elsevier.com (for print support); journalsonlinesupport-usa@elsevier.com (for online support)**.

Reprints. For copies of 100 or more of articles in this publication, please contact the Commercial Reprints Department, Elsevier Inc., 360 Park Avenue South, New York, New York 10010-1710. Tel.: +1-212-633-3874; Fax: +1-212-633-3820; E-mail: reprints@elsevier.com.

Radiologic Clinics of North America also published in Greek Paschalidis Medical Publications, Athens, Greece.

Radiologic Clinics of North America is covered in *MEDLINE/PubMed (Index Medicus), EMBASE/Excerpta Medica, Current Contents/Life Sciences, Current Contents/Clinical Medicine, RSNA Index to Imaging Literature, BIOSIS, Science Citation Index,* and *ISI/BIOMED*.

Contributors

CONSULTING EDITOR

FRANK H. MILLER, MD, FACR
Lee F. Rogers MD Professor of Medical
Education, Chief, Body Imaging Section and
Fellowship Program, Medical Director, MRI,
Department of Radiology, Northwestern
Memorial Hospital, Northwestern University
Feinberg School of Medicine, Chicago, Illinois,
USA

EDITOR

LIINA PÕDER, MD
Professor of Clinical Radiology, Obstetrics,
Gynecology, and Reproductive Sciences,
Director of Ultrasound, Department of
Radiology and Biomedical Imaging, University
of California, San Francisco, San Francisco,
California, USA

AUTHORS

MATTHIAS BARRAL, MD, PhD
Department of Radiology, Service de
Radiologie A, Hopital Cochin, APHP &
Université de Paris-Paris 5, Paris, France

SPENCER C. BEHR, MD
Associate Professor of Clinical Radiology,
Department of Radiology and Biomedical
Imaging, University of California, San
Francisco, San Francisco, California, USA

CHARIS BOURGIOTI, MD
First Department of Radiology, School of
Medicine, National and Kapodistrian University
of Athens, Aretaieion Hospital, Athens, Greece

HAILEY H. CHOI, MD
Assistant Professor of Radiology, Department
of Radiology and Biomedical Imaging,
University of California, San Francisco,
San Francisco, California, USA

JESSE COUTIER, MD
Associate Professor, Department of Radiology,
UCSF Benioff Children's Hospital,
San Francisco, California, USA

ANTHONY DOHAN, MD, PhD
Department of Radiology, Service de
Radiologie A, Hopital Cochin, APHP &
Université de Paris-Paris 5, Paris, France

RANIA FAROUK EL SAYED, MD, PhD
Head, Cairo University MRI Pelvic Floor Center
of Excellency and Research Lab Unit, Assistant
Professor, Department of Radiology, Faculty of
Medicine, Cairo University Hospitals, Cairo,
Egypt

KIREMA GARCIA-REYES, MD
Department of Radiology and Biomedical
Imaging, University of California, San
Francisco, San Francisco, California, USA

JEAN M. HANSEN, DO, MS
Assistant Professor, Department of Obstetrics/
Gynecology, Michigan Medicine, Ann Arbor,
Michigan, USA

NICOLE HINDMAN, MD
Associate Professor of Radiology and Surgery,
NYU Radiology, NYU Grossman School of
Medicine, New York, New York, USA

KYLE K. JENSEN, MD
Assistant Professor, Department of Diagnostic
Radiology, Oregon Health & Science
University, Portland, Oregon, USA

PRIYANKA JHA, MBBS
Department of Radiology and Biomedical
Imaging, University of California, San
Francisco, San Francisco, California, USA

ANNE KENNEDY, MB BCh BAO
Professor of Radiology and Imaging Sciences,
Co-director, Maternal Fetal Diagnostic Center,
University of Utah, Salt Lake City, Utah, USA

NADIA J. KHATI, MD, FACR
Associate Professor, Department of Radiology,
Abdominal Imaging Section, George
Washington University Hospital, Washington,
DC, USA

TAMMY KIM, MD
Resident, Department of Radiology,
Abdominal Imaging Section, George
Washington University Hospital, Washington,
DC, USA

MAUREEN P. KOHI, MD, FSIR
Department of Radiology and Biomedical
Imaging, University of California, San
Francisco, San Francisco, California, USA

MARIANNA KONIDARI, MD
First Department of Radiology, School of
Medicine, National and Kapodistrian University
of Athens, Aretaieion Hospital, Athens, Greece

GABRIELE MASSELLI, MD
Department of Radiology, Umberto I Hospital,
Sapienza University, Rome, Italy

KATHERINE E. MATUREN, MD, MS
Associate Professor, Department of Radiology
and Obstetrics/Gynecology, Michigan
Medicine, Ann Arbor, Michigan, USA

BRYCE A. MERRITT, MD
Clinical Fellow, Diagnostic Radiology,
Department of Radiology and Biomedical
Imaging, University of California, San
Francisco, San Francisco, California, USA

FRANK H. MILLER, MD, FACR
Lee F. Rogers MD Professor of Medical
Education, Chief, Body Imaging Section and
Fellowship Program, Medical Director, MRI,
Department of Radiology, Northwestern
Memorial Hospital, Northwestern University
Feinberg School of Medicine, Chicago, Illinois,
USA

PARDEEP K. MITTAL, MD
Professor, Department of Radiology, Medical
College of Georgia, Augusta, Georgia, USA

COURTNEY C. MORENO, MD
Associate Professor, Department of Radiology
and Imaging Sciences, Emory University
School of Medicine, Atlanta, Georgia, USA

LIA ANGELA MOULOPOULOS, MD
Professor of Radiology, Chair, First
Department of Radiology, School of Medicine,
National and Kapodistrian University of Athens,
Aretaieion Hospital, Athens, Greece

STEPHANIE NOUGARET, MD, PhD
Montpellier Cancer Research Institute,
INSERM, U1194, University of Montpellier,
Department of Radiology, Montpellier Cancer
Institute, Montpellier, France

MICHAEL A. OHLIGER, MD, PhD
Associate Professor of Radiology, Department
of Radiology and Biomedical Imaging,
University of California, San Francisco,
San Francisco, California, USA

JEFFREY DEE OLPIN, MD
Professor of Radiology, University of Utah
Health Sciences Center, Salt Lake City, Utah,
USA

LIINA PÕDER, MD
Professor of Clinical Radiology, Obstetrics,
Gynecology, and Reproductive Sciences,
Director of Ultrasound, Department of
Radiology and Biomedical Imaging, University
of California, San Francisco, San Francisco,
California, USA

SACHA PIERRE, BSc, MBBS, MRCS, FRCR
Department of Radiology, St James's
University Hospital, Leeds, United Kingdom

RANA RABEI, MD
Department of Radiology and Biomedical
Imaging, University of California,
San Francisco, San Francisco, California,
USA

JOANNA RIESS, MD
Clinical Assistant Professor, Department of
Radiology, Abdominal Imaging Section,
George Washington University Hospital,
Washington, DC, USA

JESSICA ROBBINS, MD
University of Wisconsin-Madison School of
Medicine and Public Health, Madison,
Wisconsin, USA

MEHTAB SAL, BA
Medical Student, Department of Diagnostic
Radiology, Oregon Health & Science
University, Portland, Oregon, USA

MARTINA SBARRA, MD
Radiologia Diagnostica e Interventistica
Generale, Dipartimento Diagnostica per
Immagini, Radioterapia Oncologica ed
Ematologia, Fondazione Policlinico
Universitario A. Gemelli IRCCS, Istituto di
Radiologia, Università Cattolica del Sacro
Cuore, Rome, Italy

DOROTHY SHUM, MD
Associate Professor, Department of Radiology,
University of California, San Francisco,
San Francisco, California, USA

ROYA SOHAEY, MD
Professor, Department of Diagnostic
Radiology, Oregon Health & Science
University, Portland, Oregon, USA

PHILIPPE SOYER, MD, PhD
Department of Radiology, Service de
Radiologie A, Hopital Cochin, APHP &
Université de Paris-Paris 5, Paris, France

ERICA B. STEIN, MD
Assistant Professor, Department of Radiology,
Michigan Medicine, Ann Arbor, Michigan, USA

LORETTA STRACHOWSKI, MD
Professor of Radiology, University of California,
San Francisco, San Francisco, California, USA

WENDALINE VANBUREN, MD
Assistant Professor of Radiology, Mayo Clinic,
Rochester, Minnesota, USA

SHERRY S. WANG, MBBS
Assistant Professor, Department of Radiology
and Imaging Sciences, University of Utah, Salt
Lake City, Utah, USA

MICHAEL WESTON, MB ChB, MRCP, FRCR
Department of Radiology, St James's
University Hospital, Leeds, United Kingdom

Contents

This article discusses the 4 main imaging modalities used to evaluate reproductive-aged women: ultrasound, magnetic resonance imaging, computed tomography, and fluoroscopy. For each modality, major clinical indications are described, along with important technical considerations unique to imaging reproductive-aged women. Finally, key safety issues are discussed, particularly with regard to imaging pregnant patients.

Infertility, or subfertility, is the inability to achieve a clinical pregnancy after a 1-year period of regular unprotected sexual intercourse in women younger than 35 and after 6 months in women older than 35. Although initial assessment involves a multitude of factors, including a detailed medical history, physical examination, semen analysis, and hormonal evaluation, diagnostic imaging of the female partner often plays an important role in establishing the etiology for infertility. This article provides an overview of the multimodality imaging assessment of female infertility and details the developmental and acquired pelvic abnormalities in which diagnostic imaging aids in evaluation.

Infertility, or subfertility, is the inability to achieve a clinical pregnancy after a 1-year period of regular unprotected sexual intercourse in women younger than 35 and after 6 months in women older than 35. Although initial assessment involves a multitude of factors, including a detailed medical history, physical examination, semen analysis, and hormonal evaluation, diagnostic imaging of the female partner often plays an important role in establishing the etiology for infertility. This article provides an overview of the multimodality imaging assessment of female infertility and details the developmental and acquired pelvic abnormalities in which diagnostic imaging aids in evaluation.

Benign uterine diseases are common gynecologic conditions affecting women of all ages. Ultrasonography is traditionally the first-line imaging technique but patients are increasingly referred to magnetic resonance (MR) imaging because it is more accurate for diagnosis and patient management. This article highlights the added value of MR imaging in the diagnosis of the most common benign uterine diseases, describes therapeutic options, and delineates the role of MR imaging in treatment planning.

evaluation and laboratory testing are essential, imaging plays a central role. Although various adnexal and uterine disorders may result in acute pelvic pain of gynecologic origin, other nongynecologic disorders of the gastrointestinal and genitourinary systems may likewise result in acute pelvic pain. Ultrasound is first choice for initial evaluation of acute pelvic pain of gynecologic origin. Computed tomography is performed if pelvic sonography is inconclusive, or if a suspected disorder is nongynecologic in origin.

 Video content accompanies this article at http://www.radiologic.theclinics.com.

Pelvic pain in the first trimester is nonspecific, with causes including pregnancy complications, pregnancy loss, and abnormal implantation, and symptom severity ranges from mild to catastrophic. Ultrasonography is the imaging modality of choice and essential to evaluate for the location of pregnancy, either intrauterine or not. If there is an intrauterine pregnancy, ultrasonography helps assess viability. If there is not an intrauterine pregnancy, ultrasonography helps assess for abnormal implantation, which accounts for a high percentage of maternal morbidity and mortality.

Abdominal pain is a common occurrence in pregnant women and may have a variety of causes, including those that are specific to pregnancy (eg, round ligament pain in the first trimester) and the wide range of causes of abdominal pain that affect men and women who are not pregnant (eg, appendicitis, acute cholecystitis). Noncontrast magnetic resonance (MR) imaging is increasingly performed to evaluate pregnant women with abdominal pain, either as the first-line test or as a second test following ultrasonography. The imaging appearance of causes of abdominal pain in pregnant women are reviewed with an emphasis on noncontrast MR imaging.

Placenta is a vital organ that connects the maternal and fetal circulations, allowing exchange of nutrients and gases between the two. In addition to the fetus, placenta is a key component to evaluate during any imaging performed during pregnancy. The most common disease processes involving the placenta include placenta accreta spectrum disorders and placental masses. Several systemic processes such as infection and fetal hydrops can too affect the placenta; however, their imaging features are nonspecific such as placental thickening, heterogeneity, and calcifications. Ultrasound is the first line of imaging during pregnancy, and MR imaging is reserved for problem solving, when there is need for higher anatomic resolution.

Gynecologic cancers impact women of all ages. Some women may wish to preserve their capacity for future childbearing. With appropriate patient selection, acceptable oncologic outcomes may be achieved with preservation of fertility. Determination of eligibility for fertility preservation is guided by patient factors, tumor histology, and preoperative local staging with pelvic MR imaging. The aim of this article is to educate radiologists on the current guidelines for fertility-sparing techniques in women with early stage cervical, endometrial, and ovarian malignancies.

Gynecologic malignancies are common among cancers diagnosed during pregnancy, especially those of cervical and ovarian origin. Imaging is an important part of the diagnosis, staging, and follow-up of pregnancy-associated gynecologic tumors, with sonography and magnetic resonance (MR) imaging being the most suitable modalities. MR imaging is particularly useful in cervical cancer for the evaluation of tumor size, nodal, and extrapelvic disease. Ovarian tumor is initially diagnosed with sonography; MR imaging should be performed in cases of indeterminate ultrasonography findings and for staging. Pregnancy-related changes may be responsible for erroneous diagnosis; radiologists should be aware of such pitfalls to avoid misinterpretation.

There are various complications that can occur in the postpartum period, including pain, bleeding, and infection. These include complications related to cesarean section, postpartum hemorrhage and hematomas, bladder injury, torsion and uterine dehiscence, and rupture. It is important the radiologist is aware of these entities and the associated imaging features to help guide timely and appropriate management.

Radiological guided intervention techniques are discussed in obstetric and gynecologic patients. Fallopian tube recanalization, postpartum hemorrhage control, techniques of treating uterine leiomyomas, pelvic congestion treatment, and the use of percutaneous and transvaginal ultrasonography-guided aspirations and biopsy are covered. These techniques use basic radiological interventional skills and show how they are adapted for use in the female pelvis.

PROGRAM OBJECTIVE
The objective of the *Radiologic Clinics of North America* is to keep practicing radiologists and radiology residents up to date with current clinical practice in radiology by providing timely articles reviewing the state of the art in patient care.

TARGET AUDIENCE
Practicing radiologists, radiology residents, and other healthcare professionals who provide patient care utilizing radiologic findings.

LEARNING OBJECTIVES
Upon completion of this activity, participants will be able to:
1. Review the role of imaging in the evaluation of acute pelvic pain in both pregnant and nonpregnant patients.
2. Discuss imaging modalities used to evaluate reproductive age females, specifically clinical indications and technical considerations.
3. Recognize how radiological intervention techniques are adapted for use in the female pelvis.

ACCREDITATION
The Elsevier Office of Continuing Medical Education (EOCME) is accredited by the Accreditation Council for Continuing Medical Education (ACCME) to provide continuing medical education for physicians.

The EOCME designates this journal-based CME activity for a maximum of 16 *AMA PRA Category 1 Credit*(s)™. Physicians should claim only the credit commensurate with the extent of their participation in the activity.

All other healthcare professionals requesting continuing education credit for this enduring material will be issued a certificate of participation.

DISCLOSURE OF CONFLICTS OF INTEREST
The EOCME assesses conflict of interest with its instructors, faculty, planners, and other individuals who are in a position to control the content of CME activities. All relevant conflicts of interest that are identified are thoroughly vetted by EOCME for fair balance, scientific objectivity, and patient care recommendations. EOCME is committed to providing its learners with CME activities that promote improvements or quality in healthcare and not a specific proprietary business or a commercial interest.

The planning committee, staff, authors and editors listed below have identified no financial relationships or relationships to products or devices they or their spouse/life partner have with commercial interest related to the content of this CME activity:
Matthias Barral, MD, PhD; Spencer C. Behr, MD; Charis Bourgioti, MD; Hailey H. Choi, MD; Anthony Dohan, MD, PhD; Rania Farouk El Sayed, MD, PhD; Kirema Garcia-Reyes, MD; Jean M. Hansen, DO, MS; Nicole Hindman, MD; Kyle K. Jensen, MD; Priyanka Jha, MBBS; Marilu Kelly, MSN, RN, CNE, CHCP; Nadia J. Khati, MD, FACR; Tammy Kim, MD; Marianna Konidari, MD; Pradeep Kuttysankaran; Gabriele Masselli, MD; Bryce A. Merritt, MD; Frank H. Miller, MD, FACR; Pardeep K. Mittal, MD; Courtney C. Moreno, MD; Lia Angela Moulopoulos, MD; Stephanie Nougaret, MD, PhD; Michael A. Ohliger, MD, PhD; Jeffrey Dee Olpin, MD; Liina Põder, MD; Sacha Pierre, BSc, MBBS, MRCS, FRCR; Rana Rabei, MD; Joanna Riess, MD; Jessica Robbins, MD; Mehtab Sal, BA; Martina Sbarra, MD; Dorothy Shum, MD; Roya Sohaey, MD; Philippe Soyer, MD, PhD; Erica B. Stein, MD; Loretta Strachowski, MD; Wendaline VanBuren, MD; John Vassallo; Sherry S. Wang, MBBS; Michael Weston, MB ChB, MRCP, FRCR.

The planning committee, staff, authors and editors listed below have identified financial relationships or relationships to products or devices they or their spouse/life partner have with commercial interest related to the content of this CME activity:
Jesse Coutier, MD is a consultant/advisor and owns stock in Sira Medical.

Anne Kennedy, MB BCh BAO recieves royalties from Elsevier.

Maureen P. Kohi, MD, FSIR is a consultant/advisor for Boston Scientific Corporation, Cook, Medtronic, Penumbra, Inc., and Koninklijke Philips N.V.

Katherine E. Maturen, MD, MS recieves royalties from Elsevier and Wolters Kluwer.

UNAPPROVED/OFF-LABEL USE DISCLOSURE
The EOCME requires CME faculty to disclose to the participants:
1. When products or procedures being discussed are off-label, unlabelled, experimental, and/or investigational (not US Food and Drug Administration [FDA] approved); and
2. Any limitations on the information presented, such as data that are preliminary or that represent ongoing research, interim analyses, and/or unsupported opinions. Faculty may discuss information about pharmaceutical agents that is outside of FDA-approved labelling. This information is intended solely for CME and is not intended to promote off-label use of these medications. If you have any questions, contact the medical affairs department of the manufacturer for the most recent prescribing information.

TO ENROLL

To enroll in the *Radiologic Clinics of North America* Continuing Medical Education program, call customer service at 1-800-654-2452 or sign up online at http://www.theclinics.com/home/cme. The CME program is available to subscribers for an additional annual fee of USD 330.

METHOD OF PARTICIPATION

In order to claim credit, participants must complete the following:

1. Complete enrolment as indicated above.
2. Read the activity.
3. Complete the CME Test and Evaluation. Participants must achieve a score of 70% on the test. All CME Tests and Evaluations must be completed online.

CME INQUIRIES/SPECIAL NEEDS

For all CME inquiries or special needs, please contact elsevierCME@elsevier.com.

RADIOLOGIC CLINICS OF NORTH AMERICA

RELATED SERIES

Magnetic Resonance Imaging Clinics
Neuroimaging Clinics
PET Clinics

THE CLINICS ARE AVAILABLE ONLINE!
Access your subscription at:
www.theclinics.com

RADIOLOGIC CLINICS OF NORTH AMERICA

Preface

Modern Imaging of Reproductive Age Women: Image Soundly and Wisely

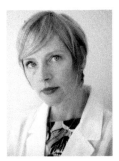

Liina Põder, MD
Editor

This issue focuses on a multimodality approach to imaging the reproductive age woman. The spectrum of diseases and physiologic changes unique to this patient population, with updated imaging guidelines, are carefully addressed. This comprehensive information is directly applicable to daily practice.

In this modern day and age, we as imagers tend to focus more on the advancements and benefits of a particular modality rather than the complementary aspect of different modalities and patients as a whole. Ultrasound remains the primary imaging modality in this patient population, yet it is important to recognize its limitations and acknowledge when and how to utilize MR imaging and computed tomography in a proper clinical setting. These modalities stand not alone nor are competitive with each other, but on the contrary, they complement each other.

I am very grateful for the expertise, time, and dedication of the talented world-class authors who have contributed to this well-composed, beautifully illustrated, and unique constellation of articles. Many of the authors are internationally known experts in their field, and I am very appreciative of the time and efforts they put into this collaboration. Many of the authors are members of the Society of Ultrasound in Radiology, the Society of Abdominal Radiology Uterine and Ovarian Disease Focused Panel members, or the European Society of Gastrointestinal and Abdominal Radiology. I would like to acknowledge these societies for advocating advancements in women's health and imaging and introducing me to these wonderful colleagues. I am appreciative of all my colleagues, at home or abroad, who teach and inspire me daily to be a better radiologist, to keep up the spirit of enthusiasm amid viewing challenging cases, and all the while being part of a patient's difficult life experience.

I would like to thank my husband, Daniel, daughter, Hanna, and our dog, Luna, for putting up with the demands of my calling as my profession. Also, I would like to acknowledge my mother, Raili Põder, who encouraged as well as inspired me to pursue this path.

Finally, and most importantly, I would like to thank *Radiologic Clinics of North America* for choosing this topic to promote sound and wise imaging of the reproductive age woman.

Liina Põder, MD
Clinical Radiology
Obstetrics, Gynecology
and Reproductive Sciences
Department of Radiology and Biomedical Imaging
University of California
San Francisco, 505 Parnassus Avenue, L-374,
San Francisco, CA 94143-0628, USA

E-mail address:
liina.poder@ucsf.edu

radiologic.theclinics.com

Imaging Safety and Technical Considerations in the Reproductive Age Female

Michael A. Ohliger, MD, PhD[a,*], Hailey H. Choi, MD[a], Jesse Coutier, MD[b]

KEYWORDS

• Female pelvis • MR imaging • CT • Ultrasound • HSG • Technique • Safety

KEY POINTS

- Ultrasound (US), magnetic resonance imaging (MR imaging), computed tomography (CT), and fluoroscopy (hysterosalpingography) are all important imaging tools for evaluating reproductive-aged women.
- US typically is the initial study of choice, followed by MR imaging for problem solving.
- CT is useful for nonlocalized symptoms or in situations, such as trauma, where rapid, comprehensive evaluation of the abdomen and pelvis is required.
- Fluoroscopy, in the form of hysterosalpingography, has important specialized applications.
- Because MR imaging and US do not use ionizing radiation, they generally are considered safer than CT. Important safety considerations remain, however, particularly when imaging pregnant patients.

INTRODUCTION

Imaging women who are reproductive age is challenging. The uterus and ovaries are deep within the pelvis; their positions and orientations are highly variable. In addition, the appearance of these organs may vary depending on several factors, including patient age and stage of menstrual cycle. Relatively rare pathologic entities must be distinguished from common benign findings and normal variants. It also is necessary to minimize the use of ionizing radiation. Finally, there are unique safety considerations when imaging pregnant patients.

The most common tools that are used to image reproductive-aged women are ultrasound (US) and magnetic resonance imaging (MR imaging). Both of these tools offer excellent anatomic detail and soft tissue contrast without exposure to ionizing radiation. US generally is used for initial evaluation whereas MR imaging typically is used for problem solving when US is either indeterminant or discordant with the overall clinical picture.[1] Computed tomography (CT) is used principally in the setting of acute pain or other situation where full abdominal and pelvic coverage is required (cancer staging, for example). The use of CT is limited, however, because it involves ionizing radiation and also because it has relatively poor soft tissue contrast in the ovaries and uterus. Finally, fluoroscopy—in the form of hysterosalpingography (HSG)—has a specialized role in evaluating the patency of the fallopian tubes.

This article describes the general approach to using each of these modalities, along with important technical considerations as well as safety issues unique to imaging women who are reproductive age. Specific diseases as well as

a Department of Radiology and Biomedical Imaging, University of California, San Francisco, Box 0628, 1001 Potrero Avenue, 1X55D, San Francisco, CA 94110, USA; b Department of Radiology, UCSF Benioff Children's Hospital, 1975 4th Street C1758P, San Francisco, CA 94158, USA
* Corresponding author.
E-mail address: Michael.ohliger@ucsf.edu

Radiol Clin N Am 58 (2020) 199–213
https://doi.org/10.1016/j.rcl.2019.10.003

specialized techniques are described in later articles. This article focuses on general approaches that can be used to improve image quality and maximize diagnostic information.

ULTRASOUND

US typically is the initial study of choice when imaging women who are reproductive age.[2,3] It is relatively inexpensive with excellent spatial resolution and soft tissue contrast. In many cases, blood flow detected on Doppler imaging is helpful for diagnosis, including vascular tumors,[4] polyps,[5] retained products of conception,[6] vascular anomalies,[7] and ovarian torsion.[8] Because US avoids the use of ionizing radiation, it generally is safe and lends itself to performing serial follow-ups and surveillance.

Ultrasound Imaging Approach

The detailed US scanning protocol is based on the exact clinical indication. Typically, both transabdominal and transvaginal images are obtained. Transabdominal images are obtained using a full urinary bladder as the acoustic window, whereas transvaginal images are obtained with the bladder empty. Although transvaginal images may have higher resolution for structures close to the US probe, transabdominal images are key for detecting extrauterine abnormalities, abdominal fluid, and hydronephrosis. When the uterus is enlarged or ovaries are superior in position, they are seen better transabdominally than transvaginally.

Measurements

Measurements of anatomic structures and masses are made along 3 axes—longitudinal, transverse, and anteroposterior—relative to the structure being imaged. Imaging relative to these axes can be challenging if the uterus has an oblique orientation or is retroverted. Color and spectral Doppler imaging is essential to detect and characterize blood flow. For example, a central vascular stalk is a helpful feature for diagnosing endometrial polyps. It is important that proper Doppler technique is used, adjusting scale, gain, and angle.

Three-dimensional reconstructions

Three-dimensional (3-D) reconstructions can be useful for many applications, including assessing the uterine contour in suspected uterine anomalies and establishing the location of intrauterine devices.[9]

Stage of menstrual cycle

With pelvic US, patient age and phase in menstrual cycle are crucial, because the endometrium and ovaries can appear different throughout a patient's life.[10] For detecting endometrial abnormalities, the early proliferative phase (immediately after menses) is the best timeframe; the endometrium is thinnest during this phase. Ovaries in a reproductive-aged woman also can undergo changes related to ovulation.

Ultrasound Safety

Heating

Because US relies on sound waves and avoids ionizing radiation, it generally is considered safe compared with alternative techniques, such as CT. No harmful effects from US have been described in humans. Based primarily on animal studies, however, there are theoretic risks from tissue heating, particularly in early gestation.[11] With this in mind, a prudent approach is to (1) perform US only when it is medically indicated[12] and (2) minimize the use of techniques associated with high-power deposition, such as power Doppler, early in pregnancy.[11]

Infection

Because US probes come in close contact with skin and mucosal surfaces, there is a risk of spreading infection between patients. When probe covers are used together with disinfectant wipes (low-level disinfection), persistent microbial DNA can be found on transvaginal probes.[13] Therefore, a meticulous cleaning program is recommended, including the use of transducer covers and high-level disinfection of transvaginal transducers and handles.[14,15]

COMPUTED TOMOGRAPHY

CT provides reliable and comprehensive evaluation of the abdomen and pelvis in a short scan time and is used frequently for the assessment of acute symptoms. Because CT requires radiation exposure and lacks the soft tissue contrast of MR imaging and US,[16] it often is not the initial study of choice in evaluating reproductive-aged women. CT is useful in the evaluation of abdominal pain when initial US is negative or equivocal. It also is useful in situations, such as cancer staging, where comprehensive evaluation of the entire abdomen and pelvis is necessary. Finally, CT is used in situations, such as major abdominal trauma, where rapid evaluation is critical and techniques, such as US, are less sensitive, particularly for parenchymal injury.

Computed Tomography Technique

CT in reproductive-aged women is performed using an approach similar to that used for other patients. Intravenous contrast generally is useful unless contraindicated. As with any patient, radiation exposure should be minimized by eliminating unnecessary contrast phases, restricting the anatomic scan coverage, and using dose-reduction techniques, such as tube current modulation[17] and iterative reconstructions.[18]

Computed Tomography Safety

CT has two major risks. First, there is risk from contrast administration, which in younger patients is predominantly allergy or allergy-like reactions.[19] There also is a risk from ionizing radiation exposure. Although the exact radiation risk from radiation in medical procedures is complex, younger patients likely are more sensitive to the effects of radiation.[20] Therefore, nonradiation alternatives, such as US and MR imaging, are preferentially used in younger patients when possible, particularly when serial examinations are needed. That said, concerns of radiation exposure should not prevent a patient from undergoing a CT examination when medically necessary.

Because of potential risks to the developing embryo or fetus, special considerations are required for using CT in pregnant patients. First, before using techniques that require x-ray exposure to the pelvis, pregnancy status should be confirmed, either through history or urine/blood testing.[21] Radiation doses less than 50 mGy convey a negligible risk for miscarriage, malignancy, or major malformation. Most radiological examinations, including single-phase CT examinations, are within this level. Caution should still be exercised, however, especially when multiple CT scans are required, including consultation with a medical physicist to verify dose.[21] Informed consent in these cases should be considered.

MAGNETIC RESONANCE IMAGING

MR imaging of the female pelvis is central to the clinical evaluation of both benign and malignant diseases.[22,23] In patients with endometrial and cervical cancers, the superior soft tissue contrast achieved by MR imaging allows for highly accurate assessment of local tumor extension as well as metastatic disease. In terms of benign disease, MR imaging is a key tool in preoperative planning for treatment of leiomyomas[24] and assessing müllerian duct anomalies.[25,26] Chemical sensitivity inherent in the MR imaging scan permits the identification of fat-containing masses, such as teratomas. Increasingly, functional techniques, such as diffusion-weighted imaging (DWI)[27,28] and dynamic contrast imaging, are permitting new insights into tumor biology.[28,29]

Pelvis Magnetic Resonance Imaging Pulse Sequences and Imaging Approach

Broadly speaking, at the authors' institution, MR imaging of the female pelvis contains 3 types of pulse sequences that are tailored to the application at hand. Pelvic MR imaging is performed using both 1.5T and 3.0T scanners. In all cases, a dedicated phased array coil is placed directly over the anatomy of interest in order to maximize sensitivity. In addition to general imaging sequences, described in this article, specialized pulses sequences and image planes may be obtained for certain applications (for example, in suspected pelvic malignancies, uterine anomalies, or abnormally invasive placenta). Those specialized approaches are discussed in other articles within this issue.

High-resolution T2-weighted imaging

The most important imaging sequence for evaluating the female pelvis is the T2-weighted fast spin-echo (FSE) without fat saturation.[30] Images have excellent tissue contrast and spatial resolution. Ovaries and uterus are well seen, along with clear delineation of important fascial planes.

Diffusion-weighted imaging

In DWI, strong magnetic field gradients are used to generate image contrast that is proportional to the amount of freedom water molecules have to move within tissues. In general, pelvic malignancies tend to be more cellular and, therefore, have higher DWI signal (and lower apparent diffusion coefficient). Low apparent diffusion coefficient can be seen, however, in both benign tumors and non-neoplastic processes, such as hemorrhage and infection.[31] DWI can aid in the detection of lymph nodes[32] and peritoneal metastases.[33]

Chemical shift imaging

T1-weighted images are obtained with fat and water in-phase and opposed-phase. Signal dropout on opposed-phase images establishes the presence of fat that is smaller than the image voxel (eg microscopic fat). Black lines, or india ink, at the interface between structures establishes the presence of bulk fat.[34]

Contrast enhancement

T1-spoiled gradient-echo sequences with fat saturation are obtained before and after administration of a gadolinium-based contrast agent (GBCA). Lesion enhancement may establish the presence of suspicious solid nodules. High T1 signal in a cystic lesion before the administration of intravenous contrast can indicate the presence of blood products in either an endometrioma or hemorrhagic cyst. Because these lesions have high T1 signal prior to administration of contrast, subtraction images may be useful in detecting enhancing nodules against an already bright background[35] (Fig. 1).

Magnetic Resonance Imaging Technique

This section addresses several common technical challenges that are encountered when performing MR imaging of the female pelvis.

T2-weighted images and fat suppression
When imaging the female pelvis with MR imaging, T2-weighted images performed without fat suppression are crucial. Fat within the pelvis allows clear delineation of fascial planes and anatomic boundaries, which are important for judging (among other things) the local extent of tumors. When fat suppression is used, high signal intensity within pelvic vessels as well as fluid in the pelvis can obscure these anatomic planes (Fig. 2).

Phase encoding direction
Unlike imaging in the abdomen, MR imaging of the female pelvis typically is performed while the patient breathes freely. This is possible because the deep pelvic organs, such as the uterus and ovary, tend to be fairly static. Considerable artifact may be generated, however, from motion of the anterior abdominal wall. When the phase encoding direction is chosen anterior-posterior (which is the direction used in the pelvis), these motion artifacts potentially obscure anatomic details within the uterus. Changing the phase encoding direction to

left-right, however, these artifacts are pushed to the side in a more benign pattern (Fig. 3).[36]

Choosing the field of view
The imaging field of view (FOV) must be chosen to match the anatomy being imaged. Many times, the FOV is made overly large in order to avoid missing things, but a large FOV leads to larger pixel sizes and coarser spatial resolution, which may make important structures, such as the uterus, difficult to evaluate. Because the uterus in particular can vary in size from one woman to another, depending on age, pregnancy, and the presence of masses, it is difficult to use a one-size-fits-all approach. Instead, the FOV can be adjusted at the time of the scan (Fig. 4).

Tailored image planes
MR imaging acquisitions in the female pelvis usually are tailored to answer specific questions, for example, assessing the depth of invasion of an endometrial mass or parametrial extension of a cervical tumor (Fig. 5). Making these choices correctly requires careful communication between radiologists and technologists and requires both parties to speak a common language and understand the physical principles involved.

Coil array positioning
Most pelvic MR imagings are acquired using an array of radiofrequency (RF) surface coils.[37] These coil arrays are composed of 8 to 32 detector coils placed over the part of the body that is being imaged (Fig. 6A). Coil arrays have increased sensitivity for objects close to the coil elements, and they experience decreased noise from regions that are not being imaged. In addition, coil arrays

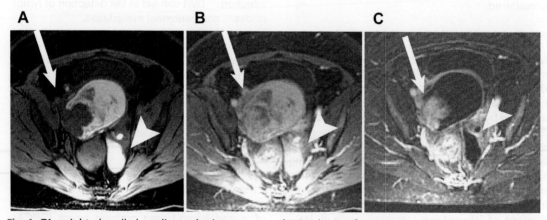

Fig. 1. T1-weighted spoiled gradient-echo images were obtained using fat saturation (A) prior to and (B) after administration of gadolinium contrast. A right-sided adnexal mass demonstrated hyperintensity on T1-weighted images both before and after contrast. (C) Subtraction images clearly showed the enhancing mass (*long arrow*). Pathology revealed endometrioid adenocarcinoma. The left fallopian tube (*arrowhead*) showed no enhancement on subtraction images and at surgery was found to be a hematosalpinx.

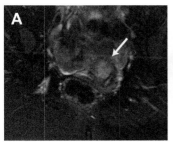 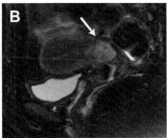

Fig. 2. T2-weighted FSE images performed using fat saturation in the (A) axial and (B) sagittal planes. A mass is seen in the cervix (arrow), but there is decreased contrast between the mass, cervical stroma, and parametrial fat. The parametrial fat has similar signal intensity to the cervical mass, which can limit the evaluation of parametrial extension.

permit the use of parallel imaging techniques that can speed up the acquisition.[38]

Because the sensitive regions of RF surface coils are highly localized, accurate positioning is critical. The positioning of surface coils can be best checked using the sagittal scout image, shown in **Fig. 6**B. In this image, the positions of the anterior and posterior surface coils

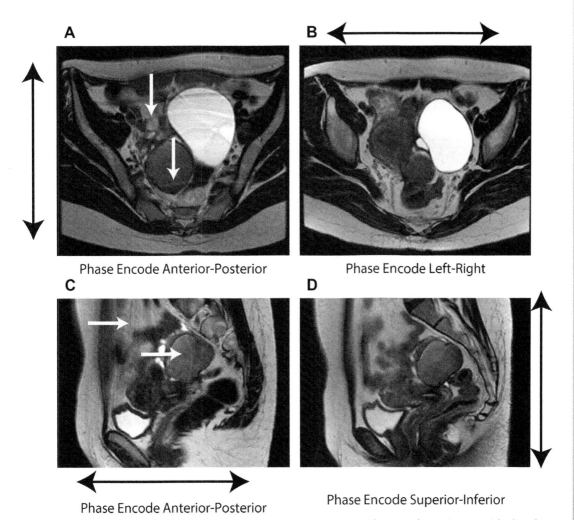

Fig. 3. (A) T2-weighted FSE image through the pelvis in a woman with an endometrioma. With the phase encoding direction in the anterior-posterior direction, artifacts due to respiratory motion are observed over the pelvis (arrows). (B) When the phase encoding direction is changed to the left-right direction, the motion is spread in a much more benign fashion. A similar effect is seen in the sagittal plane changing the phase encoding direction from (C) anterior-posterior (artifact indicated by arrows) to (D) superior-inferior.

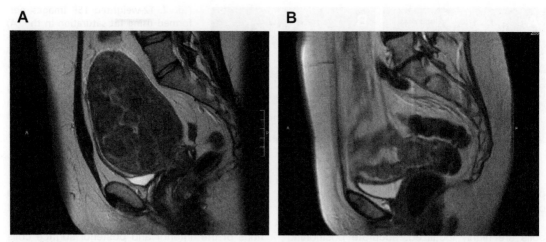

Fig. 4. (*A*) Sagittal FSE acquisition of a woman with a large myoma, in which a large FOV is necessary. (*B*) Using the same FOV in a woman with an atrophic uterus leads to a loss of spatial resolution, preventing assessment of the endometrium.

can be seen as bright spots anterior and posterior to the patient, respectively. Image slices that are obtained from outside of the sensitive volume (see **Fig. 6**B) can have severely degraded signal-to-noise ratio (SNR) compared with image slices acquired from within the sensitive volume (see **Fig. 6**B). The scout image, therefore, provides an excellent tool for checking

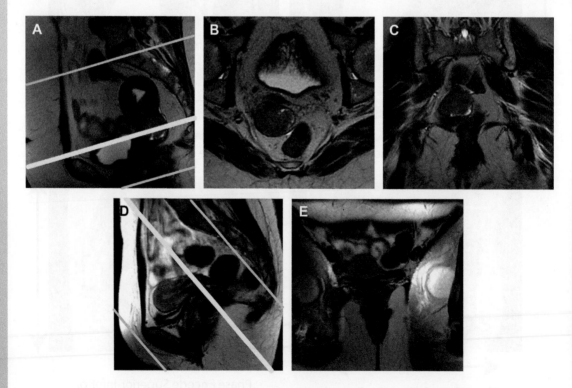

Fig. 5. (*A*) Tailored image planes (*yellow line*) are chosen perpendicular to the axis of the cervix in a patient with a cervical mass. (*B*) The axis of the plane allows precise definition of the mass with respect to cervical stroma and vaginal wall. (*C*) By contrast, a coronal image plane that extends obliquely through the tumor may give the appearance of parametrial extension. (*D*, *E*) Incorrectly obtained oblique images, where the image plane (indicated by the yellow line) is chosen perpendicular to the vagina and not the cervix or endometrium, leading to the image obtained in *E*.

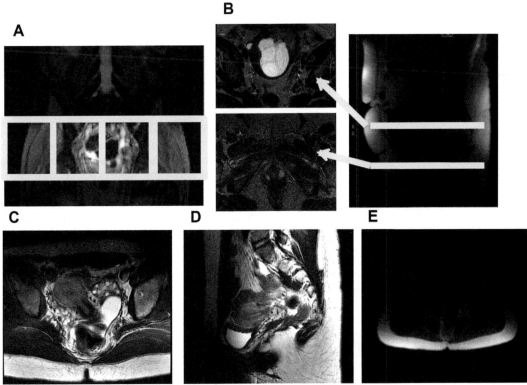

Fig. 6. (A) Schematic diagram illustrating the use of RF coil arrays to increase the sensitivity to local structures, with multiple coil elements (*yellow squares*), allowing imaging over a large FOV. (B) Two axial images in a woman with an adnexal mass showing a large difference in SNR from axial slices obtained inside (*top slice*) and outside (*bottom slice*) of the sensitive region of the coil array. The scout image (*right*) allows the sensitive region of the coil array to be seen as a region of increased coil sensitivity. Yellow lines within the scout image on the right panel illustrate the locations of the slices in the left panels. (C) Axial and (D) sagittal FSE acquisition acquired in a patient where the anterior coil elements were not used. Because diagnostic images are corrected for variations in coil sensitivity, problem is manifest by increased noise anteriorly. (E) Axial scout image from the same patient showing the anterior coil elements are clearly missing.

coil array placement and troubleshooting image quality.

Vaginal gel

Distension of the vagina with gel, which is bright on T2-weighted images, can help with assessment of cervical or vaginal lesions, including tumors and endometriosis-related implants.[39–41] Disadvantages of using gel include increased complexity and possible artifacts if air bubbles are introduced.

Antiperistaltics

Antiperistaltic agents, such as glucagon (1 mg, intravenous or intramuscular) or butylscopolamine can be used to reduce small bowel peristalsis, which can improve image quality (butylscopolamine *is not* approved for use by the US Food and Drug Administration).[41,42] The drawbacks of using these agents include expense, side effects, and

nursing required to administer the medication. Contraindications to glucagon include diabetes and known pheochromocytoma. At the authors' institution, anitperistaltics are used in situations where bowel involvement is a specific question, such as in the evaluation of deep pelvic endometriosis.

New Magnetic Resonance Imaging Approaches

In recent years, new approaches to T2-weighted imaging and DWI of the pelvis have been introduced. These new sequences are available on all MR imaging scanner platforms and have potential advantages and disadvantages.

Three-dimensional fast spin-echo

Conventional T2-weighted FSE images of the pelvis are obtained in a 2-dimensional (2-D) slice-by-slice fashion using multiple image planes. Lack of isotropic voxels makes reformatting into oblique image planes more of a challenge. Recently, 3-D approaches have become available (CUBE [GE], SPACE [Siemens], and VISTA [Philips]). In these approaches, an entire volume is acquired at once, typically with thinner slices. 3-D acquisitions are much more efficient in terms of SNR and also allow reformats into multiple image planes. These approaches can be particular useful in the assessment of uterine anomalies (Fig. 7).[26,43] Small studies comparing 3-D and 2-D techniques for cervical and endometrial cancer have found improved SNR in the 3-D sequence and no difference in accuracy of staging[44]; 3-D FSE also has been used in the assessment of endometriosis.[45]

PROPELLER

T2-weighted PROPELLER (BLADE [Siemens] and MultiVane [Philips]) uses a unique approach to filling k-space with radial blades in order to reduce motion artifacts (Fig. 8). The center of k-space is repeatedly acquired as part of each blade, which reduces motion artifacts.[46] Artifacts can occur if too few blades are acquired.[47] Small studies comparing PROPELLER to conventional FSE at 1.5T have shown a reduction in motion artifacts and improved subjective image quality.[48,49]

Novel diffusion techniques

Standard DWI is based on echo planar imaging, in which all the MR imaging data for a given slice are acquired in 1 shot and, therefore, is prone to many artifacts. In general, these artifacts are caused by errors accumulated during the acquisition. Recently, novel techniques have been introduced that seek to improve DWI by reducing the amount of data that needs to be acquired at once. These techniques operate by either reducing the required FOV[50,51] or breaking the diffusion acquisition into multiple smaller segments.[52,53]

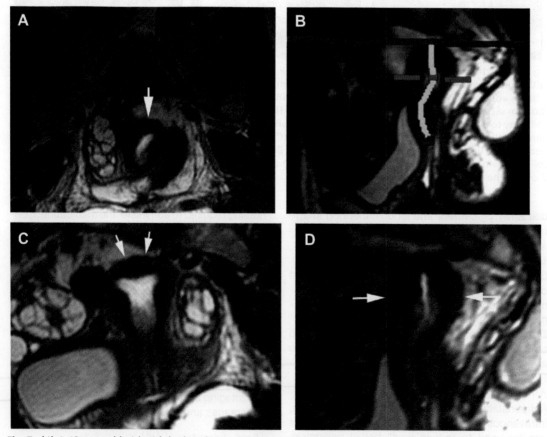

Fig. 7. (A) A 13-year-old girl with hydrosalpinx and pelvic pain. Primary coronal acquisition 3-D T2-weighted FSE image of the pelvis demonstrating the oblique orientation of the uterus (arrow). (B) Sagittal reformatted 3-D T2-weighted based on the primary data used for planning (green line, red line, and blue line) of a curved planar reformatted image of the uterus in the same patient. (C) Curved planar reformatted image aligned in the plane coronal and (D) sagittal to the uterine fundus (arrows) in the same patient.

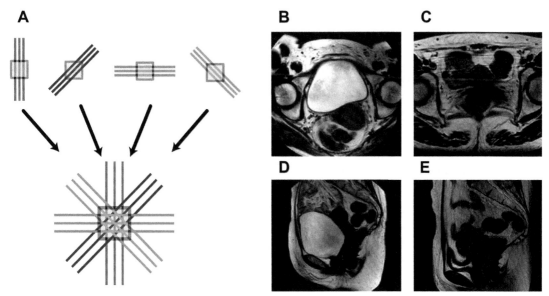

Fig. 8. (*A*) Schematic diagram illustrating the k-space filling pattern used in the PROPELLER acquisition. Each excitation acquires a series of blades, which are gradually rotated and composed to make the full *k*-space. Because each blade traverses the center of *k*-space (*pink rectangle*), the center of *k*-space is oversampled, making this technique robust to motion. (*B*) Axial and (*D*) sagittal FSE acquisitions in a patient with cervical cancer acquired using the PROPELLER sequence. The lack of motion artifact can be contrasted with (*C*) axial and (*E*) sagittal conventional 2-D FSE acquisition in the same patient who had follow-up imaging several months later.

Magnetic Resonance Imaging Safety

MR imaging is generally considered a safe imaging modality, particularly for reproductive-aged women, because it does not entail the use of ionizing radiation. Despite the lack of long-term risks associated with radiation exposure, MR imaging does pose several short-term risks. These risks include (1) magnetic objects becoming projectiles if they are inadvertently brought into the scanner room, (2) tissue heating from RF pulses, (3) peripheral nerve stimulation from magnetic field gradients, and (4) incompatible implanted devices.[54,55] These risks can be ameliorated through a formal MR imaging safety program, which includes training of personnel, screening of both personnel and patients, strict access control to the MR imaging environment, and careful attention to scan parameters that affect RF hearing and nerve stimulation. In nonpregnant women, these risks are similar to those of the general population and are discussed in other references.[54,55] The next section focuses on special issues that may arise when imaging pregnant patients using MR imaging.[56]

Magnetic Resonance Imaging and Pregnancy

For pregnant women undergoing noncontrast MR imaging, there have been no proved harmful effects to the developing embryo or fetus. Despite the lack of proven risk, are 3 main theoretic risks from MR imaging that can be considered. First, RF heating—especially during the first trimester—may potentially affect the embryo. Second, the presence of strong magnetic fields has been shown to increase double-strand DNA breaks in chick embryos. Finally, loud noises created by magnetic field gradients potentially have an effect on hearing.

Although several of these effects have been observed in animal models or isolated cells, it is uncertain how important these effects are in humans. In a large study of more than 1700 children exposed to MR imaging during the first trimester, no increase in adverse outcomes was observed.[57] A vast majority of scans were performed at a magnetic field strength of 1.5T. A second study examined 751 neonates exposed to 1.5T MR imaging at a variety of gestational ages and found no significant difference in either birth weight or hearing loss compared with a matched group of neonates who did not receive MR imaging.[58]

Fewer data are available regarding exposure to MR imaging at 3.0T. At 3.0T, both the levels of RF heating and acoustic noise potentially are greater. One recent study in a relatively small number of neonates (n = 62) found no significant difference in the rate of hearing loss in those exposed in utero to 3.0T MR imaging compared with those exposed to 1.5T MR imaging.[59]

In light of the available data, the American College of Radiology and Society for Pediatric Radiology pregnant patients "may be accepted to undergo MR examinations at stage in pregnancy" if the attending radiologist agrees that the benefit of the examination outweighs these theoretic risks.[60] In view of the fact that there may be rare risks that have not been identified in studies to date, it is prudent to perform MR imaging only in cases where the information cannot be obtained by other means; the information is used for treatment of the fetus or patient during pregnancy and where it is not possible to wait the patient delivers to obtain that information.[54]

Intravenous Contrast and Pregnancy

GBCAs are considered class C agents in pregnancy, meaning the risks to the fetus are unknown. Many GBCAs cross the placenta and are excreted into amniotic fluid. Studies in nonhuman primates have shown that although the amount of GBCA decreases with time, trace amounts of gadolinium are still found in bones and liver after delivery.[61] Furthermore, in the study, discussed previously, of neonates exposed to MR imaging during pregnancy, gadolinium-enhanced scans were associated with rheumatological-like conditions after delivery.[57] Because of the unknown risks associated with gadolinium, it is recommended that GBCAs should not be routinely administered during pregnancy and should be used only on a case-by-case basis, when the information provided by gadolinium is absolutely necessary.[60]

HYSTEROSALPINGOGRAPHY

HSG refers to fluoroscopic evaluation of the uterine cavity and fallopian tubes. HSG is used primarily for evaluating the fallopian tubes in the setting of infertility. HSG also can confirm tubal occlusion or patency after tubal ligation or reversal of tubal ligation.[62] With recent advances in reproductive medicine and a trend toward later pregnancies, HSG is becoming more common, and radiologists should be aware of several key technical and safety considerations.[62]

HSG is highly accurate in detecting tubal abnormalities. A recent meta-analysis has found HSG 94% sensitive and 92% specific in detecting tubal occlusion.[63] HSG also may be therapeutic in precipitating a pregnancy, because women were observed more likely to conceive within the first 3 months to 4 months after HSG than in other time periods,[64,65] although there are no randomized controlled studies to validate this. A recent study[65] found that women who had undergone oil-based HSG, compared with water-based HSG, had higher pregnancy rates; however, the safety of oil-based HSG should be considered, because there are cases of pulmonary and cerebral oil emboli reported in literature.[66,67]

Main contraindications to HSG include ongoing pregnancy, active pelvic infection, and severe reaction to iodinated contrast, because contrast reactions can occur even with nonvascular administration.[68]

Hysterosalpingography Technique

Timing of the examination

HSG is best performed in the follicular phase of the menstrual cycle, when the endometrium is thinnest and there are fewer chances of pregnancy. Per American College of Radiology practice guidelines,[69] HSG should be performed in day 7 to day 10 of the menstrual cycle, although some practitioners may perform the examination as late as day 12.[62] There is no consensus on timing for patients with amenorrhea or irregular menses; some possibilities include abstinence for 14 days prior to HSG[70] or urine or serum beta human chorionic gonadotropin tests.[62,69]

Premedication

For patients with a history of pelvic inflammatory disease or known tubal abnormalities, prophylactic (preprocedure) antibiotics can be considered.[71] Patients may be advised to take nonsteroidal anti-inflammatory drugs (NSAIDs) 1 hour before the examination to minimize discomfort.[62]

Preparation

Prior to the procedure, the radiologist should ensure there are no contraindications to the study and obtain informed consent. After discussion, the radiologist prepares the instruments in a sterile manner, and the patient is placed supine on the fluoroscopy table in the lithotomy position.

Procedure

HSG technique involves a speculum examination, cannulation of the cervix with aseptic technique, and fluoroscopic imaging of the uterine cavity and fallopian tubes while instilling water-soluble contrast. At the authors' institution, a 5-French or 7-French HSG catheter, clear plastic speculum, betadine, ring forceps, and water-soluble contrast are used (Fig. 9A). It is important to flush the catheter with contrast prior to examination, because injected air can mimic filling defects within the uterine cavity (Fig. 10).

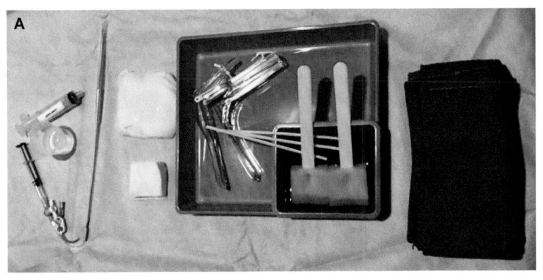

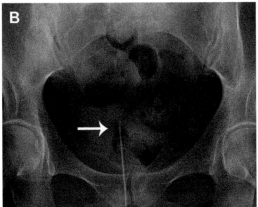
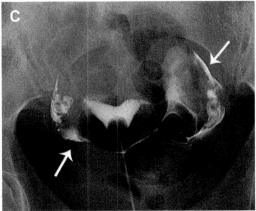

Fig. 9. (A) Tray containing materials necessary for a HSG. From left to right: HSG catheter, speculum, betadine sponges, and sterile towels. O-ring tongs are not imaged. (B) A 37-year-old woman with primary infertility who was referred for fluoroscopic HSG. Scout image of the pelvis prior to contrast instillation, demonstrating inflated balloon (arrow) placed in the lower uterine segment. (C) Spot radiograph after instillation of water-soluble contrast demonstrates free spillage from both fallopian tubes along the pelvic sidewalls (arrows).

After applying betadine to the cervix, the HSG catheter is advanced gently and the balloon is inflated within the lower uterine segment. After the speculum is removed, a supine scout view is obtained (see Fig. 9B). Under real-time fluoroscopy, contrast is instilled slowly into the uterine cavity. Fluoroscopic videos and spot radiographs are obtained to capture early uterine filling,

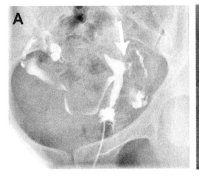
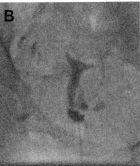

Fig. 10. (A) Spot images from an HSG showing a round filling defect in the left of the endometrial cavity (arrow) that (B) does not exist on other images obtained during filling. This likely reflects an introduced air bubble.

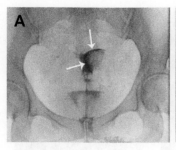
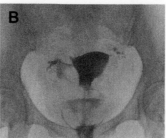

Fig. 11. A 36-year-old woman with secondary infertility referred for HSG. Early filling fluoroscopic image (*A*) demonstrates rounded filling defect (*arrows*) along the left uterine body, which corresponded to a large submucosal fibroid on prior pelvic US (not shown). The filling defect is less perceptible on a fluoroscopic image obtained after further contrast filling (*B*).

opacification of the uterine horns and fallopian tubes, and free spillage into the peritoneal cavity, with the patient in supine and bilateral oblique positions (Fig. 11). Near the end of the examination, the balloon is deflated, and fluoroscopic evaluation of the endocervical canal also is performed.

Hysterosalpingography Safety

Complications

Complications from HSG include infection, contrast reaction, and, rarely, severe bleeding and perforation. HSG has a 1.4% to 3.4% rate of infection.[71] At the authors' institution, postprocedure antibiotics are given at the discretion of referring clinicians; for this reason, the authors communicate findings of hydrosalpinx or tubal occlusion when encountered. Although nonvascular applications of iodinated contrast result in fewer complications, several anaphylactoid reactions from HSG have been reported; exposure can occur directly from the uterus and fallopian tubes, venous and lymphatic intravasation, and peritoneal spillage.[68] Severe bleeding and perforation are rare complications.[62]

Adverse effects

Many women experience discomfort (cramping) from distension of the uterine cavity, which is typically mild and self-limited, occurring during the procedure and for a few hours after.[62] This can be managed with over-the-counter NSAIDs. Patients should expect mild postprocedural bleeding, which also typically lasts less than 24 hours.[62] Rarely, women experience severe pain and vasovagal reactions during the procedure.

HSG is contraindicated in pregnancy, for potential pregnancy loss and teratogenic effects from radiation and contrast. However, in a series of 10 cases of inadvertent HSGs performed in pregnant patients from 1937 to 1964, all continued to normal pregnancy.[72]

Radiation

For an HSG with real-time fluoroscopy (0.3 minutes of average fluoroscopy time) and spot radiographs (on average, 3.2 radiographs), the average radiation dose to the female gonads is 2.7 mGy and the effective dose is 1.2 mSv.[73] To put this into perspective, the annual background radiation is 3.1 mSv sand that of a screening mammogram is 0.4 mSv.[74] In terms of biological effects for a future embryo, the risk for anomalies and fatal cancer induction depends on the age of the women; for a patient of 20 to 29 years of age, the risk for anomaly is 2.7×10^{-5} and for cancer induction is 14.5×10^{-5}, both 1000-fold lower than the background rates.[73] Although the radiation doses and theoretic risks are not large, every effort should be made to minimize radiation exposure.

SUMMARY

Multiple tools are available for imaging women who are reproductive age. US is the first-line choice in many circumstances, but MR imaging is an important problem-solving tool. CT is most valuable in people presenting with nonlocalized symptoms or trauma, where rapid comprehensive evaluation is necessary. Fluoroscopy, in the form of HSG, has important specialized applications. US and MR imaging are generally considered safe because they do not use ionizing radiation. There are still several important technical and safety considerations, however, particularly for imaging pregnant women.

DISCLOSURE

Dr Coutier is a consultant and shareholder in Sira Medical (augmented reality software company).

REFERENCES

1. Poder L, Qayyum A, Goldstein RB. Use of MR imaging for further evaluation of sonographically detected adnexal pathology. Obstet Ultrasound Gynecol Ultrasound 2006;1(2):357–83.
2. Benacerraf BR, Abuhamad AZ, Bromley B, et al. Consider ultrasound first for imaging the female pelvis. Am J Obstet Gynecol 2015;212(4):450–5.

3. Coccia ME, Rizzello F, Romanelli C, et al. Adnexal masses: what is the role of ultrasonographic imaging? Arch Gynecol Obstet 2014;290(5):843–54.

4. Brown DL, Dudiak KM, Laing FC. Adnexal masses: US characterization and reporting. Radiology 2010; 254(2):342–54.

5. Amreen S, Singh M, Choh NA, et al. Doppler evaluation of endometrial polyps. Egypt J Radiol Nucl Med 2018;49(3):850–3.

6. Sellmyer MA, Desser TS, Maturen KE, et al. Physiologic, histologic, and imaging features of retained products of conception. Radiographics 2013;33(3): 781–96.

7. Polat P, Suma S, Kantarcý M, et al. Color Doppler US in the evaluation of uterine vascular abnormalities. Radiographics 2002;22(1):47–53.

8. Chang HC, Bhatt S, Dogra VS. Pearls and pitfalls in diagnosis of ovarian torsion. Radiographics 2008; 28(5):1355–68.

9. Sakhel K, Benson CB, Platt LD, et al. Begin with the basics: role of 3-dimensional sonography as a first-line imaging technique in the cost-effective evaluation of gynecologic pelvic disease. J Ultrasound Med 2013;32(3):381–8.

10. Langer JE, Oliver ER, Lev-Toaff AS, et al. Imaging of the female pelvis through the life cycle. Radiographics 2012;32(6):1575–97.

11. Abramowicz JS. Benefits and risks of ultrasound in pregnancy. Semin Perinatol 2013;37(5):295–300.

12. Rados C. FDA cautions against ultrasound "Keepsake" images. FDA Consum 2004;38(1):12.

13. M'Zali F, Bounizra C, Leroy S, et al. Persistence of microbial contamination on transvaginal ultrasound probes despite low-level disinfection procedure. PLoS One 2014;9(4):e93368.

14. Nyhsen CM, Humphreys H, Koerner RJ, et al. Infection prevention and control in ultrasound - best practice recommendations from the European Society of Radiology Ultrasound Working Group. Insights Imaging 2017;8(6):523–35.

15. American Institute of Ultrasound in Medicine. Guidelines for Cleaning and Preparing External- and Internal-Use Ultrasound Transducers Between Patients & Safe Handling and Use of Ultrasound Coupling Gel. Available at: https://www.aium.org/accreditation/Guidelines_Cleaning_Preparing.pdf.

16. Balan P. Ultrasonography, computed tomography and magnetic resonance imaging in the assessment of pelvic pathology. Eur J Radiol 2006;58(1):147–55.

17. Kalra MK, Maher MM, Toth TL, et al. Techniques and applications of automatic tube current modulation for CT. Radiology 2004;233(3):649–57.

18. Ehman EC, Yu L, Manduca A, et al. Methods for clinical evaluation of noise reduction techniques in abdomino-pelvic CT. RadioGraphics 2014;34(4):849–62.

19. Sodagari F, Mozaffary A, Wood CG, et al. Reactions to both nonionic iodinated and gadolinium-based contrast media: incidence and clinical characteristics. Am J Roentgenol 2018;210(4):715–9.

20. Brenner DJ, Elliston CD, Hall EJ, et al. Estimated risks of radiation-induced fatal cancer from pediatric CT. Am J Roentgenol 2001;176(2):289–96.

21. American College of Radiology. ACR–SPR practice parameter for imaging pregnant or potentially pregnant adolescents and women with ionizing radiation. American College of Radiology; 2018.

22. Sala E, Rockall AG, Freeman SJ, et al. The added role of MR imaging in treatment stratification of patients with gynecologic malignancies: what the radiologist needs to know. Radiology 2013;266(3): 717–40.

23. Chilla B, Hauser N, Singer G, et al. Indeterminate adnexal masses at ultrasound: effect of MR imaging imaging findings on diagnostic thinking and therapeutic decisions. Eur Radiol 2011;21(6):1301–10.

24. Siddiqui N, Nikolaidis P, Hammond N, et al. Uterine artery embolization: pre- and post-procedural evaluation using magnetic resonance imaging. Abdom Imaging 2013;38(5):1161–77.

25. Behr SC, Courtier JL, Qayyum A. Imaging of müllerian duct anomalies. RadioGraphics 2012;32(6):E233–50.

26. Li Y, Phelps A, Zapala MA, et al. Magnetic resonance imaging of Müllerian duct anomalies in children. Pediatr Radiol 2016;46(6):796–805.

27. Namimoto T, Awai K, Nakaura T, et al. Role of diffusion-weighted imaging in the diagnosis of gynecological diseases. Eur Radiol 2009;19(3):745–60.

28. Sala E, Rockall A, Rangarajan D, et al. The role of dynamic contrast-enhanced and diffusion weighted magnetic resonance imaging in the female pelvis. Eur J Radiol 2010;76(3):367–85.

29. Wakefield JC, Downey K, Kyriazi S, et al. New MR techniques in gynecologic cancer. Am J Roentgenol 2013;200(2):249–60.

30. Hricak H, Alpers C, Crooks L, et al. Magnetic resonance imaging of the female pelvis: initial experience. AJR Am J Roentgenol 1983;141(6):1119–28.

31. Nougaret S, Tirumani SH, Addley H, et al. Pearls and pitfalls in MR imaging of gynecologic malignancy with diffusion-weighted technique. Am J Roentgenol 2013;200(2):261–76.

32. Lin G, Ho K-C, Wang J-J, et al. Detection of lymph node metastasis in cervical and uterine cancers by diffusion-weighted magnetic resonance imaging at 3T. J Magn Reson Imaging 2008;28(1):128–35.

33. Fujii S, Matsusue E, Kanasaki Y, et al. Detection of peritoneal dissemination in gynecological malignancy: evaluation by diffusion-weighted MR imaging. Eur Radiol 2008;18(1):18–23.

34. Costa DN, Pedrosa I, McKenzie C, et al. Body MR imaging using IDEAL. Am J Roentgenol 2008; 190(4):1076–84.

35. Takeuchi M, Matsuzaki K, Uehara H, et al. Malignant transformation of pelvic endometriosis: MR imaging

findings and pathologic correlation. RadioGraphics 2006;26(2):407–17.

36. Rafat Zand K, Reinhold C, Haider MA, et al. Artifacts and pitfalls in MR imaging of the pelvis. J Magn Reson Imaging 2007;26(3):480–97.

37. Roemer PB, Edelstein WA, Hayes CE, et al. The NMR phased array. Magn Reson Med 1990;16(2):192–225.

38. Deshmane A, Gulani V, Griswold MA, et al. Parallel MR imaging. J Magn Reson Imaging 2012;36(1):55–72.

39. Brown MA, Mattrey RF, Stamato S, et al. MR imaging of the female pelvis using vaginal gel. Am J Roentgenol 2005;185(5):1221–7.

40. Young P, Daniel B, Sommer G, et al. Intravaginal gel for staging of female pelvic cancersvpreliminary report of safety, distention, and gel-mucosal contrast during magnetic resonance examination. J Comput Assist Tomogr 2012;36(2):4.

41. Bazot M, Bharwani N, Huchon C, et al. European society of urogenital radiology (ESUR) guidelines: MR imaging of pelvic endometriosis. Eur Radiol 2017;27(7):2765–75.

42. Gutzeit A, Binkert CA, Koh D-M, et al. Evaluation of the anti-peristaltic effect of glucagon and hyoscine on the small bowel: comparison of intravenous and intramuscular drug administration. Eur Radiol 2012;22(6):1186–94.

43. Agrawal G, Riherd JM, Busse RF, et al. Evaluation of uterine anomalies: 3D FRFSE cube versus standard 2D FRFSE. Am J Roentgenol 2009;193(6):W558–62.

44. Hori M, Kim T, Onishi H, et al. Uterine tumors: comparison of 3D versus 2D T2-weighted turbo spin-echo MR imaging at 3.0 T—initial experience. Radiology 2011;258(1):154–63.

45. Bazot M, Stivalet A, Daraï E, et al. Comparison of 3D and 2D FSE T2-weighted MR imaging in the diagnosis of deep pelvic endometriosis: preliminary results. Clin Radiol 2013;68(1):47–54.

46. Forbes KPN, Pipe JG, Bird CR, et al. PROPELLER MR imaging: clinical testing of a novel technique for quantification and compensation of head motion. J Magn Reson Imaging 2001;14(3):215–22.

47. Kojima S, Morita S, Ueno E, et al. Aliasing artifacts with the BLADE technique: causes and effective suppression. J Magn Reson Imaging 2011;33(2):432–40.

48. Fujimoto K, Koyama T, Tamai K, et al. BLADE acquisition method improves T2-weighted MR images of the female pelvis compared with a standard fast spin-echo sequence. Eur J Radiol 2011;80(3):796–801.

49. Lane BF, Vandermeer FQ, Oz RC, et al. Comparison of Sagittal T2-Weighted BLADE and Fast Spin-Echo MR imaging of the female pelvis for motion artifact and lesion detection. Am J Roentgenol 2011;197(2):W307–13.

50. Korn N, Kurhanewicz J, Banerjee S, et al. Reduced-FOV excitation decreases susceptibility artifact in diffusion-weighted MR imaging with endorectal coil for prostate cancer detection. Magn Reson Imaging 2015;33(1):56–62.

51. Rosenkrantz AB, Chandarana H, Pfeuffer J, et al. Zoomed echo-planar imaging using parallel transmission: impact on image quality of diffusion-weighted imaging of the prostate at 3T. Abdom Imaging 2015;40(1):120–6.

52. Porter DA, Heidemann RM. High resolution diffusion-weighted imaging using readout-segmented echo-planar imaging, parallel imaging and a two-dimensional navigator-based reacquisition. Magn Reson Med 2009;62(2):468–75.

53. Foltz WD, Porter DA, Simeonov A, et al. Readout-segmented echo-planar diffusion-weighted imaging improves geometric performance for image-guided radiation therapy of pelvic tumors. Radiother Oncol 2015;117(3):525–31.

54. Kanal E, Barkovich AJ, Bell C, et al. ACR guidance document on MR safe practices: 2013. J Magn Reson Imaging 2013;37(3):501–30.

55. Sammet S. Magnetic resonance safety. Abdom Radiol (NY) 2016;41(3):444–51.

56. Ciet P, Litmanovich DE. MR safety issues particular to women. Magn Reson Imaging Clin N Am 2015;23(1):59–67.

57. Ray JG, Vermeulen MJ, Bharatha A, et al. Association between MR imaging exposure during pregnancy and fetal and childhood outcomes. JAMA 2016;316(9):952.

58. Strizek B, Jani JC, Mucyo E, et al. Safety of MR imaging at 1.5 T in fetuses: a retrospective case-control study of birth weights and the effects of acoustic noise. Radiology 2015;275(2):530–7.

59. Chartier AL, Bouvier MJ, McPherson DR, et al. The safety of maternal and fetal MR imaging at 3T. Am J Roentgenol 2019;213:1170–3.

60. ACR–SPR practice parameter for the safe and optimal performance of fetal Magnetic Resonance Imaging (MR imaging). Available at: https://www.acr.org/-/media/ACR/Files/Practice-Parameters/mr-fetal.pdf.

61. Prola-Netto J, Woods M, Roberts VHJ, et al. Gadolinium chelate safety in pregnancy: barely detectable gadolinium levels in the juvenile nonhuman primate after in utero exposure. Radiology 2018;286(1):122–8.

62. Simpson WL, Beitia LG, Mester J. Hysterosalpingography: a reemerging study. RadioGraphics 2006;26:419–31.

63. Maheux-Lacroix S, Boutin A, Moore L, et al. Hysterosalpingosonography for diagnosing tubal occlusion in subfertile women: a systematic review with meta-analysis. Hum Reprod 2014;29(5):953–63.

64. Cundiff G, Carr BR, Marshburn PB. Infertile couples with a normal hysterosalpingogram. Reproductive outcome and its relationship to clinical and laparoscopic findings. J Reprod Med 1995;40(1):19–24.

65. Dreyer K, van Rijswijk J, Mijatovic V, et al. Oil-based or water-based contrast for hysterosalpingography in infertile women. N Engl J Med 2017;376(21):2043–52.

66. Uzun O, Findik S, Danaci M, et al. Pulmonary and cerebral oil embolism after hysterosalpingography with oil soluble contrast medium. Respirology 2004;9(1):134–6.

67. Dan U, Oelsner G, Gruberg L, et al. Cerebral embolization and coma after hysterosalpingography with oil-soluble contrast medium. Fertil Steril 1990;53(5):939–40.

68. Davis PL. Anaphylactoid reactions to the nonvascular administration of water-soluble iodinated contrast media. Am J Roentgenol 2015;204(6):1140–5.

69. American College of Radiology. ACR practice parameter for the performance of hysterosalpingography. Available at: https://www.acr.org/-/media/ACR/Files/Practice-Parameters/HSG.pdf.

70. Vickramarajah S, Stewart V, van Ree K, et al. Subfertility: what the radiologist needs to know. RadioGraphics 2017;37(5):1587–602.

71. American College of Obstetricians and Gynecologists. Clinical management guidelines for obstetricians & gynecologists-prevention of infection after gynecologic procedures. Obstet Gynecol 2018;131(6):172–89.

72. Wilson RB, Lee RA, Jensen PA. Inadvertent infertility investigations in pregnant women. Fertil Steril 1966;17(1):126–32.

73. Perisinakis K, Damilakis J, Grammatikakis J, et al. Radiogenic risks from hysterosalpingography. Eur Radiol 2003;13(7):1522–8.

74. Radiologyinfo.org. Patient safety - radiation dose in X-Ray and CT exams. Available at: https://www.radiologyinfo.org/en/info.cfm?pg=safety-xray. Accessed August 4, 2019.

Imaging of Infertility, Part 1
Hysterosalpingograms to Magnetic Resonance Imaging

Bryce A. Merritt, MD[a], Spencer C. Behr, MD[b], Nadia J. Khati, MD[c],*

KEYWORDS

- Female infertility • Müllerian duct anomalies • Hysterosalpingogram • Ultrasound • Fallopian tubes
- MR imaging

KEY POINTS

- Infertility can be primary or secondary and affects up to 12% of couples of reproductive age worldwide.
- Causes of female infertility include congenital etiologies, such as Müllerian duct anomalies (MDAs), and acquired etiologies, which range from ovulatory dysfunction to cervical factors and uterine and tubal abnormalities.
- The imaging investigation of female infertility consists of a multimodality approach, and includes a combination of primarily ultrasound and hysterosalpingography (HSG), with MR imaging for problem-solving situations specifically if MDAs or deep infiltrative endometriosis are suspected.
- HSG remains the gold-standard imaging modality to assess tubal patency.

INTRODUCTION

Infertility, or subfertility, is defined as the inability to achieve a clinical pregnancy after a 1-year period of regular unprotected sexual intercourse in women younger than 35 and after 6 months in women older than 35.[1] Prospective cohort studies have estimated the prevalence of infertility in the United States ranges from 12% to 18%.[2–4] When couples undergo evaluation for infertility, the etiology is found to be 40% women and 40% men.[5] It is a unique and often multifactorial medical condition that involves a couple, rather than a single individual, requiring a comprehensive approach for diagnosis and treatment.[6] Causes of female infertility include congenital etiologies such as

Müllerian duct anomalies (MDAs) and acquired ones, which range from ovulatory dysfunction to cervical factors and uterine and tubal abnormalities. Although initial assessment involves a multitude of factors, including a detailed medical history, physical examination, semen analysis, and hormonal evaluation, diagnostic imaging of the female partner often plays an important role in establishing the etiology for infertility. This typically includes a combination of various modalities, such as ultrasound, MR imaging, and primarily hysterosalpingography (HSG), depending on the suspected etiology. In addition to these traditional imaging modalities, we review some newer imaging techniques, such as hysterosalpingo-contrast

Funding: The authors report no funding that supported this study.
[a] Diagnostic Radiology, UCSF Department of Radiology & Biomedical Imaging, 505 Parnassus Avenue, Moffitt, Suite 307H, San Francisco, CA 94143, USA; [b] UCSF Department of Radiology & Biomedical Imaging, 505 Parnassus Avenue, Moffitt, Suite 307H, San Francisco, CA 94143, USA; [c] Department of Radiology, Abdominal Imaging Section, The George Washington University Hospital, 900 23rd Street, Northwest, Washington, DC 20037, USA
* Corresponding author.
E-mail address: nkhati@mfa.gwu.edu

Radiol Clin N Am 58 (2020) 215–225
https://doi.org/10.1016/j.rcl.2019.10.010
0033-8389/20/© 2019 Elsevier Inc. All rights reserved.

sonography (HyCoSy) and virtual computed tomography (CT) and MR hysterosalpingography.

ANATOMY

The female reproductive organs consist of the cervix, uterus, fallopian tubes, and paired ovaries. During the initial 6 weeks of gestation, both male and female fetuses possess paired Müllerian (paramesonephric) and Wolffian (mesonephric) ducts. In male fetuses, the presence of Müllerian-inhibiting factor, associated with the presence of a Y chromosome, results in the regression of the Müllerian ducts. In female fetuses, the absence of Müllerian-inhibiting factor leads to concomitant regression of the Wolffian ducts and growth of paired Müllerian ducts. Embryologically, the uterus, cervix, fallopian tubes, and upper two-thirds of the vagina are formed by fusion of paired Müllerian ducts. Failure or disruption of development of the ducts, such as absence of fusion or nonresorption or partial resorption of the midline septum following fusion will result in a complex spectrum of congenital abnormalities termed Müllerian duct anomalies (MDAs), some of which may be associated with infertility. The fallopian tubes measure 10 to 12 cm and are found running along the superior aspect of the broad ligament. Each tube is composed of 4 segments: interstitial, which is the shortest and narrowest and contained within the muscular portion of the uterus; isthmic, closest to the uterine wall; and ampullary and infundibular, which is the distal funnel-shaped fimbriated portion, opening into the peritoneal cavity. The fallopian tubes are not visualized unless they are dilated or surrounded by peritoneal fluid. The paired ovaries are ellipsoid, located in the ovarian fossa along the lateral pelvic wall. They are attached to the posterior aspect of the broad ligament by the mesovarium.

IMAGING MODALITIES

The imaging investigation of female infertility consists of a multimodality approach, and includes a combination of primarily ultrasound, HSG, and MR imaging for problem-solving situations or in cases of suspected MDAs. Each of these studies will focus on and help investigate different aspects of the infertility workup process (Table 1).

Pelvic ultrasound, performed both transabdominally and transvaginally (TV), is a first screening tool to insure the presence and integrity of the female reproductive organs. It has the advantage of being readily available, fairly inexpensive, relatively easy to perform, particularly in the hands of experienced operators, and lacks ionizing radiation.

Ultrasound is excellent at diagnosing fibroids, endometrial polyps, adenomyosis/endometriosis, and imaging the ovaries to evaluate for polycystic ovaries, follicle development, and count antral follicles. Three-dimensional (3D) ultrasound is now used more routinely to assess the outside contour of the uterus in cases of suspected MDAs and has a reported 90% to 95% diagnostic accuracy.[7] It also can accurately depict intracavitary lesions, such as polyps, submucosal fibroids, septum, and synechiae. Saline infusion hysterosonography (SIS), which involves the instillation of saline or gel through the endocervical canal using a catheter, allows delineation of the endometrium and its surface.[8] This procedure can be performed using conventional 2-dimensional (2D) or 3D ultrasound. The latter consists of acquiring volumetric data that can be analyzed at a later time following the examination. This method allows for a shorter procedure time and less patient discomfort.

Dijkhuizen and colleagues[9] found that SIS had a higher diagnostic accuracy in the detection of intracavitary uterine abnormalities when comparing it with TV scanning, with SIS having a sensitivity and specificity of 100% and 85%, respectively. In a large meta-analysis, Seshadri and colleagues[10] concluded that SIS was as good as hysteroscopy in identifying all types of intracavitary uterine abnormalities, with a pooled sensitivity and specificity of 88% and 94%, respectively. Normal fallopian tubes are not detectable on ultrasound unless dilated; however, their patency can now be assessed using a contrast agent. This method was first introduced in 1984 by injecting fluid into the uterine cavity under ultrasound guidance and observing fluid in the cul-de-sac as proof of fallopian tube patency.[11] Hysterosalpingo-contrast sonography (HyCoSy), which is a newly introduced technique, uses a mixture of saline solution with air as a contrast medium and can be performed using 2D or 3D ultrasound.[12,13] The injected air appears hyperechoic and can be followed during real-time ultrasound as it traverses the fallopian tubes and spills into the peritoneal cavity, proving tubal patency. Many different contrast agents have been developed and used in Europe but are not approved by the Food and Drug Administration for intrauterine use in the United States.[7,12] HyCoSy was found to have an accuracy equivalent to HSG when compared with the criterion standard of laparoscopic chromopertubation in the determination of tubal patency with sensitivities and specificities ranging between 75% and 96% and 67% and 100%, respectively.[12] Malik and colleagues[14] evaluated 30 women with primary and secondary infertility comparing the efficacy of HSG and sonosalpingography (SSG) in the assessment of

Table 1
Studies focusing on the infertility workup process

Imaging Modalities	Advantages	Disadvantages
Ultrasound	• Usually first screening examination • Readily available, easy to perform • Inexpensive • Lacks ionizing radiation • Excellent for diagnosis of fibroids, endometrial polyps, adenomyosis/endometriosis, PCOs • 3D ultrasound can evaluate for MDAs • SIS can evaluate the uterine cavity • HyCoSy can evaluate tubal patency	• Operator dependent • 3D ultrasound requires additional training and experienced operator • Contrast agents for HyCoSy not FDA approved in the USA
HSG	• Evaluates tubal patency • Assess uterine cavity	• Uses ionizing radiation • Considered an invasive examination • Uses water or oil-based contrast medium • Cannot assess outside uterine fundal contour, hence not adequate modality for MDAs
MR imaging	• Excellent modality for MDA diagnosis; adenomyosis/DIE; leiomyomas; endometrial polyps • Great problem-solving tool for tubal/peritubal disease suspected on ultrasound or HSG • Vital role in presurgical planning for MDAs or DIE • MR-HSG has an emerging role in evaluation of tubal patency and intrauterine pathology	• Uses contrast medium • Claustrophobia • MR-HSG requires added postprocedure time and expertise
CT	• CT-HSG allows evaluation of uterus including outside fundal contour, fallopian tubes, and adnexae	• Uses ionizing radiation • Considered an invasive examination • Uses water or oil-based contrast medium • Requires added postprocessing time and expertise

Abbreviations: CT, computed tomography; 3D, 3-dimensional; DIE, deep infiltrating endometriosis; FDA, food and drug administration; HSG, hysterosalpingography; HyCoSy, hysterosalpingo-contrast sonography; MDAs, Müllerian duct anomalies; PCO, polycystic ovaries; SIS, saline infusion hysterosonography.

tubal patency. They concluded that SSG was a safe and well-tolerated procedure and could be performed instead of HSG and laparoscopy. Despite HyCoSy being a promising newer imaging technique, a large majority of patients undergoing infertility workup are still being evaluated with HSG. This study remains an essential radiologic examination and often the most commonly chosen imaging modality to assess tubal patency and morphology as well as to evaluate the uterine cavity. The examination consists of the injection of water-soluble or oil-based contrast medium into the uterine cavity under fluoroscopic guidance through a small catheter.[15–17] The decision to use water versus oil-based contrast to perform HSGs remains a debate, with a recent study showing that the use of the latter agent resulted in an increase in pregnancy rates and live births.[16] HSGs are performed in the first half of the menstrual cycle, between days 7 and 12 when the endometrium is thin and also to avoid the possibility of a pregnancy. Spot radiographs of the filled uterine cavity and opacified tubes are obtained intermittently until free spillage of contrast into the peritoneal cavity is observed, confirming tubal patency. Roma Dalfó[18] and colleagues evaluated 78 women with infertility using both HSG and hysteroscopy. They found that both tests had a high correlation, complementing each other in the diagnosis of uterine abnormalities with an overall 73% agreement. Phillips and colleagues[19] reviewed the findings of 327 infertile women who were evaluated with TV ultrasound, hysteroscopy, and HSG and concluded that the latter was superior in the diagnosis of tubal abnormalities, particularly tubal obstruction. In their meta-analysis of 20 articles, Swart and colleagues[20] came to the same conclusion, finding that HSG was a valuable diagnostic tool for diagnosing tubal obstruction. More recently, newer advanced imaging modalities have emerged using the 2D and 3D reconstruction capabilities of multidetector CT imaging and the 3D dynamic imaging capabilities of MR imaging to create virtual hysterosalpingograms.[21–23] Both imaging techniques are based on the conventional technique for performing HSGs with the added advantages of evaluating the cervix, uterine cavity and its outside contour, the entirety of fallopian tubes including their patency, and the surrounding pelvic structures such as ovaries and adnexae. Postprocessing tools include a combination of volume rendering, multiplanar reformatting, maximum intensity projection, and virtual endoscopy, all of which require added postprocedure time and expertise.

The role of MR imaging in the evaluation of female infertility is many folds: it is thought of as the gold-standard imaging modality for the diagnosis of MDAs; it is an essential imaging tool in the diagnosis and management of adenomyosis, deep infiltrative endometriosis, and leiomyomas, and is a great problem-solving examination when tubal and peritubal disease and adhesions are suspected on ultrasound or HSG.[6,24] In fact, Volondat and colleagues[25] conducted a study comparing the accuracy of HSG and MR-HSG in 26 women with infertility. They found that MR-HSG had a sensitivity and specificity of 91.7% and 92.0%, respectively for the diagnosis of both tubal patency and intrauterine pathology. In addition, MR often plays a vital role in presurgical planning.[26] Multiplanar reformatting from 3D acquisition allows for improved anatomic assessment and significantly reduced scan time. Unlike HSG, MR imaging is noninvasive and avoids the use of ionizing radiation. Unlike ultrasound, MR imaging grants a wider field of interrogation and is not limited by overlying bowel gas or patient body habitus and is usually a well-tolerated examination in the absence of claustrophobia. Standard pelvic MR imaging protocols include T1-weighted and T2-weighted images (**Table 2**).

IMAGING FINDINGS

Causes of female infertility include congenital etiologies and acquired or organic etiologies. The congenital causes are mostly represented by MDAs, which include a number of variants

Table 2
Standard pelvic MR imaging protocols

Sequences	Plane	FOV, cm	Comment
T2W SSFSE	Coronal	32–40	General overview, assessment for concurrent anatomic anomalies (eg, renal)
3D FS T2W	Coronal	18–24	Thin-cut volumetric acquisition, allows for multiplanar reconstruction to improved anatomic assessment, reduced scan time
GRE Dual-Echo T1W (In/Out)	Axial	32–40	Useful for visualization of blood products and characterization of adnexal pathology
EPI DWI	Axial	Targeted to region of interest	
3D LAVAT1WFS Pre	Axial or Sagittal	18–24	Thin-cut volumetric acquisition
Optional			
3D LAVAT1WFS Post	Axial or Sagittal	18–24	Performed for additional characterization of any unrelated or unexpected finding seen on initial noncontrast evaluation
T2W FSE	Coronal	18–24	Performed for supplemental assessment of uterine anatomy

Abbreviations: 3D, 3-dimensional; DWI, diffusion-weighted imaging; EPI, echo planar imaging; FS, fat suppressed; FSE, fast spin echo; LAVA T1WFS, liver acquisition with volume acceleration t1 weighted fat suppressed; SSFSE, single shot fast spin echo; T1W, T1-weighted; T2W, T2-weighted.

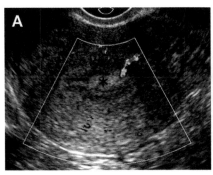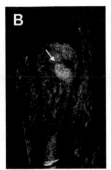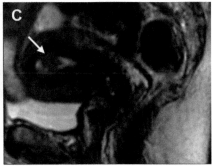

Fig. 1. Endometrial polyp. (*A*) Axial transvaginal ultrasound of the uterus demonstrates a well-defined echogenic endometrial polyp with a feeding vessel (*asterisk*). (*B*) The 3D reconstructed coronal view confirms the endometrial location of the polyp (*arrow*). (*C*) Sagittal T2-weighted non–fat-saturated MR image demonstrates the focal T2 hypointense polyp (*arrow*) arising from the posterior endometrium and extending into the adjacent endometrial canal.

according to the American Society of Reproductive Medicine classification system. Acquired causes range from ovulatory dysfunction to cervical factors and uterine and tubal abnormalities.

Acquired Causes of Infertility

Cervical abnormalities

These include cervical factor infertility, which is responsible for roughly 10% of female infertility cases and is defined as inadequate cervical mucus volume or quality, and cervical stenosis.[25] Neither of these entities require imaging for diagnosis, although the latter may be incidentally noted at the time of HSG when the cervix cannot be cannulated. Narrowing or stenosis of the cervix results in varying degrees of menstrual flow obstructive symptoms ranging from amenorrhea to dysmenorrhea, as well as preventing entry of sperm into the uterus.[27,28]

Uterine abnormalities

These are characterized by polyps, leiomyomas, adenomyosis, and synechiae. Endometrial polyps are the most common structural abnormalities of the uterine cavity and represent focal overgrowth of endometrial tissue. Among patients with

infertility, the prevalence of endometrial polyps is approximately 32%.[29] However, despite this association, limited evidence exists on the effectiveness of hysteroscopic polypectomy in improving reproductive outcomes among infertile women and the true impact of endometrial polyps on fecundity is a subject of ongoing debate.[30,31] For example, although one randomized controlled trial demonstrated improved rates of conception following hysteroscopic polypectomy,[32] a recent large-scale retrospective analysis failed to show any significant prognostic improvement following polypectomy regardless of polyp location.[33] On 2D and 3D ultrasound and SIS, endometrial polyps appear as well-defined echogenic masses within the uterine cavity and Doppler imaging may show a feeding vessel (**Fig. 1**). On HSG, polyps are best seen in the early filling phase as well-defined filling defects (**Fig. 2**) and may become difficult to differentiate from submucosal leiomyomas in the later phase when contrast fills the uterine cavity. These leiomyomas are better demonstrated at TV ultrasound (**Fig. 3**) and MR imaging as focal masses with various degrees of vascularity, distorting the endometrium or protruding into the uterine cavity. Similar to endometrial

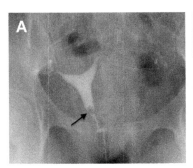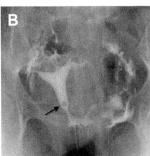

Fig. 2. Endometrial polyp on HSG. Early (*A*) and late (*B*) HSG spot radiographs show a well-defined lucent fixed, nonmobile filling defect in the lower uterine segment of the uterine cavity corresponding to a small endometrial polyp (*arrows*).

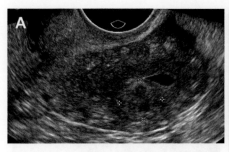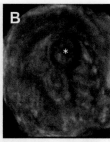

Fig. 3. Submucosal leiomyoma. Sagittal transvaginal ultrasound (A) and 3D reconstructed coronal view of the uterus (B) show an anterior submucosal leiomyoma outlined by calipers in (A). The 3D ultrasound confirms nicely the extracavitary location of the leiomyoma (asterisk).

polyps, submucosal leiomyomas can interfere with implantation of the embryo. When small in size, their appearance on HSG can overlap with that of polyps, and additional imaging may be needed to make the diagnosis. Larger submucosal leiomyomas are easier to recognize on HSG (Fig. 4). Given the excellent soft tissue contrast resolution, MR imaging is the ideal tool to characterize the size, morphology, and location of leiomyomas before myomectomy. MR imaging findings vary based on the level of degeneration of individual leiomyomas, but typically demonstrate focal masses with T2 signal intensity hypointense to that of the adjacent myometrium. Currently, there is fair evidence that hysteroscopic myomectomy for submucosal leiomyomas improves clinical pregnancy rates.[34] A single randomized controlled trial has assessed the impact of hysteroscopic myomectomy on fertility in women with submucosal leiomyomas, finding 1-year clinical pregnancy rates of 43.3% in the myomectomy group compared with 27.2% in those without surgery.[35] Subsequent systematic reviews also have supported this effect.[36]

Adenomyosis is a benign process whereby ectopic endometrial glands extend into the adjacent myometrium in a diffuse or focal fashion, referred to as an adenomyoma. It is thought that adenomyosis causes infertility due to decreased or abnormal uterine contractility slowing down sperm transport through the uterine cavity and diminished endometrial receptivity.[27,28,37–39] At imaging, adenomyosis has various appearances

and is most commonly diagnosed at ultrasound and MR imaging as patients often present with symptoms of pelvic pain and/or bleeding (Fig. 5). Both imaging examinations have varying sensitivities and specificities ranging from 53% to 89% and 67% to 89%, respectively, for ultrasound, and 78% to 88% and 67% to 93%, respectively, for MR imaging.[27] Findings at HSG can be incidental especially in women who are asymptomatic and consist of diffuse or focally grouped small contrast-filled diverticula that project beyond the uterine cavity (Fig. 6). When this is the case, MR imaging should be performed in these women to look for deep infiltrating endometriosis, given the high association of endometriosis with adenomyosis in up to 90% of women.[39] Characteristic findings on MR imaging include an enlarged globular-shaped uterus with diffuse or focal thickening of the junctional zone (>12 mm) in association with low signal intensity on T2-weighted imaging (see Fig. 4). In addition, small T2 hyperintense foci are often seen within the myometrium, corresponding to sites of punctate hemorrhage related to ectopic endometrial tissue.[40]

Synechiae are permanent adhesions or scars within the uterine cavity that may be the result of prior infection, curettage, or previous pregnancy. When associated with infertility, it is referred to as Asherman syndrome. Synechiae are best visualized at HSG and appear as irregular linear fixed filling defects within the uterine cavity.[27,28] The uterine cavity may be so scarred that it may be difficult to distend it while performing the HSG

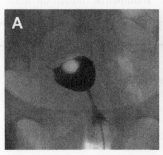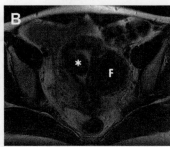

Fig. 4. Submucosal leiomyoma on HSG. (A) HSG spot radiograph shows a large well-defined lucent filling defect in the fundal aspect of the uterine cavity corresponding to a submucosal leiomyoma (asterisk) of the follow-up MR imaging (B). Note how the larger left pedunculated uterine body leiomyoma (F) cannot be visualized on the HSG.

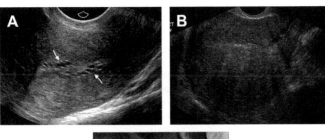
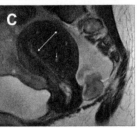

Fig. 5. Adenomyosis. Sagittal transvaginal ultrasound of the uterus in 2 different patients show (*A*) multiple small subendometrial cysts (*arrow*) and a globular uterus (*B*) with a heterogeneous thickened posterior myometrium with an indistinct endometrial/myometrial interface. (*C*) Sagittal T2-weighted non–fat-saturated MR image demonstrates an enlarged, globular uterus with thickening of the junctional zone posteriorly (*double arrow*). Also seen are multiple small T2 hyperintense foci (*single arrow*), corresponding to sites of punctate hemorrhage related to ectopic endometrial tissue.

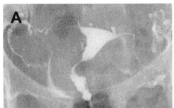
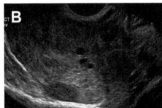

Fig. 6. Adenomyosis on HSG. (*A*) HSG spot radiograph shows small diverticular outpouchings of contrast along the uterine cavity in the fundus and right body. These correlate with small subendometrial cysts seen in the corresponding axial transvaginal ultrasound (*B*) in the same patient, and are consistent with adenomyosis and correspond to dilated ectopic endometrial glands.

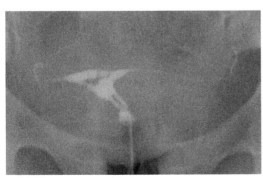
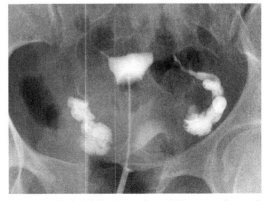

Fig. 8. Occluded fallopian tubes. HSG spot radiograph demonstrates opacification of both tubes to the most distal fimbriated ends. Note that the tubes are normal in caliber; however, are blocked given the lack spillage of contrast into the peritoneal cavity despite continued contrast injection.

Fig. 7. Synechiae. HSG spot radiograph shows irregular linear fixed filling defects within the uterine cavity.

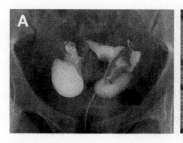 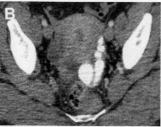

Fig. 9. Hydrosalpinx with tubal occlusion. (*A*) HSG spot radiograph demonstrates bilateral hydrosalpinges, right greater than left. No contrast spillage was seen into the peritoneal cavity. (*B*) Follow-up CT scan performed 10 days later for abdominal pain shows persistent left hydrosalpinx with retained residual contrast from the previous HSG.

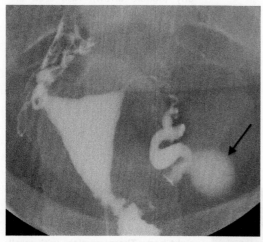

Fig. 10. Loculated spillage. HSG spot radiograph shows patent tubes bilaterally with a round well-defined collection of the contrast in the left peritubal region (*arrow*), consistent with loculated spillage due to adhesions.

(**Fig. 7**). The uterine cavity may have such a small and distorted appearance that the increased intra-uterine pressure may result in various degrees of venous and lymphatic contrast intravasation.

Fallopian tube abnormalities

These include tubal occlusion with or without hydrosalpinx, tubal polyps, and salpingitis isthmica nodosa. Occlusion of the tubes can occur anywhere along their course, but when it involves the interstitial portion it is most likely due to spam, which can be overcome by administering a spasmolytic agent or by bringing the patient back for a repeat examination.[41] True tubal blockage is usually the result of pelvic inflammatory disease (PID), endometriosis, or trauma. At HSG, occlusion is characterized by an abrupt cut-off of contrast along the tube with no spillage into the peritoneal cavity (**Fig. 8**). A hydrosalpinx develops when the occlusion occurs at the ampullary portion of the tube (**Fig. 9**). When peritubal adhesions are present, HSG shows loculated contrast surrounding the distal aspects of the tubes (**Fig. 10**). On ultrasound, CT, and MR imaging, hydrosalpinx appears as a fluid-filled convoluted tubular structure in the adnexa, separate from the adjacent ovary and extending to the uterine fundus (**Fig. 11**). The imaging characteristics of the tubes will depend on their contents, that is, simple fluid, blood, or pus. Tubal polyps, although rare, may be encountered at HSG. They represent endometrial tissue ectopically located usually within the interstitial portion of the fallopian tubes. They are most often an incidental finding at HSG and they appear as well-defined ovoid or round lucent filling defects in the tubes and do not result in tubal obstruction. Their fixed, constant presence throughout the HSG allows differentiation from air bubbles introduced during the procedure (**Fig. 12**). The general consensus is that their role as a causative factor in infertility is unknown and likely insignificant. Salpingitis isthmica nodosa results from an inflammatory process of unknown

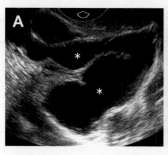 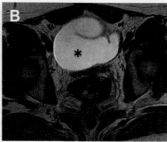

Fig. 11. Hydrosalpinx. (*A*) Pelvic sonogram shows a tubular cystic structure in the adnexa, which was avascular and separate from the adjacent ovary, compatible with a hydrosalpinx (*asterisks*). (*B*) Axial T2-weighted MR image in a different patient demonstrates a tubular hyperintense hydrosalpinx (*asterisk*).

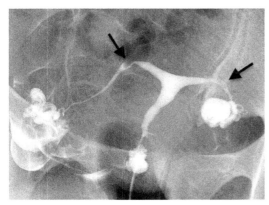

Fig. 12. Tubal polyps. HSG spot radiograph demonstrates bilateral, fixed persistent lucent filling defects in the interstitial portions of the tubes consistent with polyps (*arrows*). Note that there is no associated blockage, as evidenced by the normal opacification of the tubes, although loculated spillage is seen on the left.

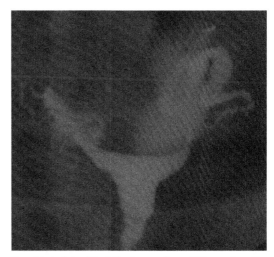

Fig. 13. Salpingitis isthmica nodosa. HSG spot radiograph demonstrates multiple small focal outpouchings of contrast in the isthmic portion of the left tube.

etiology, although it is often associated with PID, ectopic pregnancies, and infertility.[37,41] It has a characteristic appearance at HSG consisting of irregular tubes with multiple small focal outpouchings of contrast in the isthmic portion (**Fig. 13**).

Ovarian abnormalities include primary and secondary conditions. Primary conditions are usually diagnosed based on clinical and biochemical findings and consist of premature ovarian failure or nonfunctioning ovaries as well as gonadal dysgenesis. Imaging plays an insignificant role in making a diagnosis in those cases, but is rather important for identifying the secondary causes of infertility, which consist of polycystic ovarian syndrome (PCOS), endometriosis, and ovarian cancer. The latter 2 entities are covered in detail under separate articles in this issue and are beyond the scope of this article. Women with PCOS have an endocrinologic disorder characterized by hyperandrogenism and increased levels of luteinizing hormone and they may present clinically with hirsutism, obesity, and incomplete ovulatory cycles.[27] This condition affects up to 8% of women with radiological features of enlarged ovaries containing more than 12 small cysts peripherally arranged in

more than 80% of cases.[27,41] These findings are very well demonstrated on ultrasound and MR imaging, consisting of ovarian volumes greater than 20 mL, lack of a dominant follicle due to anovulation, and multiple peripherally located small cysts measuring 2 to 9 mm (**Fig. 14**). Radiologists should be cautious when making a diagnosis of PCOS when such findings are present, as approximately 20% to 30% of women may have polycystic-appearing ovaries but will lack the clinical symptoms and manifestations of the syndrome.[41]

SUMMARY/WHAT THE REFERRING PHYSICIAN NEEDS TO KNOW

- Infertility is often a multifactorial medical condition requiring a comprehensive approach for diagnosis and treatment
- The imaging investigation of female infertility consists of a multimodality approach
- MR imaging and sometimes 3D ultrasound are the imaging examination of choice when MDAs are suspected
- HSG is the gold standard study to evaluate tubal patency although HyCoSy is a promising imaging tool on the rise

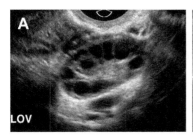
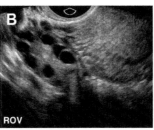

Fig. 14. Polycystic ovaries. Transvaginal pelvic ultrasound shows normal-sized left (*A*) and right (*B*) ovaries containing multiple small peripherally arranged follicles.

CONFLICT OF INTEREST

The authors report no conflicts of interests concerning the materials, methods, or results in this article.

REFERENCES

1. Practice Committee of the American Society for Reproductive Medicine. Definitions of infertility and recurrent pregnancy loss. Fertil Steril 2008;90(5 SUPPL):60.
2. Thoma ME, McLain AC, Louis JF, et al. Prevalence of infertility in the United States as estimated by the current duration approach and a traditional constructed approach. Fertil Steril 2013;99:1324–31.
3. Zinaman MJ, Clegg ED, Brown CC, et al. Estimates of human fertility and pregnancy loss. Fertil Steril 1996;65:503–9.
4. Buck Louis GM, Sundaram R, Schisterman EF, et al. Heavy metals and couple fecundity, the LIFE Study. Chemosphere 2012;87:1201–7.
5. Jeelani R, Puscheck EE. Imaging and the infertility evaluation. Clin Obstet Gynecol 2017;60(1):93–107.
6. Imaoka I, Wada A, Matsuo M, et al. MR imaging of disorders associated with female infertility: use in diagnosis, treatment, and management. Radiographics 2003;23(6):1401–21.
7. Groszmann YS, Benacerraf BR. Complete evaluation of anatomy and morphology of the infertile patient in a single visit: the modern infertility pelvic ultrasound examination. Fertil Steril 2019;105(6):1381–93.
8. Seshadri S, Khalil M, Osman A, et al. The evolving role of saline infusion sonography (SIS) in infertility. Eur J Obstet Gynecol Reprod Biol 2015;185:66–73.
9. Dijkhuizen FP, De Vries LD, Mol BW, et al. Comparison of transvaginal ultrasonography and saline infusion sonography for the detection of intracavitary abnormalities in premenopausal women. Ultrasound Obstet Gynecol 2000;15(5):372–6.
10. Seshadri S, El-Toukhy T, Douiri A, et al. Diagnostic accuracy of saline infusion sonography in the evaluation of uterine cavity abnormalities prior to assisted reproductive techniques: a systematic review and meta-analyses. Hum Reprod Update 2015;21(2):262–74.
11. Richman TS, Viscomi GN, deCherney A, et al. Fallopian tubal patency assessed by ultrasound following fluid injection. Work in progress. Radiology 1984;152(2):507–10.
12. Luciano DE, Exacoustos C, Luciano AA. Contrast ultrasonography for tubal patency. J Minim Invasive Gynecol 2014;21(6):994–8.
13. Alcázar JL, Martinez-Astorquiza Corral T, Orozco R, et al. Three-dimensional hysterosalpingo-contrast-sonography for the assessment of tubal patency in women with infertility: a systematic review with meta-analysis. Gynecol Obstet Invest 2016;81(4):289–95.
14. Malik B, Patil S, Boricha BG, et al. A comparative study of the efficacy of sonosalpingography and hysterosalpingogram to test the tubal patency in all women with primary and secondary infertility. Ultrasound Q 2014;30(2):139–43.
15. Yoder IC, Hall DA. Hysterosalpingography in the 1990s. AJR Am J Roentgenol 1991;157(4):675–83.
16. Dreyer K, van Rijswijk J, Mijatovic V, et al. Oil-based or water-based contrast for hysterosalpingography in infertile women. N Engl J Med 2017;376(21):2043–52.
17. Dun EC, Nezhat CH. Tubal factor infertility: diagnosis and management in the era of assisted reproductive technology. Obstet Gynecol Clin North Am 2012;39(4):551–66.
18. Roma Dalfó A, Ubeda B, Ubeda A, et al. Diagnostic value of hysterosalpingography in the detection of intrauterine abnormalities: a comparison with hysteroscopy. AJR Am J Roentgenol 2004;183(5):1405–9.
19. Phillips CH, Benson CB, Ginsburg ES, et al. Comparison of uterine and tubal pathology identified by transvaginal sonography, hysterosalpingography, and hysteroscopy in female patients with infertility. Fertil Res Pract 2015;1:20.
20. Swart P, Mol BW, van der Veen F, et al. The accuracy of hysterosalpingography in the diagnosis of tubal pathology: a meta-analysis. Fertil Steril 1995;64(3):486–91.
21. Carrascosa PM, Capuñay C, Vallejos J, et al. Virtual hysterosalpingography: a new multidetector CT technique for evaluating the female reproductive system. Radiographics 2010;30(3):643–61.
22. Wiesner W, Ruehm SG, Bongartz G, et al. Three-dimensional dynamic MR hysterosalpingography: a preliminary report. Eur Radiol 2001;11(8):1439–44.
23. Carrascosa P, Capuñay C, Vallejos J, et al. Two-dimensional and three-dimensional imaging of uterus and fallopian tubes in female infertility. Fertil Steril 2016;105(6):1403–20.e7.
24. Robbins JB, Broadwell C, Chow LC, et al. Müllerian duct anomalies: embryological development, classification, and MRI assessment. J Magn Reson Imaging 2015;41(1):1–12.
25. Volondat M, Fontas E, Delotte J, et al. Magnetic resonance hysterosalpingography in diagnostic work-up of female infertility—comparison with conventional hysterosalpingography: a randomised study. Eur Radiol 2019;29(2):501–8.
26. Behr SC, Courtier JL, Qayyum A. Imaging of Müllerian duct anomalies. Radiographics 2012;32(6):E233–50.
27. Steinkeler JA, Woodfield CA, Lazarus E, et al. Female infertility: a systematic approach to radiologic

imaging and diagnosis. Radiographics 2009;29: 1353–70.

28. Kaproth-Joslin K, Dogra V. Imaging of female infertility: a pictorial guide to the hysterosalpingography, ultrasonography, and magnetic resonance imaging findings of the congenital and acquired causes of female infertility. Radiol Clin North Am 2013;51(6): 967–81.

29. Hinckley MD, Milki AA. 1000 office-based hysteroscopies prior to in vitro fertilization: feasibility and findings. JSLS 2004;8(2):103–7.

30. Bosteels J, Weyers S, Puttemans P, et al. The effectiveness of hysteroscopy in improving pregnancy rates in subfertile women without other gynaecological symptoms: a systematic review. Hum Reprod Update 2010;16(1):1–11.

31. Jayaprakasan K, Polanski L, Sahu B, et al. Surgical intervention versus expectant management for endometrial polyps in subfertile women. Cochrane Database Syst Rev 2014;(8):CD009592.

32. Pérez-Medina T, Bajo-Arenas J, Salazar F, et al. Endometrial polyps and their implication in the pregnancy rates of patients undergoing intrauterine insemination: a prospective, randomized study. Hum Reprod 2005;20(6):1632–5.

33. Karakuş SS, Özdamar, Karakuş R, et al. Reproductive outcomes following hysteroscopic resection of endometrial polyps of different location, number and size in patients with infertility. J Obstet Gynaecol 2016;36(3):395–8.

34. Penzias A, Bendikson K, Butts S, et al. Removal of myomas in asymptomatic patients to improve fertility and/or reduce miscarriage rate: a guideline. Fertil Steril 2017;108(3):416–25.

35. Casini ML, Rossi F, Agostini R, et al. Effects of the position of fibroids on fertility. Gynecol Endocrinol 2006;22:106–9.

36. Pritts EA, Parker WH, Olive DL. Fibroids and infertility: an updated systematic review of the evidence. Fertil Steril 2009;91:1215–23.

37. Ledbetter KA, Shetty M, Myers DT. Hysterosalpingography: an imaging atlas with cross-sectional correlation. Abdom Imaging 2015;40(6):1721–32.

38. Sadow CA, Sahni A. Imaging female infertility. Abdom Imaging 2014;39:92–107.

39. Kissler S, Zangos S, Wiegratz I, et al. Utero-tubal sperm transport and its impairment in endometriosis and adenomyosis. Ann N Y Acad Sci 2007;1101: 38–48.

40. Valentini AL, Gul SS, Sogali BG, et al. Adenomyosis: from the sign to the diagnosis, imaging, diagnostic pitfall and differential diagnosis: a pictorial review. Radiol Med 2011;116:1267–87.

41. DeBenedectis C, Ghosh E, Lazarus E. Pitfalls in imaging of female infertility. Semin Roentgenol 2015; 50(4):273–83.

Imaging of Infertility, Part 2
Hysterosalpingograms to Magnetic Resonance Imaging

Bryce A. Merritt, MD[a], Spencer C. Behr, MD[b], Nadia J. Khati, MD[c],*

KEYWORDS

- Female infertility • Müllerian duct anomalies • Hysterosalpingogram • Ultrasonography
- Fallopian tubes • Magnetic resonance imaging

KEY POINTS

- Infertility can be primary or secondary and affects up to 12% of couples of reproductive-age worldwide.
- Causes of female infertility include congenital etiologies such as MDAs and acquired ones which range from ovulatory dysfunction to cervical factors and uterine and tubal abnormalities.
- The imaging investigation of female infertility consists of a multimodality approach, and includes a combination of primarily US and HSG, with MRI for problem-solving situations specifically if MDAs or deep infiltrative endometriosis are suspected.
- HSG remains the gold-standard imaging modality to assess tubal patency.

CONGENITAL CAUSES: MÜLLERIAN DUCT ANOMALIES

Müllerian duct anomalies (MDAs) represent a complex spectrum of congenital abnormalities resulting from failed development of the müllerian ducts, which normally give rise to the uterus, cervix, fallopian tubes, and upper third of the vagina (Table 1). In keeping with the wide spectrum of anatomic appearances of MDAs, their presenting clinical features are also varied and include primary amenorrhea, endometriosis, spontaneous abortion, intrauterine growth restriction, and preterm labor.[1] Although most women with MDAs have no issues conceiving, MDAs are associated with higher rates of spontaneous abortion, preterm delivery, and abnormal fetal lie.[2,3] In addition, although the overall prevalence of MDAs ranges from 1% to 5% in the general population, retrospective studies have shown that, among women with recurrent pregnancy loss, the prevalence of MDAs is substantially higher, ranging from 13% to 25%.[4–7] Reproductive outcomes among patients with MDAs vary significantly by subtype.[8–10] For example, 1 meta-analysis showed septate uterus to have the highest rate of spontaneous abortion (65%) of all uterine anomalies, compared with unicornuate uterus (50%), didelphys uterus (45%), and bicornuate uterus (30%).[11] Multiple classification systems have been proposed to categorize MDA subtypes.[4,12–14] Although there is no universally accepted MDA classification

Funding: The authors report no funding that supported this study.
a Diagnostic Radiology, UCSF Department of Radiology & Biomedical Imaging, 505 Parnassus Avenue, Moffitt, Suite 307H, San Francisco, CA 94143, USA; b UCSF Department of Radiology & Biomedical Imaging, 505 Parnassus Avenue, Moffitt, Suite 307H, San Francisco, CA 94143, USA; c Department of Radiology, Abdominal Imaging Section, The George Washington University Hospital, 900 23rd Street, Northwest, Washington, DC 20037, USA
* Corresponding author.
E-mail address: nkhati@mfa.gwu.edu

Table 1
Müllerian duct anomalies

MDA Subtype	Embryologic Origin	Imaging Features	Important Considerations
Uterine agenesis/ hypoplasia	Failure of müllerian duct proliferation	Spectrum of findings with most extreme form as complete absence of uterus, cervix, fallopian tubes, and upper vagina (MRKH syndrome)	• Typically present at puberty with primary amenorrhea • Important to assess for presence of hypoplastic uterus, which may require surgery in setting of associated hematometra and/ or endometriosis • Patients are invariably infertile
Unicornuate uterus	Failure of müllerian duct development	Typically fusiform banana-shaped horn located off midline; with or without a small rudimentary horn	• Renal anomalies in up to 40% of cases, typically renal agenesis ipsilateral to the absent or rudimentary horn • Important to assess for presence of endometrial tissue within rudimentary horn, which may require surgery in setting of obstruction and/or endometriosis
Bicornuate uterus	Failure of müllerian duct fusion	Two divergent communicating horns fused at the lower uterine segment; either with 1 (unicollis) or 2 cervices (bicollis) Deep external fundal cleft (>10 mm)	• Important to assess for presence of vaginal septum, which may require surgery in setting of obstruction (hematometrocolpos); however, this is rare
Uterus didelphys	Failure of müllerian duct fusion	Two divergent noncommunicating horns, each with its own cervix and (usually) proximal vagina	• Hemivaginal septum can result in obstructive symptoms, which may necessitate surgery • Obstructed hemivagina is classically associated with ipsilateral renal agenesis (OH-VIRA syndrome)
Septate uterus	Failure of septal resorption	Residual uterine septum, either partial (septum does not contact cervix) or complete (septum contacts cervix) Flat/convex external fundal cleft (<10 mm) Indentation depth > 10 mm	• Poorest reproductive outcomes of all MDAs • Hysteroscopic resection may be considered
Arcuate uterus	Failure of septal resorption	Normal external fundal contour Broad-based smooth myometrial prominence at the internal fundal contour	• Generally considered a normal anatomic variant

Abbreviations: MRKH, Mayer-Rokitansky-Küster-Hauser; OH-VIRA, obstructed hemivagina in the setting of ipsilateral renal agenesis.

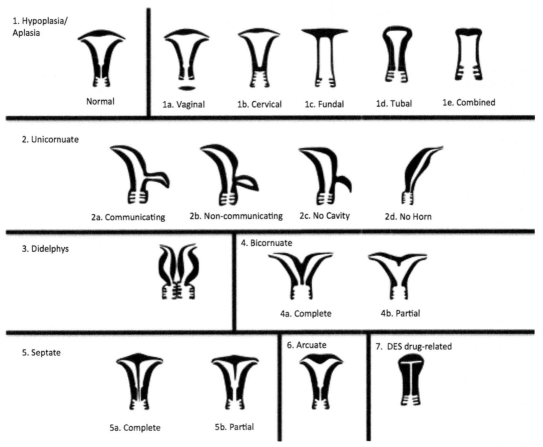

1. Hypoplasia/Aplasia

Normal | 1a. Vaginal | 1b. Cervical | 1c. Fundal | 1d. Tubal | 1e. Combined

2. Unicornuate

2a. Communicating | 2b. Non-communicating | 2c. No Cavity | 2d. No Horn

3. Didelphys

4. Bicornuate

4a. Complete | 4b. Partial

5. Septate

5a. Complete | 5b. Partial

6. Arcuate

7. DES drug-related

Fig. 1. MDA classification system as proposed by the ASRM. (*From* Li et al. Magnetic resonance imaging of Müllerian duct anomalies in children. Pediatr Radiol. 2016 May; 46(6):796-805. PMID: 27229498; with permission.)

system, the system proposed by the American Society for Reproductive Medicine (ASRM), formerly referred to as the American Fertility Society, remains the most widely used approach for categorization (Fig. 1). This system subdivides MDAs into categories that show similar anatomic appearance, clinical manifestations, and treatment.[2,12] Of note, some complex MDAs do not fit neatly into an ASRM classification subtype. In these scenarios, it is important to describe each anomaly rather than attempt to categorize the MDA according to the dominant anatomic feature.[15] In recent decades, magnetic resonance (MR) imaging has emerged as the imaging modality of choice to diagnose and classify MDAs, with reported accuracies of up to 100%.[16–19]

UTERINE AGENESIS OR HYPOPLASIA

Accounting for approximately 5% to 10% of all MDAs, early developmental failure of the müllerian ducts results in complete agenesis or hypoplasia of the uterus, cervix, fallopian tube, and upper vagina.[15] A wide spectrum of findings can be seen with this entity, with the most extreme (and most common) form showing complete absence of the uterus, cervix, fallopian tubes, and upper vagina known as Mayer-Rokitansky-Küster-Hauser syndrome.[11] Because physiologic ovarian function is usually maintained (ovaries arise from the primitive yolk sac), patients show normal secondary sexual characteristics.

Typically, these patients present at the time of puberty with primary amenorrhea.[11] MR imaging is ideal for further investigation because it can confidently differentiate uterine hypoplasia from agenesis as well as other causes of primary amenorrhea such as androgen insensitivity syndrome, which is seen in association with rudimentary testes.[20] In addition, MR imaging allows evaluation for concurrent renal anomalies, which can be seen in up to 29% of patients with uterine agenesis.[21] Sagittal T2-weighted imaging without fat saturation is the most useful sequence, showing

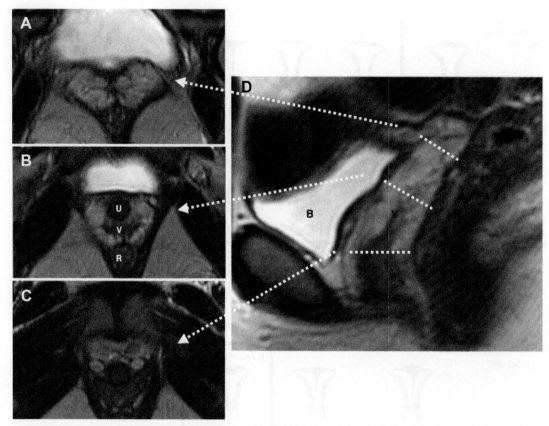

Fig. 2. Mayer-Rokitansky-Küster-Hauser syndrome. (*A–C*) Axial T2-weighted MR images at 3 levels along a hypoplastic blind-ending vagina (V) and showing its relationship to the urethra (U) and rectum (R). (*D*) Sagittal T2-weighted MR image shows absence of the upper vagina, cervix, and uterus. B, bladder.

absence of the uterus, cervix, and upper vagina in cases of complete agenesis (**Fig. 2**). In the case of partial agenesis, a rudimentary uterus may be seen as a pelvic soft tissue mass of myometrial signal intensity with no zonal anatomy. It is important to describe the presence of a hypoplastic uterus, if present, because this can be associated with the presence of a uterine cavity, which can obstruct at the time of menarche leading to cyclic hematometra and/or endometriosis, possibly requiring surgical intervention.[17] Patients with uterine agenesis or hypoplasia are invariably infertile and treatment goals in this population are primarily to enable normal sexual function, typically through the formation of a neovagina or lengthening of an existing distal vagina.[22]

UNICORNUATE UTERUS

Accounting for approximately 20% of all MDAs, complete or near-complete arrested development of 1 müllerian duct with normal development of the contralateral duct results in unicornuate uterus.[15] There are 4 subtypes commonly described, which relate to the potential presence of a rudimentary horn (RH) and its associated features: (1) communicating cavitary RH, (2) noncommunicating cavitary RH, (3) noncavitary RH, and (4) no RH. Approximately half of the cases of unicornuate uterus show a cavitary RH and, of those cases, most (70%) do not communicate with the contralateral (normal) uterine horn.[23] This scenario may manifest clinically as cyclic pelvic pain caused by an increased prevalence of endometriosis related to retrograde flow during menses in the setting of an obstructed and distended RH.[20,24,25] MR imaging is the preferred modality to assess a unicornuate uterus, which appears as a fusiform banana-shaped horn located off the midline (**Fig. 3**). It is also the most sensitive imaging modality to detect the presence of an RH, which has a varied appearance by subtype (**Fig. 4**). If there is no endometrium present within the RH, zonal anatomy is absent.[20] When a cavitary RH is present, normal zonal anatomy is typically preserved and is best appreciated on T2-weighted sequences. In such instances, it is important to comment on such findings because surgical removal is often necessary

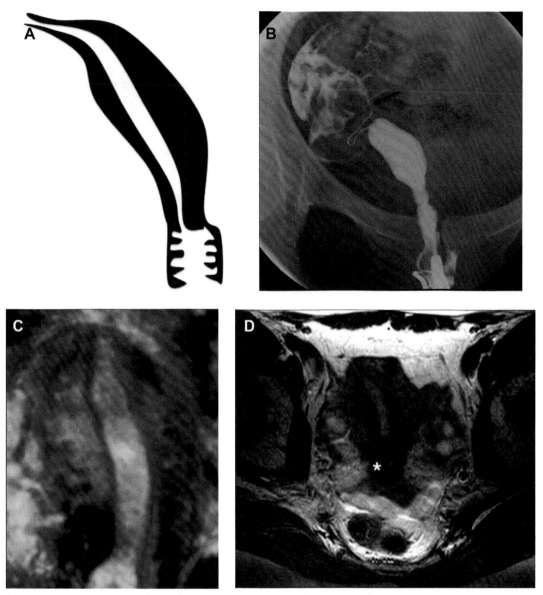

Fig. 3. Unicornuate uterus. (*A*) A right unicornuate uterus without an RH. (*B*) Hysterosalpingogram (HSG) spot image shows contrast opacifying a right tubular uterine cavity with its patent fallopian tube (*arrow*). (*C*) Three-dimensional ultrasonography image of a right unicornuate uterus without RH. (*D*) Axial T2-weighted MR image shows a right unicornuate uterus with a single cervix (*asterisk*) and no RH.

to prevent symptoms related to obstruction and/or endometriosis. In addition, resection should be performed to prevent potential complications related to pregnancy occurring within the RH, which carries an increased risk of spontaneous abortion (up to 50% of cases); preterm labor; and, most significantly, uterine rupture.[11,26,27] Ultrasonography (US) diagnosis of a unicornuate uterus and its variants can be challenging unless the clinician notices the smaller size or deviation of the uterus off midline or the presence of an adjacent smaller RH (see **Fig. 4**). Using three-

dimensional (3D) US should help confirm the diagnosis by showing its characteristic banana shape and better visualize an RH if present.[28] Unicornuate uterus has the strongest association with renal anomalies, occurring in up to 40% of cases, and classically occurs ipsilateral to the absent or rudimentary horn.[23] Although the single most common renal anomaly in these patients is unilateral renal agenesis, other anomalies, such as duplicated collecting system, horseshoe kidney, ectopic kidney, and cystic renal dysplasia, have also been described.[15,20,29] Given this association, MR

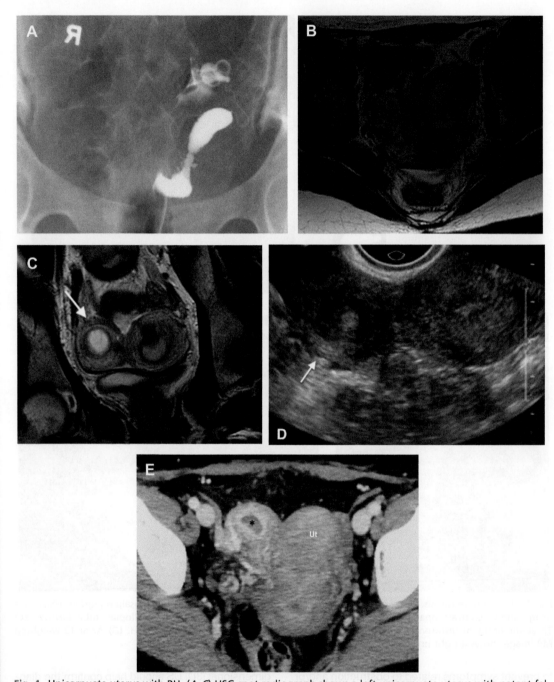

Fig. 4. Unicornuate uterus with RH. (*A–C*) HSG spot radiograph shows a left unicornuate uterus with patent fallopian tube (*A*); follow-up axial T2-weighted MR images (*B, C*) show an unexpected right cavitary noncommunicating RH in which the patient had an ectopic pregnancy (*arrow*). (*D, E*) Left unicornuate uterus with right cavitary noncommunicating RH seen (*arrow*) on pelvic sonogram (*D*) and (*E*) contrast-enhanced computed tomography scan (*asterisks*). Ut, left unicornuate uterus.

examinations protocoled for the evaluation of suspected unicornuate uterus should include at least cursory views of the upper abdomen (eg, coronal single-shot fast spin echo) to evaluate for the presence of renal anomalies.

UTERUS DIDELPHYS

Accounting for approximately 5% of all MDAs, complete failure of müllerian duct fusion results in a uterus didelphys in which each duct develops fully with duplication of the uterine horns, cervixes, and (in most cases) the proximal vagina. Duplication of the proximal vagina is often associated with a hemivaginal septum, which, if transversely oriented, can result in symptoms related to ipsilateral hemivaginal obstruction and hematometrocolpos.[11] As with other MDAs, this subtype is associated with congenital renal anomalies, usually ipsilateral to the transverse hemivaginal septum. In particular, the combination of an obstructed hemivagina in the setting of ipsilateral renal agenesis is a commonly described clinical syndrome.[30] In the absence of obstructive symptoms, patients with uterus didelphys often remain asymptomatic. However, spontaneous abortion rates of 45% and premature birth rates of 38% have been reported.[11] MR imaging shows 2 widely divergent uterine horns, each with its own cervix, with preserved uterine zonal anatomy and no communication between uterine canals (**Fig. 5**). At the uterine fundus, a deep cleft is classically seen. Per ASRM, this cleft must be greater than 10 mm deep, a finding that has been described as 100% sensitive and 99% specific in the differentiation of didelphys and bicornuate uterus from septate uterus.[31]

BICORNUATE UTERUS

Accounting for approximately 10% of all MDAs, incomplete fusion of the paired müllerian ducts results in a bicornuate uterus, which is thought to represent a milder spectrum of uterus didelphys.[11] This entity is characterized by 2 divergent uterine horns that are fused at the level of the lower uterine segment and can occur with a single cervix (unicollis) and duplicated cervixes (bicollis). Similar to uterus didelphys, bicornuate uterus is occasionally associated with the presence of a vaginal septum. Although surgical intervention is rarely indicated, vaginal septoplasty may be necessary if patients present with obstructive symptoms such as hematometrocolpos.[32,33]

On MR imaging, a bicornuate uterus invariably shows a deep (>10 mm) cleft within the external uterine fundal contour, a feature that distinguishes fusion anomalies from resorption anomalies such as septate uterus (**Fig. 6**).[31,34] Normal zonal anatomy is preserved within both uterine horns. On two-dimensional US, bicornuate and septate uteruses may have a similar appearance and using coronal reconstructed 3D US helps distinguish the two entities.[11]

As with uterus didelphys, a careful search should be made for the presence of duplicated cervixes as well as for any vaginal septa, which have been described in approximately 25% of cases.[15]

SEPTATE UTERUS

Accounting for approximately 55% of all MDAs, complete or partial failure of resorption of the uterovaginal septum results in a septate uterus.[35,36] The residual septum may be of

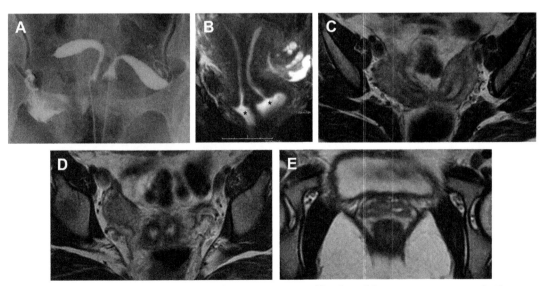

Fig. 5. Uterus didelphys. (*A*) HSG spot image shows contrast opacification of 2 separate noncommunicating uterine horns. (*B*) Coronal T2-weighted image shows 2 noncommunicating uterine cavities and distinct cervixes (*asterisks*). (*C–E*) Axial T2-weighted images show 2 adjacent, albeit separate, fundal horns (*C*), cervixes (*D*), and upper vaginas (*E*).

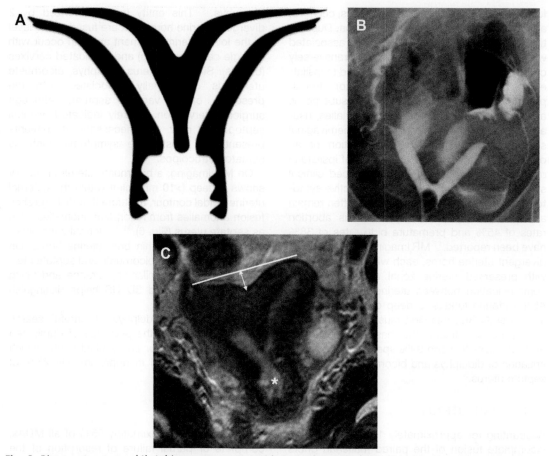

Fig. 6. Bicornuate uterus. (*A*) A bicornuate uterus with a single cervix (unicollis). (*B*) HSG spot image shows contrast opacifying 2 symmetric widely divergent fundal horns. Of note, because the external uterine fundal contour cannot be assessed fluoroscopically, US or MR imaging is necessary to distinguish this finding from septate uterus. (*C*) Axial T2-weighted MR image shows a deep external uterine fundal cleft (*double arrow*) of greater than 10 mm as well as a single cervix (*asterisk*), confirming bicornuate unicollis uterus.

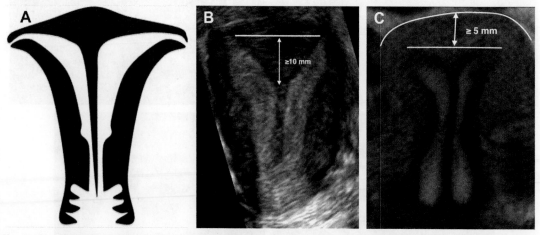

Fig. 7. Complete septate. (*A*) A complete septate uterus in which the uterine septum extends to the cervical os. (*B*) A 3D coronal US image showing an indentation depth of greater than 10 mm, distinguishing septate from arcuate uterus. (*C*) Multiplanar reformatted 3D T2-weighted image better shows the external fundal contour (*curved white line*). Specifically, the distance between the apex of the fundal contour and a line drawn between the tubal ostia is more than 5 mm, distinguishing septate uterus from bicornuate uterus and uterus didelphys.

variable length and composition, consisting of varying proportions of fibrous tissue and myometrium.[20,37] Rarely the septum can extend to the vagina, which then usually is longitudinal rather than transverse. Septate uterus is associated with the poorest reproductive outcomes, with a reported pregnancy loss up to 65% and preterm labor of up to 20%.[11] Although the precise cause of infertility in these patients remains under debate, it is thought to occur secondary to embryo implantation on a poorly vascularized septum.[36] Observational studies suggest that

hysteroscopic resection of the septum improves pregnancy outcomes by decreasing rates of spontaneous abortion, and, as a result, this procedure is frequently performed worldwide.[36,38–40] However, at present no randomized controlled trials exist to support this practice. Given the potential impact of surgical correction on fertility, accurate diagnosis of septate uterus is crucial. On imaging, septate uterus has a smooth or mildly depressed outer fundal contour, which is in contrast with the deep (>10 mm) cleft in the outer fundal contour

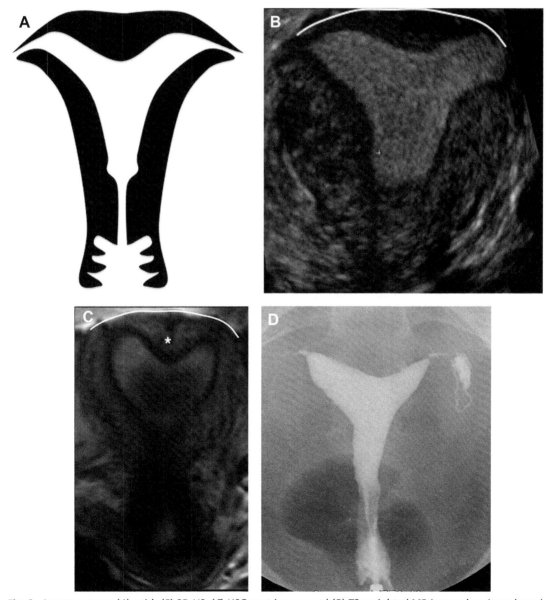

Fig. 8. Arcuate uterus (*A*), with (*B*) 3D US, (*C*) HSG spot image, and (*D*) T2-weighted MR image showing a broad-based smooth bulge at the level of the internal uterine fundal contour (*asterisk*). The normal external fundal contour (*curved white line*) can only be assessed on the 3D US and MR imaging.

seen in both bicornuate and didelphys uteri (Fig. 7).[41] Numerous societies have proposed their own diagnostic criteria for septate uterus, in which variability and inconsistency among definitions generated confusion among clinicians tasked with managing these patients. The ASRM definition considers a uterus septate when there is both an indentation depth greater than 15 mm (defined by depth from the interstitial line to the apex of the fundal indentation) as well as an indentation angle less than 90°.[34] In contrast, the European Society of Human Reproduction and Embryology (ESHRE) and the European Society for Gynaecological Endoscopy (ESGE) definition considers a uterus septate when there is an indentation/wall thickness ratio (I/WT) greater than 50%.[14] More recently, a new definition, termed Congenital Uterine Malformation by Experts (CUME) was proposed, which has settled with emerging consensus as the diagnostic criteria of choice for septate uterus. The CUME definition considers a uterus septate simply when there is an indentation depth of greater than 10 mm,[31] providing a simple and reliable tool for establishing the diagnosis. Per CUME criteria, additional ancillary features that aid in the diagnosis include an indentation angle less than 140° as well as an I/WT greater than 110%.

ARCUATE UTERUS

Often thought of as a normal variant, arcuate uterus represents the mildest MDA subtype and occurs in the setting of near-complete uterovaginal septal resorption, which results in a focal bulge at the level of the uterine internal fundal contour. Although clinical data are disparate, currently most clinicians agree that arcuate uterus is associated with minimal if any adverse reproductive outcomes.

Imaging of arcuate uterus depicts a normal external fundal contour with a broad-based smooth myometrial prominence at the internal fundal contour (Fig. 8).

DIETHYSTILBUSTEROL-EXPOSED UTERUS

Diethystilbusterol (DES) is a nonsteroidal estrogen that was prescribed from the late 1940s until 1971 to prevent miscarriages in women with a history of poor reproductive outcomes. This medication was discontinued after adverse outcomes were discovered in the female infants who were exposed to the drug in utero, which included vaginal clear-cell carcinoma and uterine hypoplasia.[42]

Although now more of historical interest (given the length of time since discontinuation), DES-exposed uteruses show a characteristic T-shaped configuration caused by a shortened upper uterine body and hypoplastic uterine cavity. In addition, so-called constriction bands are seen within the midfundal myometrium, classically appearing as areas of focal thickening at the junctional zone, which lead to an irregular and narrowed uterine canal.[11]

SUMMARY/WHAT REFERRING PHYSICIANS NEED TO KNOW

- Infertility is often a multifactorial medical condition requiring a comprehensive approach for diagnosis and treatment.
- The imaging investigation of female infertility consists of a multimodality approach.
- MR imaging and sometimes 3D US are the imaging examinations of choice when MDAs are suspected.
- Hysterosalpingogram is the gold standard study to evaluate tubal patency, although hysterosalpingo contrast sonography is a promising imaging tool that is increasingly used.

CONFLICT OF INTEREST

The authors report no conflicts of interests concerning the materials, methods, or results in this article.

REFERENCES

1. Olpin JD, Heilbrun M. Imaging of Mullerian duct anomalies. Clin Obstet Gynecol 2009;52(1):40–56.
2. Buttram VC Jr, Gibbons WE. Müllerian anomalies: a proposed classification. (An analysis of 144 cases). Fertil Steril 1979 Jul;32(1):40–6.
3. Golan A, Langer R, Bukovsky I, et al. Congenital anomalies of the müllerian system. Fertil Steril 1989;51(5):747–55.
4. Chan YY, Jayaprakasan K, Zamora J, et al. The prevalence of congenital uterine anomalies in unselected and high-risk populations: a systematic review. Hum Reprod Update 2011;17(6):761–71.
5. Grimbizis GF, Camus M, Tarlatzis BC, et al. Clinical implications of uterine malformations and hysteroscopic treatment results. Hum Reprod Update 2001;7(2):161–74.
6. Acién P. Incidence of müllerian defects in fertile and infertile women. Hum Reprod 1997;12(7):1372–6.
7. Saravelos SH, Cocksedge KA, Li TC. Prevalence and diagnosis of congenital uterine anomalies in women with reproductive failure: a critical appraisal. Hum Reprod Update 2008;14:415–29.

8. Raga F, Bauset C, Remohi J, et al. Reproductive impact of congenital Mullerian anomalies. Hum Reprod 1997;12:2277–81.

9. Woelfer B, Salim R, Banerjee S, et al. Reproductive outcomes in women with congenital uterine anomalies detected by three- dimensional ultrasound screening. Obstet Gynecol 2001;98:1099–103.

10. Lewis AD, Levine D. Pregnancy complications in women with uterine duplication abnormalities. Ultrasound Q 2010;26:193–200.

11. Troiano RN, McCarthy SM. Müllerian duct anomalies: imaging and clinical issues. Radiology 2004; 233(1):19–34.

12. American Society for Reproductive Medicine (ASRM). The American Fertility Society classifications of adnexal adhesions, distal tubal occlusion, tubal occlusion secondary to tubal ligation, tubal pregnancies, mullerian anomalies and intrauterine adhesions. Fertil Steril 1988;49(6):944–55.

13. Oppelt P, Renner SP, Brucker S, et al. The VCUAM (Vagina Cervix Uterus Adnex-associated Malformation) classification: a new classification for genital malformations. Fertil Steril 2005;84(5):1493–7.

14. Grimbizis GF, Gordts S, Di Spiezio Sardo A, et al. The ESHRE/ESGE consensus on the classification of female genital tract congenital anomalies. Hum Reprod 2013;28(8):2032–44.

15. Olpin JD, Moeni A, Willmore RJ, et al. MR imaging of müllerian fusion anomalies. Magn Reson Imaging Clin N Am 2017;25(3):563–75.

16. Deutch TD, Abuhamad AZ. The role of 3-dimensional ultrasonography and magnetic resonance imaging in the diagnosis of Mullerian duct anomalies: a review of the literature. J Ultrasound Med 2008;27: 413–23.

17. Mueller GC, Hussain HK, Smith YR, et al. Mullerian duct anomalies: comparison of MRI diagnosis and clinical diagnosis. AJR Am J Roentgenol 2007;189: 1294–302.

18. Church DG, Vancil JM, Vasanawala SS. Magnetic resonance imaging for uterine and vaginal anomalies. Curr Opin Obstet Gynecol 2009;21:379–89.

19. Pellerito JS, McCarthy SM, Doyle MB, et al. Diagnosis of uterine anomalies: relative accuracy of MR imaging, endovaginal sonography, and hysterosalpingography. Radiology 1992;183(3):795–800.

20. Behr SC, Courtier JL, Qayyum A. Imaging of müllerian duct anomalies. Radiographics 2012;32(6): E233–50.

21. Oppelt PG, Lermann J, Strick R, et al. Malformations in a cohort of 284 women with Mayer-Rokitansky-Küster-Hauser syndrome (MRKH). Reprod Biol Endocrinol 2012;10:57.

22. Garcia-Roig M, Castellan M, Gonzalez J, et al. Sigmoid vaginoplasty with a modified single Monti tube: a pediatric case series. J Urol 2014;191(5 Suppl):1537–42.

23. Epelman M, Dinan D, Gee MS, et al. Mullerian duct and related anomalies in children and adolescents. Magn Reson Imaging Clin N Am 2013;21(4): 773–89.

24. Uğur M, Turan C, Mungan T, et al. Endometriosis in association with müllerian anomalies. Gynecol Obstet Invest 1995;40(4):261–4.

25. Olive DL, Henderson DY. Endometriosis and mullerian anomalies. Obstet Gynecol 1987;69(3 pt 1): 412–5.

26. Junqueira BL, Allen LM, Spitzer RF, et al. Müllerian duct anomalies and mimics in children and adolescents: correlative intraoperative assessment with clinical imaging. Radiographics 2009;29(4): 1085–103.

27. Jayasinghe Y, Rane A, Stalewski H, et al. The presentation and early diagnosis of the rudimentary uterine horn. Obstet Gynecol 2005;105(6): 1456–67.

28. Brody JM, Koelliker SL, Frishman GN. Unicornuate uterus: imaging appearance, associated anomalies, and clinical implications. AJR Am J Roentgenol 1998;171(5):1341–7.

29. Khati NJ, Frazier AA, Brindle KA. The unicornuate uterus and its variants: clinical presentation, imaging findings, and associated complications. J Ultrasound Med 2012;31(2):319–31.

30. Li S, Qayyum A, Coakley FV, et al. Association of renal agenesis and mullerian duct anomalies. J Comput Assist Tomogr 2000;24(6):829–34.

31. Ludwin A, Martins WP, Nastri CO, et al. Congenital Uterine Malformation by Experts (CUME): better criteria for distinguishing between normal/arcuate and septate uterus? Ultrasound Obstet Gynecol 2018;51(1):101–9.

32. Miller RJ, Breech LL. Surgical correction of vaginal anomalies. Clin Obstet Gynecol 2008;51(2):223–36.

33. Rackow BW, Arici A. Reproductive performance of women with müllerian anomalies. Curr Opin Obstet Gynecol 2007;19(3):229–37.

34. Practice Committee of the American Society for Reproductive Medicine, Practice Committee of the American Society for Reproductive Medicine. Uterine septum: a guideline. Fertil Steril 2016;106(3): 530–40.

35. Steinkeler JA, Woodfield CA, Lazarus E, et al. Female infertility: a systematic approach to radiologic imaging and diagnosis. Radiographics 2009;29: 1353–70.

36. Homer HA, Li TC, Cooke ID. The septate uterus: a review of management and reproductive outcome. Fertil Steril 2000;73(1):1–14.

37. Zreik TG, Troiano RN, Ghoussoub RA, et al. Myometrial tissue in uterine septa. J Am Assoc Gynecol Laparosc 1998;5(2):155–60.

38. Venetis CA, Papadopoulos SP, Campo R, et al. Clinical implications of congenital uterine anomalies: a

meta-analysis of comparative studies. Reprod Biomed Online 2014;29(6):665–83.

39. Saygili-Yilmaz E, Yildiz S, Erman-Akar M, et al. Reproductive outcome of septate uterus after hysteroscopic metroplasty. Arch Gynecol Obstet 2003; 268(4):289–92.

40. Rikken JFW, Kowalik CR, Emanuel MH, et al. Septum resection for women of reproductive age with a septate uterus. Cochrane Database Syst Rev 2017; 1:4–6.

41. Li Y, Phelps A, Zapala MA, et al. Magnetic resonance imaging of Müllerian duct anomalies in children. Pediatr Radiol 2016;46(6):796–805.

42. Herbst AL, Ulfelder H, Poskanzer DC. Adenocarcinoma of the vagina: association of maternal stilbestrol therapy with tumor appearance in young women. N Engl J Med 1971;284(15):878–81.

Imaging Spectrum of Benign Uterine Disease and Treatment Options

Stephanie Nougaret, MD, PhD[a,b,*], Martina Sbarra, MD[c,d],
Jessica Robbins, MD[e]

KEYWORDS

- Leiomyoma • Leiomyosarcoma • Adenomyosis • MR imaging • Uterus

KEY POINTS

- Benign uterine disease mainly comprises adenomyosis and leiomyomas, common gynecologic conditions affecting women of all ages.
- Magnetic resonance (MR) imaging is the most accurate imaging modality for detection and localization of benign uterine disease and its mimics.
- MR imaging is the diagnostic tool of choice for pretreatment evaluation, assessing potential procedural risk and predicting treatment response, and monitoring treatment outcomes.

INTRODUCTION

Benign uterine diseases, such as adenomyosis and leiomyomas, are common gynecologic conditions affecting women of all ages.[1–6] Although ultrasonography (US) is the first-line imaging technique in the examination of the uterus, magnetic resonance (MR) imaging has become very useful and is the most accurate tool in lesion diagnosis and patient management.[7–13] Benign uterine disease may manifest with atypical features and can mimic malignancy, making the correct diagnosis a challenge.[10,14,15] MR imaging also assists in the triage of symptomatic patients to the most appropriate treatment modality, including surgery (hysterectomy or myomectomy), interventional procedures (uterine artery embolization), and medical therapy.[16–18] Hysterectomy is curative, but uterus-sparing therapies are a valid alternative for eligible women.

This article highlights the utility of MR imaging in the diagnosis of the most common benign uterine diseases, such as leiomyomas and adenomyosis, discusses their typical and atypical MR imaging findings, describes the therapeutic options, and delineates the role of MR imaging in treatment planning.

MAGNETIC RESONANCE IMAGING PROTOCOL

Clinical guidelines for diagnosis and management of patients with leiomyomas are extensive.[1,19,20] Recently, recommendations for MR imaging were proposed by the European Society of Urogenital Radiology (ESUR).[13]

Patient Preparation

Fasting and the use of an antiperistaltic agent such as Hyoscine Butylpromide or glucagon is useful to

[a] Montpellier Cancer Research Institute, INSERM, U1194, University of Montpellier, Montpellier, France; [b] Department of Radiology, Montpellier Cancer Institute, 208 Avenue des Apothicaires, Montpellier 34295, France; [c] Radiologia Diagnostica e Interventistica Generale, Dipartimento Diagnostica per Immagini, Radioterapia Oncologica ed Ematologia, Fondazione Policlinico Universitario A. Gemelli IRCCS, Rome, Italy; [d] Istituto di Radiologia, Università Cattolica del Sacro Cuore, Largo A. Gemelli 8-00168, Rome, Italy; [e] University of Wisconsin School of Medicine and Public Health, 750 Highland Avenue, Madison, WI 53705, USA
* Corresponding author. Department of Radiology, Montpellier Cancer Institute, 208 Ave des Apothicaires, Montpellier 34295, France.
E-mail address: stephanienougaret@free.fr

Radiol Clin N Am 58 (2020) 239–256
https://doi.org/10.1016/j.rcl.2019.10.004
0033-8389/20/© 2019 Elsevier Inc. All rights reserved.

radiologic.theclinics.com

minimize motion artifacts related to small bowel peristalsis. A moderately full bladder is recommended to reduce artifacts related to bladder filling.[13]

Imaging Protocol

High-resolution thin-section images acquired at 1.5 T or 3.0 T are recommended. The optimal protocol, according to recent ESUR guidelines, is summarized in **Table 1**.[13]

LEIOMYOMAS
Epidemiology, Pathophysiology

Leiomyomas are the most common benign uterine tumors, affecting up to 20% to 30% of reproductive-aged women.[11] They are benign neoplasms of unknown cause composed of multiple layers of smooth muscle fascicles and fibrous connective tissue anchored in the muscular wall of the uterus. These tumors may be solitary or, most frequently, multiple.[21] The size of leiomyomas is variable and influenced by estrogen and progesterone; they often grow during pregnancy and with oral contraceptive use and regress after menopause.[21] They may be asymptomatic, but 20% to 50% of women with leiomyomas present with symptoms such as menorrhagia, dysmenorrhea, pressure, urinary frequency, pelvic and back pain, and dyspareunia.[5]

Location

Leiomyomas generally involve the myometrium of the uterine corpus and are classified by their location as submucosal, intramural, and subserosal. In accordance with the International Federation of Gynecology and Obstetrics (FIGO) classification system, they can be further subdivided into 8 categories (**Fig. 1**).[22] Pedunculated lesions can become detached from the uterus, receiving blood supply from other adjacent structures, and are called parasitic leiomyomas.[23,24] Leiomyomas not related to the myometrium may be located in the cervix and in the round or broad ligaments.

Leiomyomas may occur in unusual locations, such as diffuse peritoneal leiomyomatosis, intravenous leiomyomatosis, or benign metastasizing leiomyoma. Peritoneal leiomyomatosis is characterized by multiple lesions along the peritoneal surfaces, probably caused by the iatrogenic dissemination throughout the peritoneal cavity after surgery.[25] A previous history of hysterectomy for leiomyomas or a diagnosis of uterine leiomyomas may point to the correct diagnosis. Intravenous leiomyomatosis has an aggressive intravascular growth pattern within intrauterine and systemic veins.[25]

Imaging Features

Ultrasonography
US is usually the initial imaging study.

Table 1 Protocol	
T2WI	High-resolution T2 sequences in the axial, oblique, sagittal, and coronal planes. The axial oblique T2W sequence perpendicular to the corpus of the uterus is particularly useful to evaluate the location of the lesion relative to the endometrial cavity
T1WI	Axial T1W sequence of the pelvis with and without fat suppression. Axial T1W sequence is useful to evaluate the presence of fat or blood contents and can be used to detect the presence of lymph nodes and bone marrow abnormalities
Large-FOV T1WI/T2WI	Large-FOV T1W or T2W sequence of the upper abdomen. It allows visualization of secondary signs of pelvic mass effect, such as hydronephrosis, and malignant disease, such as lymph nodes or peritoneal carcinomatosis
Contrast-enhanced T1WI	Contrast-enhanced axial T1WI of the pelvis with fat saturation. It allows further lesion characterization, vascularization, and its differentiation from an adnexal mass
Dynamic contrast injection/ MR angiography	Dynamic contrast injection/MR angiography is recommended if uterine artery embolization may be a possibility in order to evaluate uterine artery anatomy and collateral gonadal arterial supply
DWI	DWI is not mandatory but has shown added value for lesion characterization and distinction between leiomyoma and leiomyosarcoma

Abbreviations: DWI, diffusion-weighted imaging; FOV, field of view; T1W, T1-weighted; T1WI, T1-weighted imaging; T2W, T2-weighted; T2WI, T2-weighted imaging.

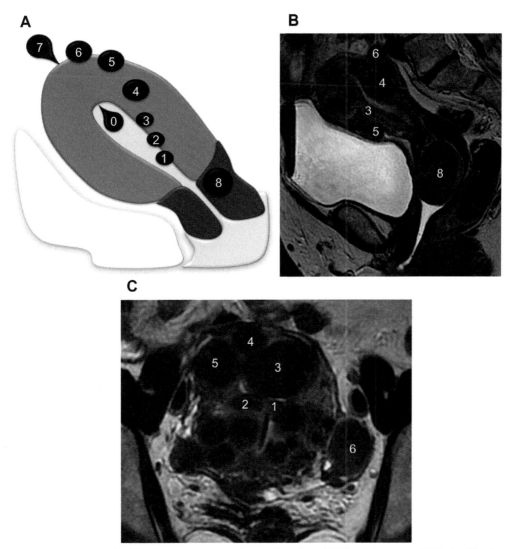

Fig. 1. Leiomyoma FIGO classification system according to location. (*A*) The leiomyoma FIGO classification: 0, pedunculated intracavitary; 1, submucosal less than 50% intramural; 2, submucosal greater than or equal to 50% intramural; 3, contacts endometrium, 100% intramural; 4, intramural; 5, subserosal greater than or equal to 50% intramural; 6, subserosal less than 50% intramural; 7, subserosal pedunculated; 8, other (specify; eg, cervical, parasitic). (*B*) Sagittal and (*C*) axial T2-weighted images show multiple leiomyomas in different locations, each labeled with its MR imaging FIGO classification.

On US, a typical leiomyoma is a well-defined mass, often shadowing at the margin and/or producing internal linear shadowing. The echogenicity varies from hypoechoic to hyperechoic in relation to the myometrium. Dystrophic calcifications can be seen particularly in postmenopausal women. On color Doppler US, circumferential blood flow around the lesion is often seen.[26]

Magnetic resonance imaging
US can be limited by coexisting pelvic diseases, uterine anomalies, unusually small or large tumors, and tumor location.[27] Thus, MR imaging is considered the most accurate imaging modality to detect, locate, and characterize myometrial lesions before patient management.[14,28] MR imaging has reported sensitivities and specificities of 94.1% and 68.7%, respectively, for uterine leiomyomas.[21,27,29]

On MR imaging, most leiomyomas, without any degeneration, are easily recognized as well-delineated round or ovoid lesions homogeneously hypointense on T2-weighted imaging (T2WI) related to the outer myometrium and isointense on T1-weighted imaging (T1WI), with heterogeneous and variable enhancement. The presence of a

T2-hyperintense rim indicates a pseudocapsule of edema caused by dilated lymphatic vessels and veins (**Fig. 2**).[29] Typical leiomyomas do not have restricted diffusion, showing a low signal intensity both on diffusion-weighted imaging (DWI) and on the corresponding apparent diffusion coefficient (ADC) map, known as the blackout phenomenon (see **Fig. 2**).[10]

There are 2 subtypes of leiomyoma.

Cellular leiomyoma is a histologic subtype characterized by more compact smooth muscle cells with little or no collagen; on MR imaging it shows higher signal intensity on T2WI and avid enhancement (**Fig. 3**).[11] The intermediate T2 signal and avid enhancement of cellular leiomyomas can make it difficult to differentiate them from leiomyosarcoma (see **Fig. 3**).[30] In a retrospective study of 51 patients with a single myometrial lesion at MR imaging, Thomassin-Naggara and colleagues[31] suggested that the evaluation of DWI and ADC (value cutoff 1.23×10^{-3} mm^2/s) may limit the misdiagnosis of uterine sarcoma as leiomyoma with diagnostic accuracy of 92.4% (see **Fig. 3**).

Lipoleiomyoma occurs in 0.03% to 0.2% of women, generally in the postmenopausal population. Lipoleiomyomas are composed of smooth muscle, adipose tissue, and fibrous tissue. The signal intensity of the fat components is typical high on T1WI and T2WI with loss of signal intensity on fat-saturated sequences.[10]

When leiomyomas enlarge and outgrow their blood supply (≥5 cm), they may degenerate.[21,27] The types of degeneration are hyaline, cystic, myxoid, hemorrhagic, and calcific (**Table 2**).

Hyaline degeneration is the most common type (60%). Leiomyomas with hyaline degeneration have low signal intensity on T2WI, an appearance similar to that of nondegenerated leiomyomas; however, they enhance to a lesser degree than standard leiomyomas (**Fig. 4**A, B).[32]

Cystic degeneration (4%) is characterized by the presence of cystic areas with high signal intensity on T2WI that do not enhance (**Fig. 4**C, D).[21]

Myxoid degeneration is rare and depends on the presence of gelatinous intralesional foci at gross examination that contain hyaluronic acid–rich mucopolysaccharides.[33] Leiomyomas with myxoid degeneration have an extremely high signal intensity on T2WI and enhance well except for foci of mucinous lakes or clefts. Delayed and prolonged

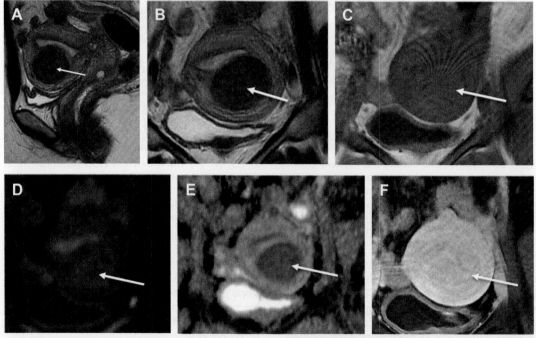

Fig. 2. Typical leiomyoma. (*A*) Sagittal and (*B*) axial T2-weighted images, (*C*) axial T1-weighted image, (*D*) axial diffusion-weighted (DW) image with (*E*) corresponding apparent diffusion coefficient (ADC) map, and (*F*) gadolinium-enhanced axial T1-weighted fat-saturated image show a myometrial lesion with endometrial contact (*arrows*) in keeping with a FIGO 3 leiomyoma. Nondegenerated leiomyoma appears as a well-defined lesion with hypointense signal intensity on T2-weighted images related to the outer myometrium (*A*, *B*), isointense signal intensity on T1-weighted image (*C*), and homogeneous contrast enhancement (*F*). The blackout phenomenon is shown, with no signs of restricted diffusion with low signal intensity on DW image (b = 1000) (*D*) and corresponding ADC map (*E*).

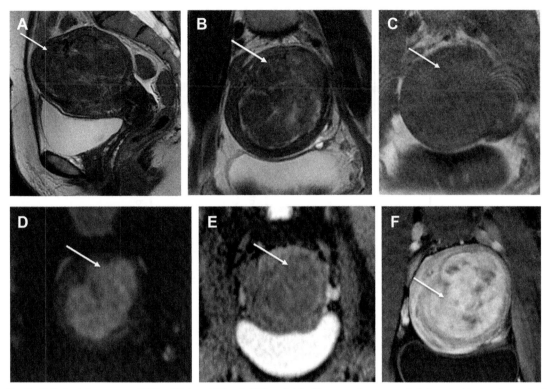

Fig. 3. Cellular leiomyoma. (*A*) Sagittal and (*B*) axial T2-weighted images show a well-delineated lesion (*arrow*) of intermediate to high signal intensity without T2 dark areas. (*C*) Axial oblique T1-weighted image shows isointense lesion without hemorrhage (*arrow*). (*D*) Axial oblique DW image (b = 1000) shows high signal intensity (*arrow*) with restriction on (*E*) corresponding ADC map (*arrow*). (*F*) Contrast-enhanced axial oblique T1-weighted fat-saturated image shows avid and heterogeneous enhancement without necrosis (*arrow*). The absence of hemorrhage and necrosis, T2 dark signal, and the presence of well-defined border favor a cellular leiomyoma rather than leiomyosarcoma; this was confirmed histologically.

contrast enhancement is caused by the presence of myxoid stroma (**Fig. 4**E, F).[34]

Hemorrhagic degeneration (red degeneration) is caused by hemorrhagic infarction resulting in coagulative necrosis and is associated with pregnancy and oral contraceptives.[35] Red degeneration may also occur after uterine artery embolization (UAE). On MR imaging, the signal intensity is variable: peripheral or diffuse hyperintensity on T1WI and inhomogeneous signal intensity on T2WI with or without the hypointense rim. The T1 hyperintensity is caused by the proteinaceous content of the blood and/or by the T1-shortening effect of methemoglobin.[12] When the hyperintensity is peripheral, it may be caused by thrombosis of the vessels that surround the lesion (**Fig. 4**G, H).[35]

Calcific degeneration is associated with end-stage hyaline degeneration and post-UAE treatment changes. On MR imaging the calcific components produce signal voids on all sequences.[10]

Smooth muscle tumor of uncertain malignant potential (STUMP) is a rare heterogeneous tumor that cannot be definitively classified histologically as leiomyoma or leiomyosarcoma.[8] Multiple subtypes have been identified according to nuclear atypia, mitotic rate, and necrosis. On MR imaging, there are no specific features, because STUMP mimics both typical leiomyoma and leiomyosarcoma. After removal they have a high rate of recurrence (7.3%–12.5%) and may recur as low-grade leiomyosarcoma; therefore, long-term follow-up is needed.[8,10]

Pitfalls to avoid on magnetic resonance imaging

- Distinction between an ovarian mass and a uterine mass: it might be hard to distinguish uterine leiomyoma from a fibrous ovarian mass. In a ovarian mass, sharp angles between the ovary and the lesion are known as the beak sign. In contrast, in a uterine mass, a normal ovary is seen separate from the mass. The claw sign (uterine tissue draped around the mass) (see **Fig. 4**C) or the bridging-vessels sign (enlarged and tortuous vessels extending from the uterus to the lesion) suggest the diagnosis of a uterine mass (see **Fig. 4**H; **Fig. 5**).

Table 2
Magnetic resonance imaging features of leiomyomas and leiomyosarcomas

	T2WI Signal	T2WI Border	T1WI	C+	DWI
Type of Leiomyoma					
Nondegenerated	Hypointense	Well defined	Isointense	Variable	Hypointense
Cellular subtype	Hyperintense	Well defined	Isointense	Vivid enhancement	Hyperintense
Lipoleiomyoma subtype	Variable: fat component (hyperintense)	Well defined	Variable: fat component (hyperintense)	Variable	Variable due to fat content
Degeneration Type					
Hyaline	Hypointense	Well defined	Isointense	Moderate enhancement	Hypointense
Cystic	Hyperintense	Well defined	Hypointense	No enhancement	Hypointense
Myxoid	Very hyperintense	Well defined	Hypointense	Delayed enhancement	Hypointense
Hemorrhagic	Variable	Well defined	Hyperintense	Variable	Variable due to blood content
Calcific	T2 hypointense	Well defined	Hypointense	No enhancement	Hypointense
Leiomyosarcoma	T2 dark areas	Nodular border	Presence of High T1 SI related to blood	Enhancement with central necrosis	High DWI/low ADC

Abbreviations: ADC, apparent diffusion coefficient; C +, contrast-enhanced imaging; DWI, diffusion-weighted imaging; T1WI, T1-weighted imaging; T2WI, T2-weighted imaging; SI, signal intensity.

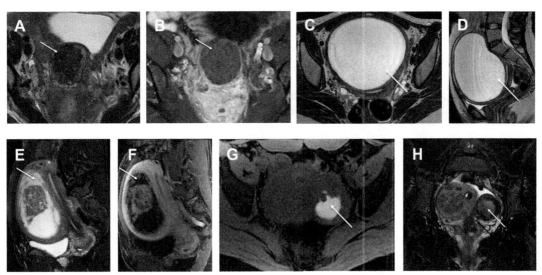

Fig. 4. Different types of leiomyoma degeneration. Hyaline degeneration. (*A*) Axial T2-weighted image and (*B*) contrast-enhanced axial T1-weighted fat-saturated image show a leiomyoma (*arrow*) with hypointense signal intensity on T2-weighted image and poor enhancement after gadolinium injection, suggesting hyaline degeneration. Cystic degeneration. (*C*) Axial T2-weighted image and (*D*) sagittal T2-weighted image show a large, well-defined cystic lesion (*arrow*) with high T2 signal intensity, consistent with cystic leiomyoma because of its uterine origin (claw sign). Myxoid degeneration. (*E*) Sagittal T2-weighted fat-saturated image and (*F*) contrast-enhanced sagittal T1-weighted fat-saturated image show a leiomyoma (*arrow*) presenting areas with high signal intensity on T2-weighted image and enhancement after gadolinium injection, with the exception of the nonenhancing mucinous lakes, suggesting a myxoid leiomyoma. Hemorrhagic degeneration. (*G*) Axial T1-weighted fat-saturated image and (*H*) axial T2-weighted fat-saturated image show a left parauterine lesion (*white arrow*) with a component of very high signal intensity on T1-weighted image and low signal intensity on T2-weighted image, suggesting intralesional hemorrhage. The lesion is a hemorrhagic subserosal pedunculated leiomyoma (MR imaging FIGO 7) with enlarged and tortuous vessel (*black arrow, H*) that extends from the uterus to the mass (bridging vessel sign), indicating the uterine origin of the lesion.

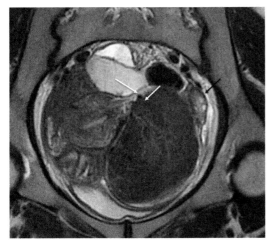

Fig. 5. Indeterminate origin of a mass: ovarian versus uterine. Axial T2-weighted image shows a well-defined left parauterine mass with low signal intensity that could resemble either a uterine leiomyoma or ovarian fibroma. In this case, the left ovary (*black arrow*) is normal and separate from the mass. Enlarged and tortuous vessels extended from the uterus to supply the mass (*white arrows*, bridging vessels sign), suggesting the diagnosis of uterine leiomyoma.

- Focal myometrial contractions: contractions may appear as low-T2-signal myometrial masses and may simulate uterine leiomyomas. Because they are transient and usually do not persist during the entire examination they can be easily differentiated from leiomyomas (Fig. 6).
- Endometrial polyp: submucosal leiomyoma may be mistaken for an endometrial polyp. Polyps have heterogeneous or high signal on T2WI, in contrast with pedunculated submucosal leiomyomas, which are low signal on T2WI and have a stalk that arises from the myometrium.
- Adenomyomas: discussed later.
- Leiomyosarcomas: it is critical to differentiate a benign leiomyoma from leiomyosarcoma. Although leiomyosarcomas arise de novo and have no biological link to leiomyomas,[36] they may present with symptoms and imaging features similar to leiomyomas. Large size and rapid growth are unreliable signs of malignancy.[36] Growth of a uterine mass after menopause and increased lactate dehydrogenase (LDH [level]), particularly LDH isozyme

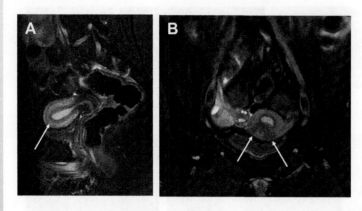

Fig. 6. Transient myometrial contraction. (A) Sagittal and (B) axial T2-weighted fat-saturated images. Axial T2-weighted image shows hypointense bands perpendicular to the junctional zone (JZ) in the anterior myometrium (arrows, B). This finding was absent on previous sagittal T2-weighted image that shows normal uterus with thin and distinct JZ (arrow, A), confirming the diagnosis of transient myometrial contraction.

type 3, is suspicious for leiomyosarcoma.[36] Endometrial sampling may aid diagnosis of uterine sarcoma but sensitivity is limited because of the myometrial origin of the tumor.[36,37] Although no single MR imaging feature can reliably distinguish leiomyosarcomas from atypical leiomyomas, a combination of MR imaging features may improve the diagnostic performance of MR imaging for the correct diagnosis of leiomyosarcoma. In a study from Lakhman and colleagues,[14] the combination of 3 or more of 4 discriminative features, including nodular borders, hemorrhage (high signal intensity on T1WI), T2-weighted (T2W) dark areas, and central areas of nonenhancement, was associated with an improved sensitivity and specificity for the diagnosis of leiomyosarcoma (Fig. 7). Uterine sarcoma also shows rapid early enhancement of the solid components and restricted diffusion.[8] Diffusion restriction alone is insufficient for diagnosis because there is considerable overlap in ADC values between leiomyomas and leiomyosarcoma; leiomyomas may show restricted diffusion, especially cellular leiomyomas (see Fig. 3D, E).[38] Notably, the presence of restricted diffusion and a T2 blackout effect is highly specific for a leiomyoma (see Fig. 2).[15] More recently, Thomassin-Naggara and colleagues[31] reported that, using a recursive model combining T2 signal intensity, b1000 images, and ADC map with a cutoff value 1.23, MR imaging achieved 92.4% accuracy in distinguishing benign and uncertain

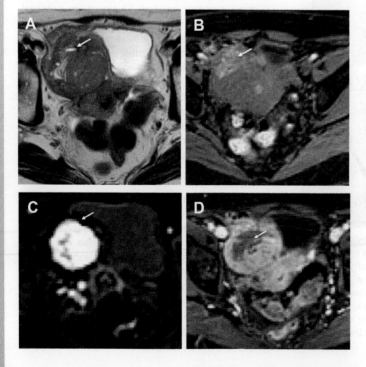

Fig. 7. Leiomyosarcoma. (A) Axial T2-weighted image, (B) axial T1-weighted image, (C) axial DW image, and (D) gadolinium-enhanced axial T1-weighted fat-saturated image. Axial T2-weighted image shows dark T2 area (arrow, A) and ill-defined border. Hemorrhage is seen on the axial T1-weighted image (arrow, B). (C) Axial oblique DW image (b = 1000) shows high signal intensity (arrow). (D) Contrast-enhanced axial oblique T1-weighted fat-saturated image shows heterogeneous enhancement with central necrosis (arrow). These combined features are suggestive of leiomyosarcoma, which was confirmed histologically.

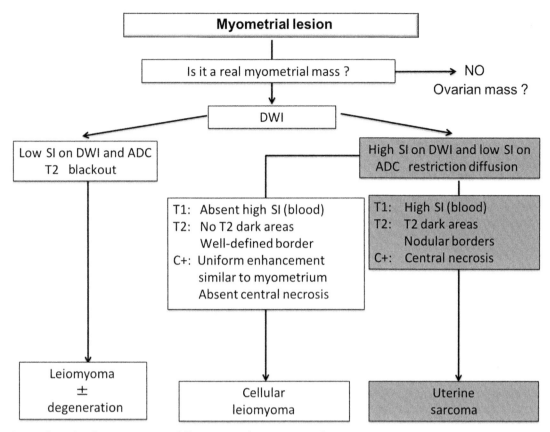

Fig. 8. The role of MR imaging in differentiating leiomyoma and uterine sarcoma.

or malignant myometrial tumors. The investigators concluded that DWI may be of interest to distinguish between uterine sarcomas and benign leiomyomas.[31] **Fig. 8** shows an algorithm to help differentiate leiomyoma and leiomyosarcoma.

Treatment Options

Depending on the spectrum of symptoms that patients are experiencing, they may benefit from conservative management. Asymptomatic leiomyomas do not require treatment. Nonsteroidal antiinflammatory medications may diminish symptoms of dysmenorrhea, but it is unclear whether these effects extend to women with dysmenorrhea caused by leiomyomas.[39] Oral contraceptives or gonadotropin-releasing hormone (GnRH) agonists may be used to reduce menstrual bleeding associated with leiomyomas.[39,40] GnRH agonists may also reduce the size of leiomyomas.[39] Although some investigators advocate the use of levonorgestrel-releasing intrauterine devices (IUDs) as a means to reduce menstrual bleeding with leiomyomas, the data to support its effectiveness are limited.[39,41] Because submucosal leiomyomas increase the risk of IUD expulsion

and bleeding complications, they are a relative contraindication for the use of an IUD.[40]

Women with refractory abnormal bleeding or those experiencing bulk symptoms, such as pelvic fullness, constipation, or urinary symptoms, may be eligible for surgical management. Uterine-sparing myomectomy can be considered for patients with 3 or fewer dominant symptomatic leiomyomas less than 8 cm in diameter.[40] Hysteroscopic myomectomy is optimal for the treatment of submucosal leiomyomas that are predominantly intracavitary, are less than 4 cm in size, and have at least 5 mm of intact myometrium overlying the leiomyoma, whereas laparoscopic or open myomectomy is preferred for subserosal or intramural leiomyomas.[40] If the patient no longer desires childbearing, hysterectomy, via abdominal, laparoscopic, or vaginal approach, is a consideration. Although there is risk inherent with surgical intervention, hysterectomy yields the highest degree of symptom improvement.[42]

UAE is a minimally invasive uterine-sparing treatment option for leiomyomas resulting in abnormal bleeding, anemia, and/or bulk symptoms. UAE is an alternative to myomectomy, but, unlike myomectomy, it is also useful in patients with multiple (>3) and large (>10 cm) leiomyomas.[43] UAE offers the opportunity to preserve fertility, improves or eliminates bulk symptoms and bleeding, is durable, and has a low complication rate.[44,45] There is a roughly 10% to 15% treatment failure rate in which patients require additional treatment with hysterectomy, myomectomy, or repeat UAE.[45,46]

Some centers use UAE before myomectomy. In this scenario, UAE is performed 24 to 48 hours before standard myomectomy. Compared with myomectomy alone, this combined technique decreases the risk of bleeding requiring transfusion, minimizes the risk of conversion to hysterectomy, and results in a shorter postoperative hospital stay.[47]

ADENOMYOSIS
Epidemiology, Clinical Symptoms, and Pathophysiology

Adenomyosis is a common benign gynecologic condition. It is defined as ectopic endometrial glands and stroma in the myometrium more than 2.5 mm from the endometrium-myometrium interface.[5,48–51] Although it is estimated that up to one-third of patients with adenomyosis are asymptomatic, the symptoms of adenomyosis are common but are nonspecific, including dysmenorrhea, menorrhagia, and abnormal vaginal bleeding. Adenomyosis is associated with female infertility, possibly in part because of the overlapping pathophysiology and association with endometriosis.[52] The cause of adenomyosis is still unclear.[4] Exposure to estrogen, prior uterine surgery, and parity are known risk factors.

Ultrasonography Imaging Features

Multiple US features have been associated with adenomyosis, including myometrial heterogeneity with thin linear shadowing (so-called venetian blinds) alternating with increased echogenicity, globular uterine enlargement, asymmetric thickening of the myometrium (pseudowidening sign), and isolated or clustered small anechoic cysts.[53–63] The US appearance of adenomyomas may be similar to uterine leiomyoma. Leiomyomas usually have a well-defined border and peripheral color flow, whereas adenomyomas tend to be ill-defined, show less mass effect, and have diffuse and central color flow.[59]

Magnetic Resonance Imaging Features

MR imaging is highly accurate for the diagnosis of adenomyosis. In a prospective cohort, Stamatopoulos and colleagues[64] described a sensitivity of 46.1%, specificity of 99.2%, and positive predictive value of 92.3% of MR imaging in the diagnosis of adenomyosis. An MR imaging classification of adenomyosis was recently proposed by Bazot and Darai,[65] including definitions of different forms of adenomyosis.

Classic magnetic resonance imaging appearance of adenomyosis

- Subendometrial cysts are a direct sign of adenomyosis correlated with the presence of endometrial glands within the myometrium. These microcysts typically show water signal on T1WI and T2WI. Hemorrhagic content may accumulate within the cysts and show T1-hyperintense signal.[4] They are mainly located in the superficial myometrium and are highly specific (98%). However, they are only detected in 50% of cases (Fig. 9).[66–70]
- Thickening of the junctional zone (JZ) is an indirect sign related to myometrial hypertrophy, secondary to the presence of ectopic endometrial glands within the myometrium. A JZ thickness of greater than 12 mm has a diagnostic accuracy of 85%, specificity of 96%, and sensitivity of 63% to predict adenomyosis.[67] The JZ differential sign was described by Dueholm and colleagues[71] as the difference between maximal and minimal thicknesses in the anterior and posterior uterine JZ; a differential of greater than 5 mm may be a more reliable marker than a JZ thickness of greater than 12 mm (see Fig. 9).
- Because adenomyosis may show variable degrees of enhancement, intravenous contrast does not enhance the diagnostic capacity of MR imaging.

Subtypes of adenomyosis

- Adenomyoma is a masslike confluence of ectopic endometrial glands within the myometrium, distinct from the JZ. The distinction from leiomyoma may be challenging; adenomyomas are usually ill-defined low-signal T2W masses that may contain punctate foci of high T2 signal (Fig. 10).[7,69,72,73]
- Hemorrhagic cystic adenomyosis (adenomyotic cyst) is a rare subtype of adenomyosis and is frequently symptomatic with dysmenorrhea and menorrhagia. This lesion develops following spontaneous hemorrhage of ectopic endometrial glands.[74] The hemorrhage is contained by a partial or complete rim of myometrial tissue, resulting in a cystlike appearance with high signal on T1WI and a low-signal rim on T2WI. The cyst may be submucosal, intramural, or subserosal (Fig. 11).[74,75]

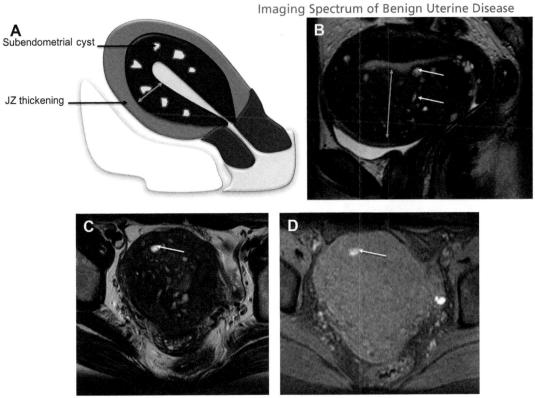

Fig. 9. Adenomyosis. (*A*) Classic features of adenomyosis: subendometrial cysts and diffuse thickening (*orange arrow*) of the JZ. (*B*) Sagittal T2-weighted image shows an enlarged uterus with the classic MR imaging appearance of adenomyosis as thickening of the JZ, particularly of the anterior myometrium (*orange arrow*) with multiple foci with high T2 signal (*white arrows*). (*C*) Axial T2-weighted image and (*D*) axial T1-weighted fat-saturated image show a high-T2 and high-T1 focus within the anterior myometrium (*arrow, C, D*) caused by hemorrhagic content.

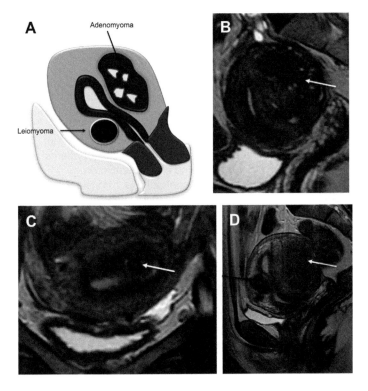

Fig. 10. Adenomyoma. (*A*) The different features of adenomyoma and leioemyoma. An adenomyoma is T2 dark with internal bright foci caused by endometrial glands, whereas a typical leiomyoma is homogeneously dark with a bright peripheral rim caused by perilesional edema that generally causes more adjacent mass effect than adenomyoma. (*B*) Sagittal and (*C*) axial T2-weighted images show an ill-defined, low-signal-intensity mass with embedded hyperintense foci in the posterior myometrium (*arrow, B*) suggesting an adenomyoma. (*C*) Axial oblique T2-weighted image shows a well-defined, low-signal-intensity mass with embedded hyperintense foci bulging into the endometrium (*arrow, C*) suggesting a subendometrial adenomyoma. (*D*) Sagittal T2-weighted image shows an enlarged uterus, with the coexistence of an adenomyoma, as ill-defined hypointense masslike lesion with embedded hyperintense punctate foci in the posterior myometrium (*white arrow*), and a leiomyoma as well-defined very hypointense mass in the anterior myometrium causing adjacent mass effect (*black arrow*).

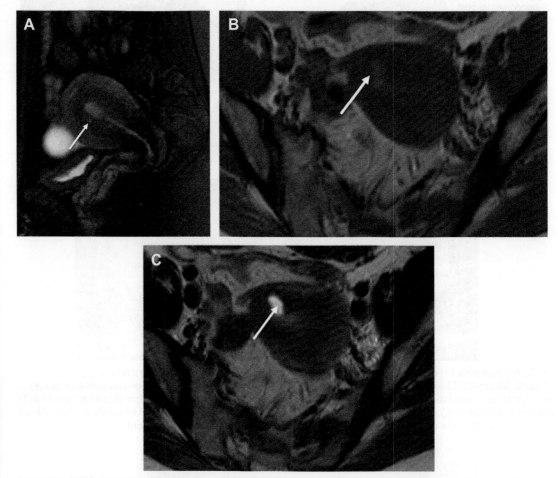

Fig. 11. Hemorrhagic cystic adenomyosis. (*A*) Sagittal T2-weighted fat-saturated image shows diffuse thickening of the JZ and a single intramural focus of high signal intensity in the anterior myometrium (*arrow*). (*B, C*) The cystlike focus is better seen on (*B*) axial T1-weighted image and (*C*) axial T2-weighted image, characterized by T1 and T2 high signal (*arrow, B, C*), confirming hemorrhagic content.

- External adenomyosis arises in the outer part of the uterus, most likely in the posterior myometrium, disrupting the serosa but not affecting the JZ. It is usually associated with deep endometriosis. On MR imaging, it appears as an ill-defined subserosal posterior T2-hypointense mass/pseudomass and may contain T2-hyperintense small cystic areas.

- Adenomyomatous polyp or polypoid adenomyoma presents as a polypoid mass in the lower uterine endometrium or endocervix, and accounts for about 2% of all endometrial polyps. On MR imaging, it is a hypointense polypoid mass associated with T2-hyperintense foci.[76–78]

Magnetic resonance imaging differential diagnosis

- Cyclic physiologic changes of the uterus (pseudothickening of the JZ): thickness of the JZ is hormone dependent and changes according to the menstrual cycle. Preferably, MR imaging should not be performed during menstruation to avoid this pitfall.[72,75]

- Nonmeasurable JZ: the JZ may not be measurable in postmenopausal patients and in women using contraceptive drugs.[2,9,79–84]

- Myometrial contractions: transient uterine contractions are hypointense T2W bands perpendicular to the JZ or focal thickening of the JZ and can mimic focal adenomyosis.[85] Repeating the acquisition of images within a few minutes may show their transient nature; cine MR imaging may also help (see **Fig. 6**).

- Endometrial cancer: adenomyosis can be seen in 20% of patients with endometrial cancer.[3] Evaluation of myometrial invasion may become difficult with the coexistence of adenomyosis because it may be responsible for a pseudowidening of the endometrium being mistaken

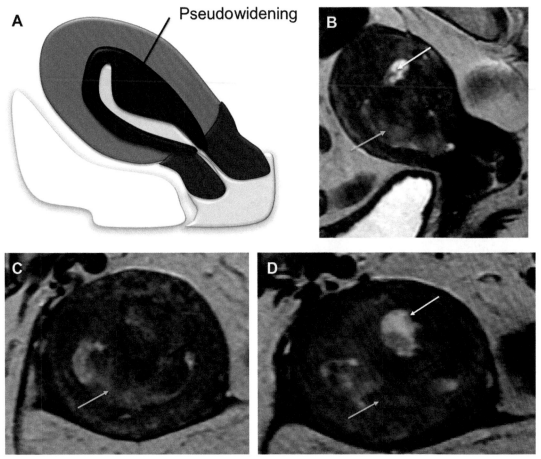

Fig. 12. Pseudowidening of the JZ with coexisting endometrial cancer. (*A*) The pseudowidening of the JZ. Sagittal (*B*) and (*C*) axial oblique T2-weighted images show an intermediate T2 signal within the endometrial cavity (*orange arrow*) with diffuse thickening of the JZ bulging in the endometrial cavity (pseudowidening of the JZ, *black arrow*). Note the large cystic area on (*B, D*) consistent with a subendometrial cyst (*white arrow*). On fused T2-DW image (*D*) signal hyperintensity is solely seen at the level of the intermediate T2 signal corresponding with the endometrial cancer (*orange arrow*). No areas of restricted diffusion are seen within the pseudowidening of the JZ. In this case, DWI was particularly helpful to delineate the cancer.

for myometrial invasion (**Fig. 12**).[3,86–88] Because endometrial cancer frequently extends into the ectopic endometrial tissue in adenomyosis, the true degree of myometrial invasion may be difficult to evaluate in the setting of concomitant adenomyosis. DWI may help to define the depth of myometrial invasion; adenomyosis does not restrict diffusion, whereas endometrial cancer does (**Fig. 13**).[89]

- Leiomyoma: traditionally, adenomyomas present as a T2 hypointense mass with ill-defined borders, minimal mass effect, and with multiple bright foci. In contrast, leiomyoma, besides also being T2 hypointense, also has a well-defined border, adjacent mass effect, and large vessels surrounding the lesion (see **Fig. 10**).[90]

Treatment Options

Medical therapy for adenomyosis relies on hormonal suppression. Oral contraceptives and GnRH agonists both induce amenorrhea and thus reduce symptoms of pain and bleeding. Symptoms tend to recur with cessation of therapy.[91] Levonorgestrel-releasing IUDs may be slightly more efficacious than oral contraceptives in reducing pain and uterine bleeding[92] and seem to improve quality-of-life measures similarly or slightly more than hysterectomy.[93] Traditionally, the standard treatment of symptomatic adenomyosis has been hysterectomy.[91] However, uterine-sparing techniques, including either complete or partial adenomyomectomy via open or laparoscopic approaches, can be considered in women wishing to maintain fertility, those who

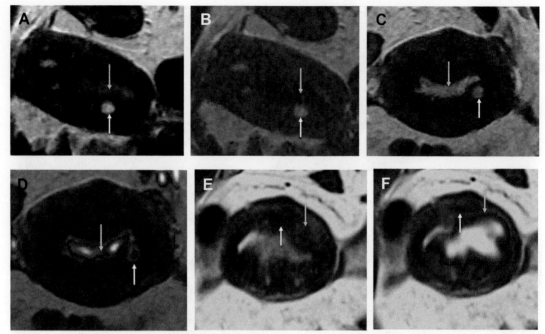

Fig. 13. Endometrial cancer with coexisting adenomyosis in 3 different patients (*A–F*). Axial oblique T2-weighted images (*A, C*) show an intermediate T2 signal corresponding to endometrial cancer within the endometrial cavity (*orange arrows*) with a diffuse thickening of the JZ and single subendometrial cysts (*white arrows*) in two patients. The subendometrial cyst in (*C*) shows the same signal as the endometrial thickening, which is confirmed on DWI (*D*) with an high signal. In the first case, the endometrial cancer does not extend into the adenomyosis; in the second case, tumor extends into the adenomyosis. DWI was again particularly helpful to delineate the cancer. (*E*) Axial oblique T2-weighted image shows an intermediate T2 signal within the endometrial cavity and within the myometrium (very ill-defined) (*orange arrow*) with diffuse thickening of the JZ (*white arrow* in *E* and *F*). (*F*) DWI shows a large very-well-defined area of hyperintense signal consistent with an endometrial cancer with deep myometrial invasion (*orange arrow*); again DWI was helpful to differentiate the tumor from the thickening of the JZ.

cannot tolerate a large operation, or in those wishing to consider a more conservative approach. Complete adenomyomectomy is effective in the setting of a focal adenomyoma. Partial adenomyomectomy, removal of a portion of the clinically recognizable adenomyosis, is used in the setting of diffuse adenomyosis when complete resection would effectively result in a functional hysterectomy. All of the uterine-sparing operative techniques yield improvements in pain in 82% to 85% of patients, reduction in abnormal uterine bleeding in 50% to 69% of patients, and preserve fertility in 43% to 47%.[94]

In select patients, UAE can be used to treat adenomyosis with or without leiomyomas. Symptom relief may not be as great or as durable as expected in the setting of isolated leiomyomas,[95] and patients with combined adenomyosis and leiomyomas tend to experience greater symptom relief from UAE than patients with pure adenomyosis.[96,97] Ultimately, with UAE, hysterectomy can be avoided in up to 85% of patients with symptomatic adenomyosis.[96,97]

SUMMARY

Benign uterine diseases, including adenomyosis and leiomyomas, are common conditions affecting women of all ages. US is often the initial imaging study obtained; however, MR imaging is the preferred modality for additional lesion characterization and provides critical information to assist in selecting the appropriate therapies for symptomatic patients. Treatment options for adenomyosis and leiomyomas include medical, surgical, and minimally invasive techniques such as UAE.

DISCLOSURE

Nothing to disclose.

REFERENCES

1. American Association of Gynecologic Laparoscopists (AAGL): Advancing Minimally Invasive Gynecology Worldwide. AAGL practice report: practice guidelines for the diagnosis and management of

submuccous leiomyomas. J Minim Invasive Gynecol 2012;19(2):152–71.

2. Brosens JJ, de Souza NM, Barker FG. Uterine junctional zone: function and disease. Lancet 1995; 346(8974):558–60.

3. Habiba M, Pluchino N, Petignat P, et al. Adenomyosis and endometrial cancer: literature review. Gynecol Obstet Invest 2018;83(4):313–28.

4. Krentel H, Cezar C, Becker S, et al. From clinical symptoms to MR imaging: diagnostic steps in adenomyosis. Biomed Res Int 2017;2017:1514029.

5. Munro MG. Uterine polyps, adenomyosis, leiomyomas, and endometrial receptivity. Fertil Steril 2019; 111(4):629–40.

6. Vannuccini S, Petraglia F. Recent advances in understanding and managing adenomyosis. F1000Res 2019;8 [pii:F1000 Faculty Rev-283].

7. Agostinho L, Cruz R, Osorio F, et al. MRI for adenomyosis: a pictorial review. Insights Imaging 2017; 8(6):549–56.

8. Bolan C, Caserta MP. MR imaging of atypical fibroids. Abdom Radiol (NY) 2016;41(12):2332–49.

9. Brown HK, Stoll BS, Nicosia SV, et al. Uterine junctional zone: correlation between histologic findings and MR imaging. Radiology 1991;179(2):409–13.

10. DeMulder D, Ascher SM. Uterine leiomyosarcoma: can MRI differentiate leiomyosarcoma from benign leiomyoma before treatment? AJR Am J Roentgenol 2018;211(6):1405–15.

11. Deshmukh SP, Gonsalves CF, Guglielmo FF, et al. Role of MR imaging of uterine leiomyomas before and after embolization. Radiographics 2012;32(6): E251–81.

12. Dudiak CM, Turner DA, Patel SK, et al. Uterine leiomyomas in the infertile patient: preoperative localization with MR imaging versus US and hysterosalpingography. Radiology 1988;167(3):627–30.

13. Kubik-Huch RA, Weston M, Nougaret S, et al. European Society of Urogenital Radiology (ESUR) guidelines: MR imaging of leiomyomas. Eur Radiol 2018; 28(8):3125–37.

14. Lakhman Y, Veeraraghavan H, Chaim J, et al. Differentiation of uterine leiomyosarcoma from atypical leiomyoma: diagnostic accuracy of qualitative MR imaging features and feasibility of texture analysis. Eur Radiol 2017;27(7):2903–15.

15. Sato K, Yuasa N, Fujita M, et al. Clinical application of diffusion-weighted imaging for preoperative differentiation between uterine leiomyoma and leiomyosarcoma. Am J Obstet Gynecol 2014;210(4):368.e1–8.

16. Dubuisson J. The current place of mini-invasive surgery in uterine leiomyoma management. J Gynecol Obstet Hum Reprod 2019;48(2):77–81.

17. Lewis TD, Malik M, Britten J, et al. A comprehensive review of the pharmacologic management of uterine leiomyoma. Biomed Res Int 2018;2018: 2414609.

18. Owen C, Armstrong AY. Clinical management of leiomyoma. Obstet Gynecol Clin North Am 2015;42(1): 67–85.

19. Stokes LS, Wallace MJ, Godwin RB, et al. Quality improvement guidelines for uterine artery embolization for symptomatic leiomyomas. J Vasc Interv Radiol 2010;21(8):1153–63.

20. Burke CT, Funaki BS, Ray CE Jr, et al. ACR Appropriateness Criteria(R) on treatment of uterine leiomyomas. J Am Coll Radiol 2011;8(4):228–34.

21. Murase E, Siegelman ES, Outwater EK, et al. Uterine leiomyomas: histopathologic features, MR imaging findings, differential diagnosis, and treatment. Radiographics 1999;19(5):1179–97.

22. Munro MG, Critchley HO, Broder MS, et al, FIGO Working Group on Menstrual Disorders. FIGO classification system (PALM-COEIN) for causes of abnormal uterine bleeding in nongravid women of reproductive age. Int J Gynaecol Obstet 2011; 113(1):3–13.

23. Araki H, Yoshizako T, Yoshida R, et al. MR imaging of parasitic leiomyoma with red degeneration. Magn Reson Med Sci 2019. [Epub ahead of print].

24. Garrido Oyarzun MF, Saco A, Castelo-Branco C. Anterior abdominal wall parasitic leiomyoma: case report. Gynecol Endocrinol 2018;34(2):103–6.

25. Fasih N, Prasad Shanbhogue AK, Macdonald DB, et al. Leiomyomas beyond the uterus: unusual locations, rare manifestations. Radiographics 2008; 28(7):1931–48.

26. Van den Bosch T, Dueholm M, Leone FP, et al. Terms, definitions and measurements to describe sonographic features of myometrium and uterine masses: a consensus opinion from the Morphological Uterus Sonographic Assessment (MUSA) group. Ultrasound Obstet Gynecol 2015;46(3):284–98.

27. Hricak H, Tscholakoff D, Heinrichs L, et al. Uterine leiomyomas: correlation of MR, histopathologic findings, and symptoms. Radiology 1986;158(2): 385–91.

28. Dueholm M, Lundorf E, Hansen ES, et al. Accuracy of magnetic resonance imaging and transvaginal ultrasonography in the diagnosis, mapping, and measurement of uterine myomas. Am J Obstet Gynecol 2002;186(3):409–15.

29. Mittl RL Jr, Yeh IT, Kressel HY. High-signal-intensity rim surrounding uterine leiomyomas on MR images: pathologic correlation. Radiology 1991; 180(1):81–3.

30. Nougaret S, Horta M, Sala E, et al. Endometrial cancer MRI staging: updated guidelines of the European Society of Urogenital Radiology. Eur Radiol 2019;29(2):792–805.

31. Thomassin-Naggara I, Dechoux S, Bonneau C, et al. How to differentiate benign from malignant myometrial tumours using MR imaging. Eur Radiol 2013; 23(8):2306–14.

32. Arleo EK, Schwartz PE, Hui P, et al. Review of leiomyoma variants. AJR Am J Roentgenol 2015; 205(4):912–21.

33. Prayson RA, Hart WR. Pathologic considerations of uterine smooth muscle tumors. Obstet Gynecol Clin North Am 1995;22(4):637–57.

34. Ueda H, Togashi K, Konishi I, et al. Unusual appearances of uterine leiomyomas: MR imaging findings and their histopathologic backgrounds. Radiographics 1999;19(Spec No):S131–45.

35. Kawakami S, Togashi K, Konishi I, et al. Red degeneration of uterine leiomyoma: MR appearance. J Comput Assist Tomogr 1994;18(6):925–8.

36. Ricci S, Stone RL, Fader AN. Uterine leiomyosarcoma: epidemiology, contemporary treatment strategies and the impact of uterine morcellation. Gynecol Oncol 2017;145(1):208–16.

37. Rieber A, Aschoff A, Nussle K, et al. MRI in the diagnosis of small bowel disease: use of positive and negative oral contrast media in combination with enteroclysis. Eur Radiol 2000;10(9):1377–82.

38. Namimoto T, Yamashita Y, Awai K, et al. Combined use of T2-weighted and diffusion-weighted 3-T MR imaging for differentiating uterine sarcomas from benign leiomyomas. Eur Radiol 2009;19(11):2756–64.

39. American College of Obstetricians and Gynecologists. ACOG practice bulletin. Alternatives to hysterectomy in the management of leiomyomas. Obstet Gynecol 2008;112(2 Pt 1):387–400.

40. Marret H, Fritel X, Ouldamer L, et al. Therapeutic management of uterine fibroid tumors: updated French guidelines. Eur J Obstet Gynecol Reprod Biol 2012;165(2):156–64.

41. Sangkomkamhang US, Lumbiganon P, Laopaiboon M, et al. Progestogens or progestogen-releasing intrauterine systems for uterine fibroids. Cochrane Database Syst Rev 2013;(2):CD008994.

42. Spies JB, Bradley LD, Guido R, et al. Outcomes from leiomyoma therapies: comparison with normal controls. Obstet Gynecol 2010;116(3):641–52.

43. Smeets AJ, Nijenhuis RJ, van Rooij WJ, et al. Uterine artery embolization in patients with a large fibroid burden: long-term clinical and MR follow-up. Cardiovasc Intervent Radiol 2010;33(5):943–8.

44. Lohle PN, Voogt MJ, De Vries J, et al. Long-term outcome of uterine artery embolization for symptomatic uterine leiomyomas. J Vasc Interv Radiol 2008; 19(3):319–26.

45. Goodwin SC, Spies JB, Worthington-Kirsch R, et al. Uterine artery embolization for treatment of leiomyomata: long-term outcomes from the FIBROID registry. Obstet Gynecol 2008;111(1):22–33.

46. Pelage JP, Cazejust J, Pluot E, et al. Uterine fibroid vascularization and clinical relevance to uterine fibroid embolization. Radiographics 2005;25(Suppl 1):S99–117.

47. McLucas B, Voorhees WD 3rd. The effectiveness of combined abdominal myomectomy and uterine artery embolization. Int J Gynaecol Obstet 2015; 130(3):241–3.

48. Tetikkurt S, Celik E, Tas H, et al. Coexistence of adenomyosis, adenocarcinoma, endometrial and myometrial lesions in resected uterine specimens. Mol Clin Oncol 2018;9(2):231–7.

49. Vercellini P, Parazzini F, Oldani S, et al. Adenomyosis at hysterectomy: a study on frequency distribution and patient characteristics. Hum Reprod 1995; 10(5):1160–2.

50. Vavilis D, Agorastos T, Tzafetas J, et al. Adenomyosis at hysterectomy: prevalence and relationship to operative findings and reproductive and menstrual factors. Clin Exp Obstet Gynecol 1997; 24(1):36–8.

51. Weiss G, Maseelall P, Schott LL, et al. Adenomyosis a variant, not a disease? Evidence from hysterectomized menopausal women in the Study of Women's Health Across the Nation (SWAN). Fertil Steril 2009; 91(1):201–6.

52. Tskhay VB, Schindler AE, Mikailly GT. Diffuse massive adenomyosis and infertility. Is it possible to treat this condition? Horm Mol Biol Clin Investig 2019;37(1) [pii:/j/ hmbci.2019.37.issue-1/hmbci-2018-0026/hmbci-2018-0026.xml].

53. Andres MP, Borrelli GM, Ribeiro J, et al. Transvaginal ultrasound for the diagnosis of adenomyosis: systematic review and meta-analysis. J Minim Invasive Gynecol 2018;25(2):257–64.

54. Atzori E, Tronci C, Sionis L. Transvaginal ultrasound in the diagnosis of diffuse adenomyosis. Gynecol Obstet Invest 1996;42(1):39–41.

55. Dueholm M. Transvaginal ultrasound for diagnosis of adenomyosis: a review. Best Pract Res Clin Obstet Gynaecol 2006;20(4):569–82.

56. Dueholm M, Lundorf E. Transvaginal ultrasound or MRI for diagnosis of adenomyosis. Curr Opin Obstet Gynecol 2007;19(6):505–12.

57. Hanafi M. Ultrasound diagnosis of adenomyosis, leiomyoma, or combined with histopathological correlation. J Hum Reprod Sci 2013;6(3):189–93.

58. Konrad J, Merck D, Wu JY, et al. Improving ultrasound detection of uterine adenomyosis through computational texture analysis. Ultrasound Q 2018; 34(1):29–31.

59. Sharma K, Bora MK, Venkatesh BP, et al. Role of 3D ultrasound and doppler in differentiating clinically suspected cases of leiomyoma and adenomyosis of uterus. J Clin Diagn Res 2015;9(4): QC08–12.

60. Van den Bosch T, Van Schoubroeck D. Ultrasound diagnosis of endometriosis and adenomyosis: state of the art. Best Pract Res Clin Obstet Gynaecol 2018;51:16–24.

61. Atri M, Reinhold C, Mehio AR, et al. Adenomyosis: US features with histologic correlation in an in-vitro study. Radiology 2000;215(3):783–90.

62. Van den Bosch T, de Bruijn AM, de Leeuw RA, et al. Sonographic classification and reporting system for diagnosing adenomyosis. Ultrasound Obstet Gynecol 2019;53(5):576–82.

63. Cunningham RK, Horrow MM, Smith RJ, et al. Adenomyosis: a sonographic diagnosis. Radiographics 2018;38(5):1576–89.

64. Stamatopoulos CP, Mikos T, Grimbizis GF, et al. Value of magnetic resonance imaging in diagnosis of adenomyosis and myomas of the uterus. J Minim Invasive Gynecol 2012;19(5):620–6.

65. Bazot M, Darai E. Role of transvaginal sonography and magnetic resonance imaging in the diagnosis of uterine adenomyosis. Fertil Steril 2018;109(3):389–97.

66. Reinhold C, Atri M, Mehio A, et al. Diffuse uterine adenomyosis: morphologic criteria and diagnostic accuracy of endovaginal sonography. Radiology 1995;197(3):609–14.

67. Reinhold C, McCarthy S, Bret PM, et al. Diffuse adenomyosis: comparison of endovaginal US and MR imaging with histopathologic correlation. Radiology 1996;199(1):151–8.

68. Reinhold C, Tafazoli F, Mehio A, et al. Uterine adenomyosis: endovaginal US and MR imaging features with histopathologic correlation. Radiographics 1999;19(Spec No):S147–60.

69. Reinhold C, Tafazoli F, Wang L. Imaging features of adenomyosis. Hum Reprod Update 1998;4(4):337–49.

70. Tafazoli F, Reinhold C. Uterine adenomyosis: current concepts in imaging. Semin Ultrasound CT MR 1999;20(4):267–77.

71. Dueholm M, Lundorf E, Hansen ES, et al. Magnetic resonance imaging and transvaginal ultrasonography for the diagnosis of adenomyosis. Fertil Steril 2001;76(3):588–94.

72. Tamai K, Togashi K, Ito T, et al. MR imaging findings of adenomyosis: correlation with histopathologic features and diagnostic pitfalls. Radiographics 2005;25(1):21–40.

73. Novellas S, Chassang M, Delotte J, et al. MRI characteristics of the uterine junctional zone: from normal to the diagnosis of adenomyosis. AJR Am J Roentgenol 2011;196(5):1206–13.

74. Troiano RN, Flynn SD, McCarthy S. Cystic adenomyosis of the uterus: MRI. J Magn Reson Imaging 1998;8(6):1198–202.

75. Takeuchi M, Matsuzaki K. Adenomyosis: usual and unusual imaging manifestations, pitfalls, and problem-solving MR imaging techniques. Radiographics 2011;31(1):99–115.

76. Takeuchi M, Matsuzaki K, Harada M. MR manifestations of uterine polypoid adenomyoma. Abdom Imaging 2015;40(3):480–7.

77. Patel N, Hatfield J, Sohaey R, et al. MRI of prolapsed polypoid adenomyoma: expanding the differential diagnosis for the broccoli sign. Clin Imaging 2018;52:177–9.

78. Sajjad N, Iqbal H, Khandwala K, et al. Polypoid adenomyoma of the uterus. Cureus 2019;11(2):e4044.

79. McCarthy S, Scott G, Majumdar S, et al. Uterine junctional zone: MR study of water content and relaxation properties. Radiology 1989;171(1):241–3.

80. Scoutt LM, Flynn SD, Luthringer DJ, et al. Junctional zone of the uterus: correlation of MR imaging and histologic examination of hysterectomy specimens. Radiology 1991;179(2):403–7.

81. Masui T, Katayama M, Kobayashi S, et al. Changes in myometrial and junctional zone thickness and signal intensity: demonstration with kinematic T2-weighted MR imaging. Radiology 2001;221(1):75–85.

82. Lesny P, Killick SR. The junctional zone of the uterus and its contractions. BJOG 2004;111(11):1182–9.

83. Fusi L, Cloke B, Brosens JJ. The uterine junctional zone. Best Pract Res Clin Obstet Gynaecol 2006;20(4):479–91.

84. Kiguchi K, Kido A, Kataoka M, et al. Uterine peristalsis and junctional zone: correlation with age and postmenopausal status. Acta Radiol 2017;58(2):224–31.

85. Ozsarlak O, Schepens E, de Schepper AM, et al. Transient uterine contraction mimicking adenomyosis on MRI. Eur Radiol 1998;8(1):54–6.

86. Hertlein L, Rath J, Zeder-Goss C, et al. Coexistence of adenomyosis uteri and endometrial cancer is associated with an improved prognosis compared with endometrial cancer only. Oncol Lett 2017;14(3):3302–8.

87. Aydin HA, Toptas T, Bozkurt S, et al. Impact of coexistent adenomyosis on outcomes of patients with endometrioid endometrial cancer: a propensity score-matched analysis. Tumori 2018;104(1):60–5.

88. Erkilinc S, Taylan E, Gulseren V, et al. The effect of adenomyosis in myometrial invasion and overall survival in endometrial cancer. Int J Gynecol Cancer 2018;28(1):145–51.

89. Jha RC, Zanello PA, Ascher SM, et al. Diffusion-weighted imaging (DWI) of adenomyosis and fibroids of the uterus. Abdom Imaging 2014;39(3):562–9.

90. Mark AS, Hricak H, Heinrichs LW, et al. Adenomyosis and leiomyoma: differential diagnosis with MR imaging. Radiology 1987;163(2):527–9.

91. Garcia L, Isaacson K. Adenomyosis: review of the literature. J Minim Invasive Gynecol 2011;18(4):428–37.

92. Shaaban OM, Ali MK, Sabra AM, et al. Levonorgestrel-releasing intrauterine system versus a low-dose combined oral contraceptive for treatment of adenomyotic uteri: a randomized clinical trial. Contraception 2015;92(4):301–7.

93. Ozdegirmenci O, Kayikcioglu F, Akgul MA, et al. Comparison of levonorgestrel intrauterine system versus hysterectomy on efficacy and quality of life in patients with adenomyosis. Fertil Steril 2011;95(2):497–502.

94. Grimbizis GF, Mikos T, Tarlatzis B. Uterus-sparing operative treatment for adenomyosis. Fertil Steril 2014;101(2):472–87.

95. Froeling V, Scheurig-Muenkler C, Hamm B, et al. Uterine artery embolization to treat uterine adenomyosis with or without uterine leiomyomata: results of symptom control and health-related quality of life 40 months after treatment. Cardiovasc Intervent Radiol 2012;35(3):523–9.

96. de Bruijn AM, Smink M, Hehenkamp WJK, et al. Uterine artery embolization for symptomatic adenomyosis: 7-year clinical follow-up using UFS-Qol questionnaire. Cardiovasc Intervent Radiol 2017; 40(9):1344–50.

97. de Bruijn AM, Smink M, Lohle PNM, et al. Uterine artery embolization for the treatment of adenomyosis: a systematic review and meta-analysis. J Vasc Interv Radiol 2017;28(12):1629–42.e1.

Imaging of Benign Adnexal Disease

Nadia J. Khati, MD*, Tammy Kim, MD, Joanna Riess, MD

KEYWORDS

- Benign ovarian cysts • Ovarian mass • Ultrasonography • Magnetic resonance imaging
- Benign adnexal masses

KEY POINTS

- Most adnexal masses are benign.
- The primary imaging modality for evaluating ovarian and adnexal masses is ultrasonography.
- Determining the ovarian or extraovarian origin of a lesion is essential for accurate differential diagnosis and proper management.
- When an adnexal mass is indeterminate on ultrasonography, contrast magnetic resonance (MR) imaging is the problem-solving imaging modality of choice.
- Adding diffusion-weighted imaging to conventional MR studies may help characterize certain benign ovarian and adnexal lesions.

 Video content accompanies this article at http://www.radiologic.theclinics.com.

INTRODUCTION

Adnexal disease involves the ovaries, fallopian tubes, and surrounding structures, and is common. Adnexal lesions may be found in symptomatic patients (eg, pelvic pain or palpable pelvic mass) or may be incidentally discovered when imaging for other unrelated conditions. Most adnexal masses are benign, with a reported incidence of up to 20%. This article reviews a variety of benign ovarian and adnexal conditions in premenopausal and postmenopausal women in addition to lesions discovered during pregnancy. Malignant ovarian disease is beyond the scope of this article and will be covered separately under a different article in this issue. Diagnosis and management of benign adnexal masses can be challenging, and this article addresses those issues, as well as examining the new proposed guidelines recently introduced by the American College of Radiology (ACR) Ovarian-Adnexal Reporting and Data System (O-RADS) Committee and the newly published ADNEx Scoring System.

IMAGING MODALITIES

The primary imaging modality for evaluating ovarian and adnexal masses is ultrasonography (US), which allows accurate identification in roughly 90% of cases (Table 1).[1] It has the advantage of being readily available, inexpensive, easy to perform (particularly when in the hands of experienced operators), and lacks ionizing radiation. The Women's Imaging ACR Appropriateness Criteria Committee rates US with duplex Doppler as usually appropriate when initially assessing for a gynecologic or nongynecologic cause in women presenting with acute pelvic pain[2] or when an

Funding: The authors report no funding that supported this study.
Department of Radiology, Abdominal Imaging Section, The George Washington University Hospital, 900 23rd Street, Northwest, Washington, DC 20037, USA
* Corresponding author.
E-mail address: nkhati@mfa.gwu.edu

Radiol Clin N Am 58 (2020) 257–273
https://doi.org/10.1016/j.rcl.2019.10.009

Table 1
Imaging modalities

Imaging Modalities	Advantages	Disadvantages
US	Easy to perform Widely available Low cost No ionizing radiation Excellent screening tool	Operator dependent Some degree of expertise needed for interpretation Some masses may remain indeterminate
MR imaging	Problem-solving tool for indeterminate US findings Excellent soft tissue resolution Can be used in pregnant patients	Not readily available Costly Limited by patient size and claustrophobia
CT	Used for malignancy staging	Ionizing radiation Poor soft tissue discrimination of adnexae
PET/CT	No role in evaluation of benign adnexal disease	Ionizing radiation

Abbreviations: CT, computed tomography; MR, magnetic resonance.

adnexal mass is clinically suspected.[3] No other imaging modality had shown better diagnostic capabilities than US as a first-line diagnostic imaging tool when an adnexal mass was suspected.[4]

Combining a transabdominal and transvaginal (TV) approach allows identification of large pelvic masses extending into the lower abdomen as well as deep-seated pelvic masses in the cul-de-sac. TV US has a reported sensitivity and specificity of 93.5% and 91.5% respectively in differentiating benign from malignant adnexal masses.[5] Although three-dimensional (3D) US is being used increasingly in the diagnostic work-up of female pelvic disease, two-dimensional (2D) US remains the principal technique used in daily practice. Color Doppler is a paramount adjunct to gray-scale imaging. However, its sensitivity in distinguishing between benign and malignant lesions remains low, varying between 50% and 80%, with a slightly higher specificity ranging

between 80% and 90%.[6] Real-time contrast-enhanced US can improve characterization of otherwise indeterminate ovarian lesions found on conventional 2D gray-scale US by observing both the degree and timing of enhancement of solid components. Zhang and colleagues[7] found that transabdominal contrast-enhanced US evaluation of malignant ovarian masses showed both faster and more enhancement than benign lesions. They also observed that the pattern of enhancement was more inhomogeneous in 44 out of 48 of their malignant ovarian lesions compared with only 5 out of 72 benign masses.[7] In their study of 51 ovarian lesions, Szymanski and colleagues[6] showed similar results using contrast-enhanced TV US, confirming that the presence of neovascularity in lesions could predict malignancy. Hu and colleagues[8] combined TV 2D and 3D contrast-enhanced US to differentiate small benign from malignant adnexal masses and achieved a diagnostic sensitivity of 100%.

Computed tomography (CT) is not the preferred imaging modality in the initial evaluation of the female pelvis and it is not ideal for imaging pregnant patients or for follow-up of any known adnexal disorder other than in cases of staging and preoperative planning for ovarian cancer. The Women's Imaging ACR AC Committee rates the use of CT with or without intravenous contrast as usually not appropriate in the initial evaluation of a suspected gynecologic adnexal mass or follow-up of a known adnexal mass.[2,3] This is principally because its soft tissue discrimination of the adnexal region is extremely poor and it also exposes the female pelvis to potentially harmful ionizing radiation. However, the increasing use of multidetector CT imaging in everyday clinical practice has led to incidental discovery of many adnexal lesions in patients being imaged for other reasons. It is therefore important to recognize CT findings that are particular to certain adnexal disorders and, more importantly, to recommend the appropriate next imaging modality because this is common practice. "Management of Incidental Adnexal Findings on CT and MRI: A White Paper of the American College of Radiology Incidental Findings Committee" revised guidelines are in press at the time of completion of this article.

Contrast-enhanced CT has been found to have a diagnostic accuracy comparable with US and magnetic resonance (MR) imaging in differentiating malignant from benign lesions.[9]

MR imaging is an excellent cross-sectional imaging tool to better characterize adnexal masses that are indeterminate on US either based on atypical sonographic features or the inconclusive organ of origin. It is also ideal for imaging pregnant patients given its lack of ionizing radiation to the fetus. Approximately 5% to 25% of adnexal masses are still classified as indeterminate following US evaluation.[10] MR imaging is particularly helpful because of its superior soft tissue contrast and resolution and its multiplanar imaging capabilities, with reported overall accuracy of up to 95% in differentiating benign from malignant ovarian masses.[11] The acquisition of different series, such as T1-weighted and T2-weighted sequences, chemical shift sequences, and fat-suppressed sequences, allows identification of specific tissue types, such as fluid, hemorrhage, fat, or solid/fibrotic components. The adjunct of intravenous (IV) contrast with dynamic imaging allows the evaluation of vascularity and enhancement of septations, internal mural nodules, or papillary projections. MR imaging with IV contrast has been found to be the next best imaging study when an incidentally found ovarian mass remains indeterminate on US, being a highly specific test given its ability to diagnose benign disease.[12] Functional MR imaging techniques such as diffusion-weighted and perfusion-weighted sequences have been reported to be valuable in distinguishing benign from malignant ovarian lesions.[13,14] In 2016, the European Society of Urogenital Radiology (ESUR) published new recommendations for MR imaging characterization of indeterminate ovarian masses on US.[10] They recommended combining the use of diffusion-weighted imaging (DWI) with a high b value with T2-weighted sequences to diagnose certain solid benign ovarian and adnexal lesions. They found that lesions that were hypointense on T2 and DWI regardless of their enhancement pattern had a high likelihood of being benign, an observation that is particularly helpful during pregnancy given that MR contrast is contraindicated.

There is no documented role in the literature for the use of PET/CT imaging in the initial evaluation or follow-up of a known or suspected benign adnexal mass in premenopausal or postmenopausal and pregnant women.

IMAGING DIAGNOSIS OF BENIGN OVARIAN AND ADNEXAL LESIONS

Across imaging modalities, adnexal masses can be classified as cystic, solid, or mixed solid/cystic. In 2010 and 2019, the Society of Radiologists in Ultrasound (SRU) published diagnostic guidelines and follow-up recommendations for asymptomatic ovarian and adnexal cystic lesions in premenopausal and postmenopausal women, excluding solid masses.[15,16] Table 2 summarizes their recommendations.

BENIGN OVARIAN LESIONS
Simple Ovarian Cysts

Most simple cysts are benign functional cysts. When an US diagnosis of simple cyst is made, a benign process is established in 98.7% and 100% of premenopausal and postmenopausal women respectively.[17,18] Furthermore, Valentin and colleagues[19] evaluated the risk of malignancy of 1148 unilocular cysts at TV imaging and found it to be 0.96% overall in premenopausal and postmenopausal women.

Most simple cysts in premenopausal women are either follicular or corpus luteum cysts measuring less than or equal to 3 cm and resolve without intervention. During the menstrual cycle, follicular

Table 2
Society of Radiologists in Ultrasound consensus guidelines for follow-up of incidental ovarian cysts

Ovarian Lesion	Premenopausal	Postmenopausal
Follow-up		
Simple cyst	>5 cm and ≤7 cm: none >7 cm: additional imaging at 2–6 mo for further characterization or 6–12 mo for growth assessment	>3 cm and ≤5 cm: none >5 cm: additional imaging at 3–6 mo for further characterization or 6–12 mo for growth assessment
Hemorrhagic cyst	≤5 cm: none >5 cm: 6–12 wk to confirm resolution	Early menopause: any size should be followed up to confirm resolution Late menopause: consider surgical evaluation
Endometrioma	First follow-up at 6–12 wk then yearly unless removed surgically	First follow-up at 6–12 wk then yearly unless removed surgically
Dermoid cyst	Follow-up yearly unless surgically removed	Follow-up yearly unless surgically removed

cysts enlarge progressively through the proliferative phase with 1 dominant follicle becoming mature and largest by ovulation time. If ovulation fails, the follicle continues to enlarge, becoming a functional cyst that can reach up to 20 cm. Simple cysts have an imperceptible smooth wall, with no internal septations, mural nodularity, or papillary projections. They are anechoic on US, showing posterior acoustic enhancement, and are avascular on color Doppler. On CT and MR imaging, cysts have simple fluid attenuation density and intensity respectively. Corpus luteum cysts are seen after ovulation and represent the residua of an involuting follicle (Fig. 1).

Other simple cystic ovarian lesions include serous cystadenomas, theca lutein cysts, and polycystic ovaries. Serous cystadenomas are subtypes of epithelial ovarian tumors and represent up to 25% of all benign ovarian neoplasms. They are often seen in women 40 to 50 years of age and are one of the most common simple cystic ovarian lesions found in postmenopausal women at surgery.[20] They present on imaging as unilateral or bilateral unilocular cysts, may be as large as 50 cm, and persist on follow-up imaging[20] (Fig. 2). Theca lutein cysts consist of multiple unilocular cysts and are the result of increased levels of beta-human chorionic gonadotropin (β-hCG) in the setting of gestational trophoblastic disease, multiple pregnancies, or ovarian hyperstimulation during assisted reproduction therapy. US shows bilateral ovarian enlargement caused by the presence of numerous unilocular follicles of varying size (Fig. 3). On CT and MR imaging, the ovaries may have a spoke-wheel appearance with the follicles arranged peripherally surrounding the more central ovarian stroma. The cysts regress spontaneously later in the pregnancy or after delivery. In the setting of hyperreactio luteinalis, which is a result of hypersensitivity to circulating hCG levels in the absence of ovulation induction treatment, the ovaries have a similar appearance. The

diagnosis is usually suggested by the timing, occurring in the third trimester, as well as by the presence of maternal virilization, seen in up to 25% of cases.[21] Polycystic ovaries also contain multiple cysts; however, their appearance differs from theca lutein cysts based on the number and size of the individual cysts. Ovarian volumes do not necessarily help in differentiating between the 2 entities because polycystic ovaries may or may not be enlarged. According to the American College of Obstetricians and Gynecologists (ACOG) guidelines, the imaging diagnosis of polycystic ovaries is made if 1 or both ovaries contain 12 or more small follicles measuring 2 to 9 mm and if the ovarian volume is greater than 10 cm^3.[22] Although roughly 23% of premenopausal women have polycystic-appearing ovaries, only about 5% to 10% have symptoms of polycystic ovarian syndrome (PCOS), which is an endocrinologic disorder with chronic anovulation caused by an imbalance in follicle-stimulating and luteinizing hormones. Patients with PCOS often present with infertility, amenorrhea, obesity, and hirsutism.[23] The US and MR imaging appearance of polycystic ovaries is characteristic, with numerous peripherally arranged small follicles in a classic string-of-pearls pattern (Fig. 4).

Not Simple Ovarian Cysts

Endometriomas are characterized by the presence of active ectopic endometrial tissue outside the uterus and may have a range of appearances on imaging. They have been referred to as chocolate cysts because of their dark, thick, gelatinous content, which represents aged blood products. The classic US findings are those of a unilocular thick-walled homogeneous cyst containing multiple low-level ground-glass echoes (Fig. 5). This appearance was described in 95% of endometriomas by Patel and colleagues[24] in a retrospective review of 252 adnexal masses. Additional

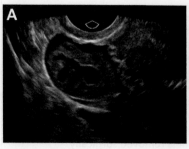 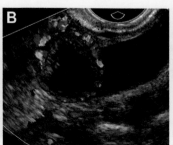 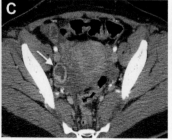

Fig. 1. Corpus luteum cyst. Sonogram in a premenopausal woman showing a corpus luteum cyst with a thick crenulated wall (A) with a surrounding rim of blood flow on color Doppler (B). (C) Contrast-enhanced CT scan shows a right corpus luteum cyst (arrow) with rim-enhancing wall, not to be mistaken for an abscess.

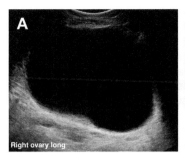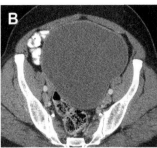

Fig. 2. Serous cystadenoma. (*A*) Pelvic sonogram showing a large right unilocular cyst in a postmenopausal woman that persisted on follow-up imaging. (*B*) Corresponding CT scan showing the large serous cystadenoma.

sonographic findings described in typical endometriomas include hyperechoic foci in the cyst wall or multilocularity. Endometriomas may have a more atypical appearance in pregnancy and postmenopausal women. These appearances include multiple septations, fluid-fluid levels, and central calcifications (**Fig. 6**A).[25,26] Decidualized endometriomas seen during pregnancy may develop solid vascular mural nodules mimicking neoplasms (**Fig. 6**B).[25,27] Some helpful distinguishing imaging features that have been suggested for making a prospective diagnosis include vascular solid nodules with smooth lobulated margins noted early in pregnancy and without showing significant change in size, and a similar appearance to the decidualized endometrium.[28,29] It is important to recognize these less

common atypical features in order not to overdiagnose or overlook malignant transformations of endometriomas into endometrioid carcinomas or clear cell carcinomas, which can occur in up to 1%.[30] Malignant transformations should be suspected if a known endometrioma shows rapid enlargement and interval development of solid vascular components. On MR imaging, endometriomas have homogeneous high signal intensity on T1-weighted fat-suppressed sequences and low signal on T2-weighted sequences, referred to as T2 shading (see **Fig. 5**). They may have a T2 dark fibrous wall that enhances after contrast administration without any mural nodularity or enhancement of central contents. When such a lesion shows these MR characteristics, a diagnosis of endometrioma can be made with a higher

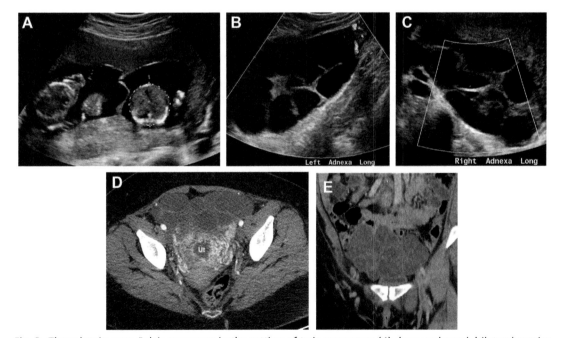

Fig. 3. Theca lutein cysts. Pelvic sonogram in the setting of twin pregnancy (*A*) shows enlarged, bilateral ovaries (*B*, *C*) with a spoke-wheel appearance. Contrast-enhanced axial (*D*) and coronal (*E*) CT scan in a different patient shows bilateral theca lutein cysts in the setting of gestational trophoblastic disease. Ut, uterus.

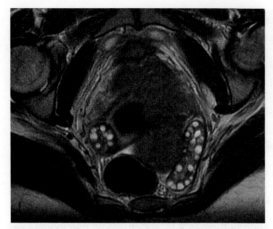

Fig. 4. Polycystic ovaries. Axial T2-weighted MR image shows polycystic ovaries containing greater than 12 small follicles arranged peripherally.

than 90% specificity.[31] Malignant transformation is better diagnosed on dynamic subtraction images (**Fig. 7**). Compared with hemorrhagic cysts' signal intensity on MR imaging, endometriomas tend to have higher T1 and lower T2 signal characteristics, which is thought to be caused by their higher protein concentration and increased viscosity.[32] In addition, Corwin and colleagues[33] showed that findings of a T2 dark spot on MR imaging within cystic adnexal masses helped establish a diagnosis of endometrioma with a specificity of 93% and a positive predictive value of 98%. However, distinguishing between the 2 entities on conventional MR imaging can be challenging at times given the overlapping imaging characteristics of blood products, and it has been suggested that using apparent diffusion coefficient (ADC) values would be helpful in making that distinction. In their study of 25 women, Balaban and colleagues[34] observed that endometriomas had significantly lower ADC values compared

with hemorrhagic cysts, with a higher sensitivity and specificity at *b* 1000.

Hemorrhagic cysts are thought to be the result of bleeding into corpus luteum cysts. Patients usually present with acute pelvic pain and US allows a definitive diagnosis in most cases (**Fig. 8**). Most hemorrhagic cysts resolve over time and do not need additional confirmatory imaging. However, when incidentally discovered on MR imaging, they may have similar signal characteristics to endometriomas with a few discriminating features: hemorrhagic cysts are often more heterogeneous than endometriomas and they are less T1 hyperintense and less T2 hypointense.[35] When they rupture, they can result in hemoperitoneum of variable amount in the pelvis and upper abdomen (**Fig. 9**). It is important to exclude the possibility of a ruptured ectopic pregnancy in this setting given that patients may present with similar symptoms and imaging findings. Hemorrhagic cysts are not encountered in late menopausal women because they no longer ovulate and, if similar-appearing cysts are found at imaging, these patients need surgical evaluation to exclude a neoplastic lesion.[15] However, these cysts can still occur in perimenopausal and early postmenopausal women; in this patient population a 6-week to 12-week interval follow-up with US is recommended to ensure resolution.[15]

Mixed Solid and Cystic Masses

Dermoid cysts represent up to 25% of all benign ovarian neoplasms and are the most common benign germ cell tumors encountered in premenopausal women. They represent the most commonly diagnosed benign ovarian neoplasm during pregnancy.[21] These congenital ovarian masses are derived from at least 2 of the 3 germ cell layers (ectoderm, mesoderm, and endoderm) and are also referred to as mature cystic

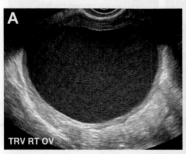
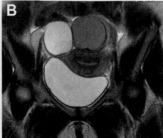
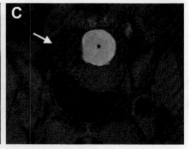

Fig. 5. Endometrioma. (*A*) Pelvic sonogram shows a typical endometrioma as a unilocular homogeneous cyst with posterior acoustic enhancement containing multiple low-level ground-glass echoes. Coronal T2 (*B*) and T1 fat-suppressed (*C*) MR images show the classic T2-shading appearance of a left endometrioma with hemosiderin ring and T2 dark spot. The endometrioma (*asterisk*) is hyperintense on T1 fat-suppressed sequence. Note the adjacent simple cyst in the right ovary (*arrow*).

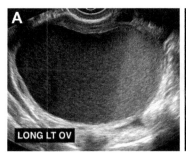
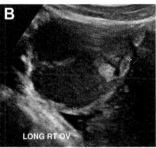

Fig. 6. Atypical endometriomas. (*A*) Pelvic sonogram shows an atypical endometrioma with a fluid-fluid level mimicking the appearance of a dermoid cyst. (*B*) Pelvic sonogram in a pregnant woman shows a decidualized endometrioma with solid echogenic mural nodules.

teratomas given their mature tissue composition. The ectoderm component usually is the dominant one. Dermoid cysts can be unilateral or bilateral and may reach up to 40 cm in size.[36] The US features are characteristic (**Fig. 10**). The presence of a fat-fluid level is a less common finding, as is the presence of calcifications representing bone or teeth. Dermoid cysts are easily recognized on CT by the presence of fat and calcifications (see **Fig. 10**). Typical MR imaging findings are caused by the presence of macroscopic fat and consist of a T1-hyperintense cystic lesion that shows signal decrease on the T1 fat-suppressed sequences (**Fig. 11**), a feature that helps differentiate them from endometriomas and other hemorrhagic ovarian masses, which remain hyperintense.[35,37] In most cases, this imaging characteristic is sufficient to make a confident diagnosis of a dermoid cyst. However, when these cysts have very small amounts of fat and no calcified elements, using the ADC values and DWI can help establish a diagnosis. These lesions have high signal intensity on DWI and low ADC values, presumably because of their keratinoid substance, which seems to be present in almost all of these entities.[38] Their T2 signal characteristics are variable. Dermoid cysts may contain low-signal-intensity calcifications. The most common complications include torsion, rupture causing chemical peritonitis, and

infection.[39] Malignant transformation can occur in up to 2%, occurring in larger lesions and postmenopausal women and resulting in squamous cell carcinomas.[40]

Solid Masses

Fibromas and thecomas are sex-cord stromal tumors and often have overlapping histologic features resulting in fibrothecomas, which are the most common solid benign ovarian tumors. These tumors occur in middle-aged women and there may be associated increased estrogen levels causing uterine enlargement, endometrial hyperplasia, and polyps. In the setting of Meigs syndrome, patients have associated ascites or pleural effusions. Their appearance is similar to fibroids on all imaging modalities because of their dense collagen and fibroblast content. On US, fibrothecomas are heterogeneous, solid masses with marked posterior acoustic shadowing and are hypovascular on Doppler imaging (**Fig. 12**A). When such findings are seen in the adnexa, it is important to differentiate them from pedunculated or broad ligament fibroids. The multiplanar imaging capabilities of MR imaging help resolve that dilemma by showing their ovarian origin as well as their characteristic T2 hypointensity (**Fig. 12**). They may have low or intermediate signal on

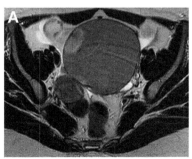
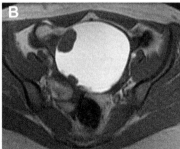
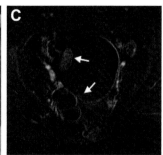

Fig. 7. Malignant transformation of endometrioma. Axial T2-weighted (*A*) and T1-weighted (*B*) MR images show an endometrioma with multiple solid mural nodules. (*C*) Axial T1 fat-suppressed postcontrast subtraction MR image shows enhancement of the mural nodules (*arrows*).

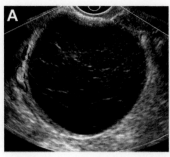 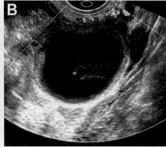

Fig. 8. Hemorrhagic cyst. Pelvic sonogram shows a well-defined cyst containing multiple avascular thin intersecting lines corresponding with fibrin strands (*A*). On follow-up imaging, the clot retracts with angular and concave margins (*B*).

T1-weighted sequences and show delayed hypoenhancement relative to myometrium and fibroids.[20,36,39] Fibrothecomas may have cystic and/or edematous changes caused by cystic degeneration resulting in areas of high T2 signal. The thecoma component may have a high fat content, better appreciated on chemical shift or fat-suppressed sequences.[20,37]

Cystadenofibromas are rare, representing less than 2% of all ovarian neoplasms. They are benign epithelial tumors with different subtypes depending on the epithelial component (mucinous, serous, clear cell, endometrioid, or mixed), with a peak incidence in women in their 40s and 50s. On imaging, their appearance is variable depending on which of the cystic or fibrous components predominates, and ranges from purely cystic, mixed solid, and cystic to purely solid. In their retrospective evaluation of 23 pathologically proven cystadenofibromas, Alcázar and colleagues[41] found that the most common appearance on TV US was that of a unilocular complex cystic mass, with 56.5% having solid nodules or papillary projections. Goldstein and colleagues[42] found that 69% of cystadenofibromas (91% serous cystadenofibromas and 9% mucinous cystadenofibromas) in their study were unilocular cysts with 1 or more avascular solid mural projections (**Fig. 13**A). On MR imaging, the solid fibrous components have the typical low T2 signal and

show less enhancement than myometrium. The presence of a thickened cyst wall with dark T2 signal is reported to be suggestive of the diagnosis (**Fig. 13**B).[43]

Brenner tumors are solid benign ovarian tumors representing 2% to 5% of surface epithelial benign masses.[36,44] However, there are borderline and malignant types.[20] Benign types are usually small and unilateral and discovered incidentally in older women. The US appearance is that of a solid hypoechoic mass, mimicking fibromas (**Fig. 14**). One helpful differentiating imaging finding is the presence of central or peripheral calcifications within Brenner tumors resulting in posterior acoustic shadowing on US or readily visualized on CT.[20,36] As with other fibrous tumors, they are hypointense on T1-weighted and T2-weighted sequences with rapid avid enhancement, which is a helpful distinguishing feature from the hypovascular fibrothecomas. They are reported to be lower in signal intensity on T2 than other solid ovarian tumors.[20,44] They can be associated with other surface epithelial tumors within the same ovary, most commonly mucinous cystadenomas in 30% of cases,[20] leading to a mass with cystic changes and areas of high signal intensity on T2-weighted sequences. Borderline and malignant Brenner tumors have significantly different appearances than benign ones, containing solid and cystic components with multiple locules and papillary elements.

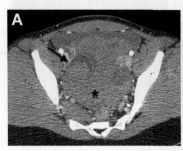 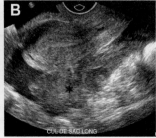

CUL DE SAC LONG

Fig. 9. Ruptured hemorrhagic cyst. (*A*) Contrast-enhanced CT in a patient with acute right lower quadrant pain shows hemoperitoneum (*asterisk*) caused by a ruptured right ovarian hemorrhagic cyst (*arrow*). (*B*) Pelvic sonogram in the same patient shows the hemoperitoneum in the cul-de-sac (*asterisk*).

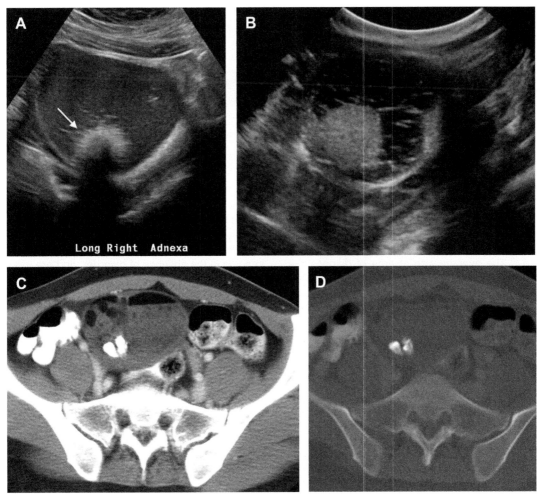

Fig. 10. Dermoid cyst. (*A*) Pelvic sonogram shows well-defined dermoid cyst containing a shadowing echogenic dermoid plug or Rokitansky nodule corresponding with hair and sebaceous material (*arrow*) and (*B*) dermoid mesh consisting of echogenic lines and dots representing hair. CT scan of the pelvis shows a dermoid cyst with a fat-fluid level (*C*) containing teeth better seen on bone windows (*D*).

BENIGN ADNEXAL LESIONS
Paraovarian Cysts

Paraovarian cysts account for 10% to 20% of all adnexal masses and are most commonly seen in premenopausal women in their 30s to 40s.[45,46] They are thought to arise from the mesovarium or mesosalpinx, which are congenital remnants in the broad ligament.[47,48] Identification of a separate ovary is important for diagnosis (**Fig. 15**). In a study by Kim and colleagues,[46] of 42 patients with surgically proven paraovarian cysts, the ovary was detected 76% of the time on transabdominal US

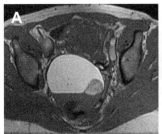
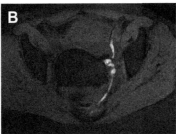

Fig. 11. Dermoid cyst. T1-weighted (*A*) axial MR image shows a right dermoid cyst with a fat-fluid level that shows signal drop on the T1 fat-suppressed sequence (*B*).

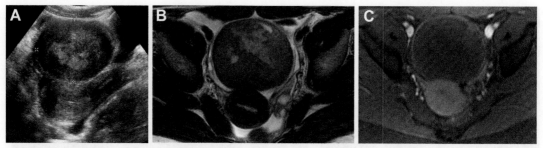

Fig. 12. Fibrothecoma. Pelvic sonogram shows a well-defined fibrothecoma that is heterogeneous in echotexture (*A*). MR imaging shows a well-defined heterogeneous T2-hypointense fibroma (*B*) with hypoenhancement relative to myometrium following contrast administration (*C*).

scanning. An exophytic ovarian cyst may mimic a paraovarian cyst, which can be separated from the ovary by applying pressure during US scanning.[48] The average size at time of diagnosis is approximately 8 cm.[46] Patients may be asymptomatic or present with abdominal pain, irregular menses, or abdominal distention.[49] Paraovarian cysts are infrequently complicated by torsion or hemorrhage, which can appear as thickening of the cyst wall along the mesosalpinx with internal echogenic debris.[47] They are almost always benign, and the rate of malignancy is less than 1% for simple adnexal cysts up to 10 cm in women of any age.[50] Although rare, solid components within the cyst may represent a benign or malignant neoplasm such as cystadenoma or cystadenocarcinoma.[46] Although there is limited utility of CT, MR imaging more clearly shows a paraovarian cyst as a homogeneous structure separate from the ovary with high T2 and low T1 signal in the absence of torsion or hemorrhage.[47]

Hydrosalpinx, Hematosalpinx, Pyosalpinx, Tubo-ovarian Abscess

The fallopian tubes course along the superior aspect of the broad ligament, extending from the uterus to the ovaries laterally and measure approximately 10 to 12 cm long and 1 to 4 mm in diameter.[51] They are not typically visualized on imaging in the absence of disorder, and are more easily seen when pathologically thickened, dilated, or surrounded by fluid.[52] Common causes of hydrosalpinx include chronic pelvic inflammatory disease (PID) and endometriosis, with other causes including tubal ligation, hysterectomy, and obstructing malignancy.[53,54] Patients may be asymptomatic or present with pelvic pain or infertility. On US, hydrosalpinx is characterized by a tubular cystic structure separate from the ovary with internal projections/incomplete septations. The distended tube folds on itself and may appear as a sausagelike C-shaped or S-shaped structure. In the axial plane, longitudinal folds may form a pathognomonic cogwheel appearance[55] (Video 1). However, these folds should not be mistaken for mural nodules, such as are seen in ovarian neoplasms. Lack of peristalsis and location distinguish hydrosalpinx from pelvic bowel loops. A retrospective study by Patel and colleagues[56] examining preoperative US of surgically removed cystic adnexal masses described a waist sign as a potential useful imaging finding in making the diagnosis of hydrosalpinx. Hydrosalpinx is often

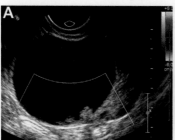
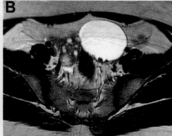
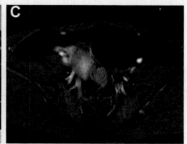

Fig. 13. Cystadenofibroma. (*A*) Pelvic sonogram shows a unilocular cystadenofibroma with multiple small avascular solid mural projections. (*B*) Axial T2 MR image of the same lesion shows the typical low T2 signal of the solid fibrous mural projections. Axial T1 fat-suppressed postcontrast MR image shows minimal enhancement of the mural nodules (*C*).

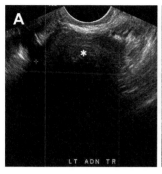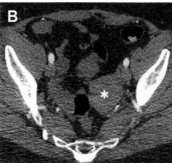

Fig. 14. Brenner tumor. (*A*) Pelvic sonogram shows an ill-defined solid hypoechoic adnexal mass with significant posterior acoustic shadowing (*asterisk*). (*B*) The corresponding CT scan shows the solid left ovarian Brenner tumor (*asterisk*) mimicking a fibroma.

incidentally seen on CT as a tubular fluid-density adnexal structure. MR may be performed when US remains indeterminate, allowing better depiction of the tubular morphology given its multiplanar imaging capabilities. Hydrosalpinx appears as a T2-hyperintense and T1-hypointense tubular structure with thin walls and internal folds. In contrast with PID, there is no significant wall enhancement or sign of surrounding inflammation such as tethering or loculations.[56]

Hematosalpinx results from blood products filling an obstructed and dilated fallopian tube. Endometriosis is the most common cause, although it may also be seen in the context of tubal ectopic pregnancy, PID, adnexal torsion, malignancy, and trauma.[57] Blood products appear as homogeneous low-level echoes on US, hyperdense on CT, and hyperintense signal on T1-weighted fat-suppressed sequences (**Fig. 16**). In addition, blood products in the fallopian tubes may cause adhesions that pull the ipsilateral ovary toward the midline, known as the kissing-ovary sign. Occasionally, this encases the ovary, mimicking a complex cystic mass.[58,59] Because the US and CT imaging findings of hydrosalpinx, pyosalpinx, and hematosalpinx may overlap, MR imaging findings may be more helpful for characterization of hematosalpinx in equivocal cases (see **Fig. 16**).

PID is a spectrum of disease involving the upper female genital tract, which includes endometritis, salpingitis, pyosalpinx, and tubo-ovarian abscess (TOA). PID results from an ascending infection from the vagina and cervix, often with *Neisseria gonorrhoeae* and *Chlamydia trachomatis* as causative organisms but is polymicrobial in 30% to 40% of cases.[55] Progression of infection and inflammation in PID can result in destruction of normal pelvic structures to form an abscess involving the fallopian tube and ovary, known as TOA. This complication occurs in up to one-third of patients hospitalized for acute salpingitis.[60] Although less common, rupture of TOA can result in life-threatening peritonitis.[60] A detailed description of the imaging findings of PID and TOA is beyond the scope of this article and this will be covered separately under a different article in this issue.

Broad Ligament Fibroid

Extrauterine fibroids are rare but can create diagnostic dilemmas.[61,62] Broad ligament fibroids adhere to an extrauterine structure, recruit a secondary blood supply, and lose their original association with the uterus. On US, broad ligament fibroids appear as well-circumscribed lesions with varying echogenicity, depending on the presence of degeneration or calcifications[63] (**Fig. 17**). TV US is especially helpful to visualize the fibroid separate from the ovary. There are some case reports of broad ligament fibroids causing pseudo-Meigs syndrome with increased CA-125 (cancer antigen 125) levels, both of which may raise suspicion for ovarian malignancy.[64,65] On MR, broad ligament fibroids have low to intermediate T1 and low

Fig. 15. Paraovarian cyst. Pelvic sonogram shows a thin-walled, rounded, well-circumscribed anechoic cyst, adjacent to/separate from the ovary (*arrow*).

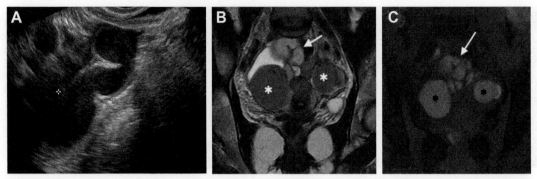

Fig. 16. Hematosalpinx. (*A*) Pelvic sonogram shows a dilated fallopian tube with homogeneous low-level echoes, consistent with a hematosalpinx. Coronal T2 (*B*) and T1 fat-suppressed MR images (*C*) show a hematosalpinx in a different patient as a convoluted T1-hyperintense and T2-hypointense tubular structures (*arrows*). The patient also had bilateral endometriomas (*asterisks*).

T2 signal intensity that follows smooth muscle (**Fig. 18**). More dedicated description of fibroids is presented in Stephanie Nougaret and colleagues' article, "Imaging Spectrum of Benign Uterine Disease and Treatment Options," elsewhere in this issue.

Peritoneal Inclusion Cysts

The peritoneum is made up of layers of cells of mesodermal origin. It is discontinuous in women at the distal ends of the fallopian tubes, allowing communication between the intraperitoneal and extraperitoneal spaces, which contain the ovaries and uterus, respectively.[66] The peritoneum plays a role in fluid and lymph resorption, which is compromised in the presence of injury or inflammation.[47] Peritoneal inclusion cysts (PICs) form when ovarian exudates are trapped within adhesions, which may result from mechanical injury or inflammation. PICs are most commonly found in premenopausal women with a history of prior surgery, trauma, PID, and endometriosis.[67] Higher concentrations of ovarian steroid hormones in the loculated fluid of PICs, compared with that of plasma, strongly supports that the fluid is ovarian in origin.[68] They may range in size from a few millimeters to larger masses that extend into the abdomen. The varied nomenclature for PICs reflects evolving understanding regarding their pathogenesis and prognosis. Alternate names include peritoneal pseudocysts, entrapped ovarian cysts, inflammatory cysts of the pelvic peritoneum and benign cystic mesothelioma.[69,70] Although it is largely described as a nonneoplastic entity caused by mesothelial proliferation, a few cases of metaplasia and malignant transformation have been described.[71]

Proper imaging diagnosis is crucial to prevent unnecessary surgery, especially because PICs are known to recur in up to 30% to 50% of patients following surgery.[72] Most PICs have an indolent course and are managed conservatively with follow-up imaging and pain medications as needed. Oral contraceptives or gonadotropin-releasing hormone agonist therapy may also be considered to suppress ovulation.[73–75] For symptomatic PICs, US-guided fine-needle aspiration or ethanol ablation have also been proposed as less invasive treatment options.[76,77]

US is the first imaging modality of choice, with identification of an uninvolved ovary being key to diagnosis. A study by Guerriero and colleagues[78] showed a specificity of 96% and sensitivity of 62% for detecting PICs on TV US. A typical US appearance is a multiloculated

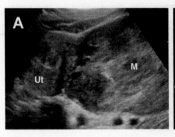

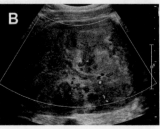

Fig. 17. Broad ligament fibroid. (*A*) Pelvic sonogram shows a large heterogeneous, left solid adnexal mass (M) with disorganized central vascularity on color Doppler (*B*).

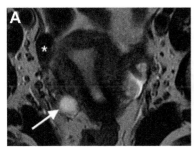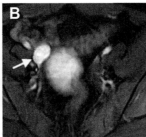

Fig. 18. (*A*) Axial T2-weighted MR image from a different patient shows a small, hypointense, well-circumscribed mass in the right adnexa (*asterisk*), separate from the right ovary (*arrow*). (*B*) There is homogeneous enhancement (*arrow*) on axial T1-weighted fat-suppressed postcontrast MR image.

cystic adnexal lesion with thin internal septations and an intact ovary. The ovary often has a central or eccentric location surrounded by weblike thin septations, creating a pathognomonic spider-in-web pattern (**Fig. 19**).[78] When septations are not extensive, they may appear similar to a paraovarian cyst. A common imaging pitfall is the presence of irregular and thickened septations, most commonly from underlying endometriosis, which can mimic a malignant ovarian neoplasm.[78] Solid components, mural nodularity, and papillary projections should suggest a malignant process.[79] MR imaging may be helpful in complex cases, when the ovary is not clearly visualized on US (**Fig. 20**). Absence of a true wall may be more readily apparent on MR, because PICs conform to surrounding structures rather than displacing them. Presence of concurrent endometriosis may explain more atypical findings of PICs, including T1 signal hyperintensity and more thickened and irregular-appearing septations. The absence of typical US and MR findings may necessitate laparoscopy or surgery.

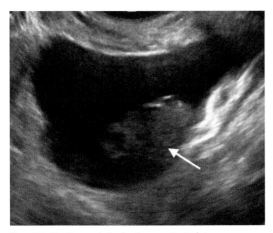

Fig. 19. Peritoneal inclusion cyst. Pelvic sonogram shows a cystic structure surrounding the left ovary (*arrow*).

IMAGING GUIDELINES AND THEIR IMPACT ON MANAGEMENT OF PATIENTS: INTERNATIONAL OVARIAN TUMOR ANALYSIS; SOCIETY OF RADIOLOGISTS IN ULTRASOUND/AMERICAN COLLEGE OF RADIOLOGY, OVARIAN-ADNEXAL REPORTING AND DATA SYSTEM RECOMMENDATIONS; AND ADNEx MAGNETIC RESONANCE SCORING SYSTEM

To date, many different societies and committees have been created in an attempt to simplify and standardize the terminology used in the description of ovarian and adnexal masses across medical specialties. The goal was to produce more structured reports that would allow a more consistent multidisciplinary approach to patient management, including follow-up imaging procedures when needed and appropriate treatment guidance. Some of these groups include, but are not limited to, the International Ovarian Tumor Analysis group (IOTA); the ESUR; the Society of Radiologists in Ultrasound (SRU)/ACR committee, and the most recently created O-RADS committee. Given that US is the primary imaging modality used in the diagnostic work-up of known or suspected ovarian or adnexal masses, the terminology is not surprisingly focused on gray-scale as well as color and power Doppler features. The IOTA group's goal in 2000 was to focus on generating a list of descriptive terms to be used for describing ovarian and adnexal lesions in a standardized manner (location, size, internal components, solid or cystic nature, and presence or absence of vascularity).[80] Subsequently, in 2010 and 2019 the SRU/ACR consensus committee published diagnostic guidelines and follow-up recommendations with additional imaging or surgical evaluation for ovarian and adnexal cystic lesions in premenopausal and postmenopausal women, excluding solid masses.[15,16] Their diagnostic and follow-up guidelines are summarized in **Table 2**. The O-RADS was created in 2015 under the guidance of the ACR in an attempt to emulate the BI-

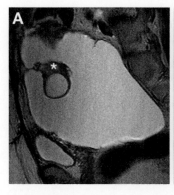 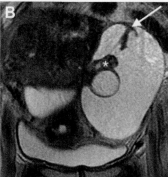

Fig. 20. (*A*) Sagittal T2-weighted and (*B*) coronal T2-weighted MR images in a different patient show a cystic lesion containing internal septations (*arrow in B*), encircling the left ovary (*asterisk in both*).

RADS (Breast Imaging Reporting and Data System), which had been widely successful since their establishment in 1993 and is now in its fifth edition. The committee was able to tabulate a long list of descriptive terms with their corresponding definitions elaborating on the IOTA terminology. The goal of the O-RADS committee was to overcome the limitations of previous groups and to create a universal standardized US lexicon in order to simplify interpretation of findings, improve communication with referring physicians, and eventually allow better patient management.[81] As such, lesions would be given O-RADS scores varying from 0 to 5, with 5 corresponding with the group with highest risk. Each of these numeric groups would have corresponding imaging and clinical management recommendations for premenopausal and postmenopausal women. Larger-scale implementation with multicenter testing with retrospective and prospective studies is needed at this time to evaluate the efficiency and usefulness of these newly established O-RADS. More recently, the ADNEx MR scoring system was published by Sadowski and colleagues.[82] This scoring system was developed by integrating additional MR sequences such as diffusion and perfusion series into the imaging algorithm of sonographically indeterminate adnexal lesions. Using universal terminology, lesions would be described based on their anatomic and functional MR appearance and given a numeric score from 1 to 5 with 5 corresponding with highest specificity for malignancy with a positive predictive value for malignancy of 96%. This scoring system seems promising and a multicenter prospective study is underway throughout Asia, Europe, and the United States.

SUMMARY/WHAT REFERRING CLINICIANS NEED TO KNOW

- Ovarian and adnexal masses are common, encountered in symptomatic patients, or incidentally discovered in patients being examined or imaged for other unrelated conditions.
- When a pelvic mass is suspected on physical examination or incidentally discovered on CT, US evaluation is the next best step in patient management.
- If an adnexal mass remains indeterminate on US, multiparametric MR imaging with contrast is a useful problem-solving imaging modality.
- Further implementation of the recent O-RADS (US) and ADNEx (MR imaging) reporting systems will help stratify lesions into risk categories and improve communication with referring physicians, eventually allowing better patient management.

CONFLICT OF INTEREST

The authors report no conflicts of interests concerning the materials, methods, or results in this article.

SUPPLEMENTARY DATA

Supplementary data related to this article can be found online at https://doi.org/10.1016/j.rcl.2019.10.009.

REFERENCES

1. Brown DL, Dudiak KM, Laing FC. Adnexal masses: US characterization and reporting. Radiology 2010; 254(2):342–54.
2. Bhosale PR, Javitt MC, Atri M, et al. ACR appropriateness criteria® acute pelvic pain in the reproductive age group. Ultrasound Q 2016;32(2): 108–15.
3. Atri M, Alabousi A, Reinhold C, et al. ACR appropriateness criteria® clinically suspected adnexal mass, no acute symptoms. J Am Coll Radiol 2019; 16(5):S77–93.

4. American College of Obstetricians and Gynecologists' Committee on Practice Bulletins—Gynecology. Practice bulletin No. 174: evaluation and management of adnexal masses. Obstet Gynecol 2016;128(5):e210–26.

5. Biggs WS, Marks ST. Diagnosis and management of adnexal masses. Am Fam Physician 2016;93(8): 676–81.

6. Szymanski M, Socha MW, Kowalkowska ME, et al. Differentiating between benign and malignant adnexal lesions with contrast-enhanced transvaginal ultrasonography. Int J Gynaecol Obstet 2015; 131(2):147–51.

7. Zhang X, Mao Y, Zheng R, et al. The contribution of qualitative CEUS to the determination of malignancy in adnexal masses, indeterminate on conventional US - A multicenter study. PLoS One 2014;9(4): e93843.

8. Hu R, Xiang H, Mu Y, et al. Combination of 2- and 3-dimensional contrast-enhanced transvaginal sonography for diagnosis of small adnexal masses. J Ultrasound Med 2014;33(11):1889–99.

9. Zhang J, Mironov S, Hricak H, et al. Characterization of adnexal masses using feature analysis at contrast-enhanced helical computed tomography. J Comput Assist Tomogr 2008;32(4):533–40.

10. Forstner R, Thomassin-Naggara I, Cunha TM, et al. ESUR recommendations for MR imaging of the sonographically indeterminate adnexal mass: an update. Eur Radiol 2017;27(6):2248–57.

11. Valentini AL, Gui B, Miccò M, et al. Benign and suspicious ovarian masses—MR imaging criteria for characterization: pictorial review. J Oncol 2012; 2012:1–9.

12. Anthoulakis C, Nikoloudis N. Pelvic MRI as the "gold standard" in the subsequent evaluation of ultrasound-indeterminate adnexal lesions: a systematic review. Gynecol Oncol 2014;132(3):661–8.

13. Thomassin-Naggara I, Toussaint I, Perrot N, et al. Characterization of complex adnexal masses: value of adding perfusion- and diffusion-weighted MR imaging to conventional MR imaging. Radiology 2011; 258(3):793–803.

14. Thomassin-Naggara I, Daraï E, Cuenod CA, et al. Contribution of diffusion-weighted MR imaging for predicting benignity of complex adnexal masses. Eur Radiol 2009;19(6):1544–52.

15. Levine D, Brown DL, Andreotti RF, et al. Management of asymptomatic ovarian and other adnexal cysts imaged at US. Ultrasound Q 2010;26(3): 121–31.

16. Levine D, Patek MD, Suh-Burgmann, et al. Simple adnexal cysts: SRU consensus conference update on follow-up and reporting. Radiology 2019;293(2): 359–71.

17. Modesitt SC, Pavlik EJ, Ueland FR, et al. Risk of malignancy in unilocular ovarian cystic tumors less than 10 centimeters in diameter. Obstet Gynecol 2003; 102(3):594–9.

18. Dørum A, Blom GP, Ekerhovd E, et al. Prevalence and histologic diagnosis of adnexal cysts in postmenopausal women: an autopsy study. Am J Obstet Gynecol 2005;192(1):48–54.

19. Valentin L, Ameye L, Franchi D, et al. Risk of malignancy in unilocular cysts: a study of 1148 adnexal masses classified as unilocular cysts at transvaginal ultrasound and review of the literature. Ultrasound Obstet Gynecol 2013;41(1):80–9.

20. Griffin N, Grant LA, Sala E. Adnexal masses: characterization and imaging strategies. Semin Ultrasound CT MR 2010;31(5):330–46.

21. Glanc P, Salem S, Farine D. Adnexal masses in the pregnant patient a diagnostic and management challenge. Ultrasound Q 2008;24(4):225–40.

22. Lee TT, Rausch ME. Polycystic ovarian syndrome: role of imaging in diagnosis. Radiographics 2012; 32(6):1643–57.

23. Ackerman S, Irshad A, Lewis M, et al. Ovarian cystic lesions. a current approach to diagnosis and management. Radiol Clin North Am 2013;51(6):1067–85.

24. Patel MD, Feldstein VA, Chen DC, et al. Endometriomas: diagnostic performance of US. Radiology 2013;210(3):739–45.

25. Asch E, Levine D. Variations in appearance of endometriomas. J Ultrasound Med 2007;26(8): 993–1002.

26. Van Holsbeke C, Van Calster B, Guerriero S, et al. Endometriomas: their ultrasound characteristics. Ultrasound Obstet Gynecol 2010;35(6):730–40.

27. Yacobozzi M, Nguyen D, Rakita D. Adnexal masses in pregnancy. Semin Ultrasound CT MR 2012;33(1): 55–64.

28. Poder L, Coakley FV, Rabban JT, et al. Decidualized endometrioma during pregnancy: recognizing an imaging mimic of ovarian malignancy. J Comput Assist Tomogr 2008;32(4):555–8.

29. Morisawa N, Kido A, Kataoka M, et al. Magnetic resonance imaging decidualized endometriotic cysts: comparative study with ovarian cancers associated with endometriotic cysts. J Comput Assist Tomogr 2014;38(6):879–84.

30. Perera DS, Prabhakar HB. Imaging of the adnexal mass. Clin Obstet Gynecol 2015;58(1):28–46.

31. Siegelman ES, Oliver ER. MR imaging of endometriosis: ten imaging pearls. Radiographics 2012;32(6): 1675–91.

32. Outwater E, Schiebler ML, Owen RS, et al. Characterization of hemorrhagic adnexal lesions with MR imaging: blinded reader study. Radiology 1993; 186(2):489–94.

33. Corwin MT, Gerscovich EO, Lamba R, et al. Differentiation of ovarian endometriomas from hemorrhagic cysts at MR imaging: utility of the T2 dark spot sign. Radiology 2013;271(1):126–32.

34. Balaban M, Idilman IS, Toprak H, et al. The utility of diffusion-weighted magnetic resonance imaging in differentiation of endometriomas from hemorrhagic ovarian cysts. Clin Imaging 2015;39(5):830–3.

35. Masch WR, Daye D, Lee SI. MR imaging for incidental adnexal mass characterization. Magn Reson Imaging Clin N Am 2017;25(3):521–43.

36. Heilbrun ME, Olpin J, Shaaban A. Imaging of benign adnexal masses: characteristic presentations on ultrasound, computed tomography, and magnetic resonance imaging. Clin Obstet Gynecol 2009; 52(1):21–39.

37. Vargas HA, Barrett T, Sala E. MRI of ovarian masses. J Magn Reson Imaging 2013;37(2):265–81.

38. Nakayama T, Yoshimitsu K, Irie H, et al. Diffusion-weighted echo-planar MR imaging and ADC mapping in the differential diagnosis of ovarian cystic masses: usefulness of detecting keratinoid substances in mature cystic teratomas. J Magn Reson Imaging 2005;22(2):271–8.

39. Sala EJS, Atri M. Magnetic resonance imaging of benign adnexal disease. Top Magn Reson Imaging 2003;14(4):305–27.

40. Park SB, Lee JB. MRI features of ovarian cystic lesions. J Magn Reson Imaging 2014;40(3):503–15.

41. Alcázar JL, Errasti T, Mínguez JA, et al. Sonographic features of ovarian cystadenofibromas: spectrum of findings. J Ultrasound Med 2001;20(8):915–9.

42. Goldstein SR, Timor-Tritsch IE, Monteagudo A, et al. Cystadenofibromas: can transvaginal ultrasound appearance reduce some surgical interventions? J Clin Ultrasound 2015;43(6):393–6.

43. Montoriol PF, Mons A, Da Ines D, et al. Fibrous tumours of the ovary: aetiologies and MRI features. Clin Radiol 2013;68(12):1276–83.

44. Imaoka I, Wada A, Kaji Y, et al. Developing an MR imaging strategy for diagnosis of ovarian masses. Radiographics 2006;26(5):1431–48.

45. Kishimoto K, Ito K, Awaya H, et al. Paraovarian cyst: MR imaging features. Abdom Imaging 2002;27(6): 685–9.

46. Kim JS, Woo SK, Suh SJ, et al. Sonographic diagnosis of paraovarian cysts: value of detecting a separate ipsilateral ovary. AJR Am J Roentgenol 1995;164(6):1441–4.

47. Moyle PL, Kataoka MY, Nakai A, et al. Nonovarian cystic lesions of the pelvis. Radiographics 2010; 30(4):921–38.

48. Laing FC, Allison SJ. US of the ovary and adnexa: to worry or not to worry? Radiographics 2012;32(6): 1621–39.

49. Athey P, Cooper N. Sonographic features of parovarian cysts. Am J Roentgenol 1985;144(1):83–6.

50. Ekerhovd E, Wienerroith H, Staudach A, et al. Preoperative assessment of unilocular adnexal cysts by transvaginal ultrasonography: a comparison between ultrasonographic morphologic imaging and histopathologic diagnosis. Am J Obstet Gynecol 2001;184(2):48–54.

51. Simpson WL, Beitia LG, Mester J. Hysterosalpingography: a reemerging study. Radiographics 2007; 26(2):419–31.

52. Benjaminov O, Atri M. Sonography of the abnormal fallopian tube. Am J Roentgenol 2004;183(3): 737–42.

53. Horrow MM. Ultrasound of pelvic inflammatory disease. Ultrasound Q 2004;20(4):171–9.

54. Mitchell DG, Mintz MC, Spritzer CE, et al. Adnexal masses: MR imaging observations at 1.5 t, with US and CT correlation. Obstet Gynecol Surv 1987; 42(8):531–2.

55. Rezvani M, Shaaban AM. Fallopian tube disease in the nonpregnant patient. Radiographics 2011; 31(2):527–48.

56. Patel MD, Acord DL, Young SW. Likelihood ratio of sonographic findings in discriminating hydrosalpinx from other adnexal masses. Am J Roentgenol 2006; 186(4):1033–8.

57. Atri M, Ascher SM. Fallopian tubes: hematosalpinx. In: Hricak H, Akin O, Sala E, et al, editors. Diagnostic imaging: gynecology. Salt Lake City (UT): Amirsys-Elsevier; 2006. p. 50–5.

58. Shalev E, Yarom I, Bustan M, et al. Transvaginal sonography as the ultimate diagnostic tool for the management of ectopic pregnancy: experience with 840 cases. Fertil Steril 1998;69(1):62–5.

59. Ghezzi F, Raio L, Cromi A, et al. "Kissing ovaries": a sonographic sign of moderate to severe endometriosis. Fertil Steril 2005;83(1):143–7.

60. Summary B, Aral SO, Brunham RC, et al. Pelvic inflammatory disease: guidelines for prevention and management. MMWR Recomm Rep 1991;40(RR-5):1–25.

61. Szklaruk J, Tamm EP, Choi H, et al. MR imaging of common and uncommon large pelvic masses. Radiographics 2003;23(2):403–24.

62. Wallach EE, Buttram VC, Reiter RC. Uterine leiomyomata: etiology, symptomatology, and management. Fertil Steril 1981;36(4):433–45.

63. Fasih N, Prasad Shanbhogue AK, Macdonald DB, et al. Leiomyomas beyond the uterus: unusual locations, rare manifestations. Radiographics 2008; 28(7):1931–48.

64. Brown RSD, Marley JL, Cassoni AM. Pseudo-Meigs' syndrome due to broad ligament leiomyoma: a mimic of metastatic ovarian carcinoma. Clin Oncol 1998;10(3):198–201.

65. Pallavee P, Ghose S, Samal S, et al. Fibroid after hysterectomy: a diagnostic dilemma. J Clin Diagn Res 2014;8(7):7–8.

66. Levy AD, Shaw JC. From the archives of the AFIP primary peritoneal tumors: imaging features with pathologic correlation. Radiographics 2008;28: 583–607.

67. Sohaey R, Gardner TL, Woodward PJ, et al. Sonographic diagnosis of peritoneal inclusion cysts. J Ultrasound Med 1995;14(12):913–7.

68. Hoffer FA, Kozakewich H, Colodny A, et al. Peritoneal inclusion cysts: ovarian fluid in peritoneal adhesions. Radiology 2014;169(1):189–91.

69. Jain KA. Imaging of peritoneal inclusion cysts. Am J Roentgenol 2000;174(6):1559–63.

70. Kim JS, Lee HJ, Woo SK, et al. Peritoneal inclusion cysts and their relationship to the ovaries: evaluation with sonography. Radiology 2014;204(2):481–4.

71. González-Moreno S, Yan H, Alcorn KW, et al. Malignant transformation of "Benign" cystic mesothelioma of the peritoneum. J Surg Oncol 2002;79(4):243–51.

72. Ross MJ, Welch WR, Scully RE. Multilocular peritoneal inclusion cysts (So-called cystic mesotheliomas). Cancer 1989;64(6):1336–46.

73. Nozawa S, Iwata T, Yamashita H, et al. Gonadotropin-releasing hormone analogue therapy for peritoneal inclusion cysts after gynecological surgery. J Obstet Gynaecol Res 2000;26(6):389–93.

74. Kurachi H, Murakami T, Maeda T, et al. Value of gonadotropin-releasing hormone agonist in diagnosing peritoneal pseudocysts. Acta Obstet Gynecol Scand 1996;75(3):294–7.

75. Letterie GS, Yon JL. Use of a long-acting GnRH agonist for benign cystic mesothelioma. Obstet Gynecol 1995;85(5 Pt 2):901–3.

76. Takeuchi K, Kitazawa S, Kitagaki S, et al. Conservative management of post-operative peritoneal cysts associated with endometriosis. Int J Gynaecol Obstet 1998;60(2):151–4.

77. Lipitz S, Seidman DS, Schiff E, et al. Treatment of pelvic peritoneal cysts by drainage and ethanol instillation. Obstet Gynecol 1995;86(2):297–9.

78. Guerriero S, Ajossa S, Mais V, et al. Role of transvaginal sonography in the diagnosis of peritoneal inclusion cysts. J Ultrasound Med 2004;23(9):1193–200.

79. Veldhuis WB, Akin O, Goldman D, et al. Peritoneal inclusion cysts: clinical characteristics and imaging features. Eur Radiol 2013;23(4):1167–74.

80. Timmerman D, Valentin L, Bourne TH, et al. Terms, definitions and measurements to describe the sonographic features of adnexal tumors: a consensus opinion from the International Ovarian Tumor Analysis (IOTA) group. Ultrasound Obstet Gynecol 2000;16(5):500–5.

81. Andreotti RF, Timmerman D, Benacerraf BR, et al. Ovarian-Adnexal reporting lexicon for ultrasound: a white paper of the ACR Ovarian-Adnexal Reporting and Data System Committee. J Am Coll Radiol 2018;15(10):1415–29.

82. Sadowski EA, Robbins JB, Rockall AG, et al. A systematic approach to adnexal masses discovered on ultrasound: the ADNEx MR scoring system. Abdom Radiol (NY) 2018;43(3):679–95.

Imaging Spectrum of Endometriosis (Endometriomas to Deep Infiltrative Endometriosis)

Nicole Hindman, MD[a],*, Wendaline VanBuren, MD[b]

KEYWORDS

• Endometriosis • Adenomyosis • Endometrioma • Deep infiltrating endometriosis

KEY POINTS

- Endometriosis is a common disease.
- In women of reproductive age with pelvic pain, dysmenorrhea, dyspareunia, or infertility, endometriosis as a cause should be considered.
- Detection of endometriosis on imaging can be subtle; therefore, a targeted approach to imaging evaluation is recommended.
- Targeted ultrasound and MR imaging techniques are effective in the detection of endometriosis.

INTRODUCTION

Endometriosis is a common, benign disorder defined as the presence of endometrial tissue at extrauterine sites, typically involving the pelvis. The cause and pathogenesis of endometriosis are incompletely understood and appear to be due to multifactorial causes, including the presence of ectopic endometrial tissue, altered immunity, disrupted cell proliferation and apoptosis, and disordered endocrine signaling and genetics.[1] The prevalence estimates of endometriosis vary, with 1% of all women who undergo major gynecologic surgery having evidence of endometriosis, and 9% to 50% of all women undergoing laparoscopy for infertility having evidence of endometriosis.[2,3] It is estimated that there is a 10% prevalence of endometriosis in women of reproductive age.[4] The classic symptoms of endometriosis are dysmenorrhea, pelvic pain, dyspareunia, and/or infertility.

Typically, once endometriosis is clinically suspected, patients are evaluated on physical examination for tenderness in commonly involved pelvic regions (cul-de-sac, rectovaginal space, uterine body, and uterosacral ligaments). Laboratory tests are limited in the diagnosis of endometriosis (CA-125 has a detection rate of only 54% in patients with severe endometriosis[5] and is neither sensitive nor specific for the diagnosis). The gold standard for diagnosis of endometriosis has traditionally been surgical visualization and biopsy; however, in recent years, diagnostic laparoscopy (surgery performed in order to diagnose endometriosis, not to treat endometriosis) is becoming less common at university hospitals.[6] Replacement of diagnostic laparoscopy by noninvasive imaging is due to the improvement in diagnostic capability of preoperative imaging (typically ultrasound [US] and MR imaging) for the detection of endometriosis.[6]

Endometriosis typically manifests in 3 ways: ovarian endometriomas, superficial peritoneal implants, and deep infiltrating endometriosis (DIE). DIE is defined as a solid endometriotic implant more than 5 mm deep to the peritoneum.[7] Both ovarian endometriomas and DIE can be detected

[a] NYU Radiology, NYU School of Medicine, 550 First Avenue, New York, NY 10010, USA; [b] Mayo Clinic, 200 1st Street Southwest, Rochester, MN 55905, USA
* Corresponding author.
E-mail address: Nicole.Hindman@nyulangone.org

Radiol Clin N Am 58 (2020) 275–289
https://doi.org/10.1016/j.rcl.2019.11.001
0033-8389/20/© 2019 Elsevier Inc. All rights reserved.

accurately with imaging. Accurate imaging is important for confirming the presence of disease and for guiding treatment decisions.

Treatment of endometriosis is complicated and includes conservative approaches combined with medical therapies or surgical intervention. The treatment decisions are individualized and consider the patient's clinical presentation, duration and type of symptoms, the disease extent, and location as determined by imaging, the patient's age, reproductive wishes, medication cost/side effects, and surgical cost/patient candidacy for surgery.[8–10] The American Society for Reproductive Medicine Practice Committee states that "endometriosis should be viewed as a chronic disease that requires a lifelong management plan with the goal of maximizing the use of medical treatment and avoiding repeated surgical procedures."[11] To that end, many patients are stratified for medical treatment with or without surgical treatment based on the severity of the symptoms or imaging findings and desire for child-bearing, with first-line medical therapy typically including nonsteroidal anti-inflammatory drugs and hormonal (contraceptive) agents, with more severe symptoms being treated with gonadotropin-releasing hormones and/or surgery (again, based on clinical symptoms, disease severity, and patient factors). The resection of endometriomas and endometriotic implants at the time of surgery is important for symptom control and preservation of fertility.[12] Thorough preoperative planning is essential for complete endometriosis excision.

In this article, the authors review the optimal imaging protocols for US and MR imaging of suspected endometriosis, review the compartmental approach to dictating these examinations (with a focus on mapping of disease before surgical intervention), discuss the diagnostic criteria (sensitivity and specificity of US and MR) for endometriosis detection by anatomic site, discuss the differential diagnosis, and review pearls and pitfalls in diagnosis and what the referring physician needs to know.

NORMAL ANATOMY AND IMAGING TECHNIQUE

Endometriosis most commonly occurs in the following locations in the pelvis: the ovaries, uterus, fallopian tubes, uterosacral ligaments, broad ligaments, round ligaments, cul-de-sac, bladder, ureters, rectovaginal septum, and rectosigmoid colon.[13–16] The frequency of endometriotic implants in each of these locations, with the corresponding sensitivity and specificity of detection in these regions by specialized endometriosis US and MR, is listed in **Table 1**.[14–17]

These anatomic regions can be subdivided according to functional and clinical relevance into anterior, middle, and posterior compartments.[18] The anterior compartment includes the insertion site of the ureters, the bladder, the vesicouterine pouch, and the vesicovaginal pouch. The middle compartment contains the uterine body, fallopian tube, and uterine ligaments. The posterior compartment contains the uterosacral ligaments, rectovaginal septum, anterior rectal wall, and sigmoid colon. A cartoon depiction of the regions typically involved by deep endometriosis is shown in **Fig. 1**. The corresponding normal anatomy for the anterior compartment, middle compartment, and posterior compartments is shown for US (**Fig. 2**) and MR imaging (**Fig. 3**).

Ultrasound

Transvaginal ultrasound (TVUS) is typically the initial imaging evaluation performed in patients with pelvic pain and infertility or when there is clinical suspicion for endometriosis. This examination is very accessible compared with MR imaging, and the sensitivity and specificity for detection of ovarian endometriomas and lesions in the rectal wall are high. However, there is controversy in the lack of reproducibility in the community of the US technique described by specialized tertiary care centers, and the inability of nontertiary care centers to reproduce the high sensitivity and specificity rates reported in the literature.

The best means of detection of deep endometriosis on US require a more involved US protocol than that which is traditionally used for screening TVUS. This "specialized endometriosis" US protocol involves techniques described by the American Institute of Ultrasound in Medicine (AIUM)[19] and the International Deep Endometriosis Analysis (IDEA) groups,[20] including use of a targeted physical examination before obtaining the images, the routine TVUS protocol combined with a dedicated targeted compartmental transvaginal sonogram (described in **Box 1**), with attention primarily to the posterior compartment (uterosacral ligaments, rectovaginal septum, and rectum), with use of the "sliding organ" maneuver[21] to detect subtle adhesions (see **Box 1**), with additional more specialized techniques also considered (tenderness-guided transvaginal sonography; rectal-water transvaginal sonography). For detection of uterovesicular adhesions/implants, the sliding maneuver is as follows: the transvaginal probe is placed in the anterior fornix and the uterus is moved between the probe and 1 hand of the operator that is placed over the suprapubic region. If the posterior bladder slides freely over the anterior uterine wall, then the

Table 1
Frequency of endometriosis by pelvic location at surgical laparoscopy, and corresponding sensitivity and specificity of ultrasound and MR imaging for detection

Location	Frequency Present in This Location at Laparoscopic Evaluation, %[13–15]	Specialized Endometriosis US Detection[24,48,49]	MR Imaging Detection[24,50,51]
Retrocervical region/ uterosacral ligaments	60–85	53%–64% sensitivity 93%–97% specificity	86% sensitivity 84% specificity
Uterus	40	n/a	86% sensitivity 84% specificity
Ovaries	20–40	83% sensitive 89% specific	90% sensitive 98% specific
Bladder	3–20	55% sensitivity 93.5% specificity	75%–87% sensitive 99%–100% specific
Rectosigmoid colon	9.9–37	90% sensitive 96% specific	85%–91% sensitive 72%–89% specific
Rectovaginal septum	11	81% sensitive 95% specific	81% sensitive 86% specific
Vagina	14.5–30	57% sensitive 99% specific	77%–79% sensitive 76%–93% specific
Round ligaments	0.3–14	n/a	20%–40% sensitive 30% specific
Ureters	0.01–1	Limited data: 92% sensitivity 100% specificity	83% sensitive 98.6% specific

Abbreviation: n/a, not applicable.

sliding sign is positive and the uterovesical region is classified as nonobliterated. If the bladder does not slide freely over the anterior uterine wall, then the sliding sign is negative and the uterovesical region is classified as obliterated.

In specialized tertiary care centers where attention to this meticulous technique is followed, US has the potential for high sensitivity and specificity (as high as 95% sensitivity and 96% specificity)[14,15,17,22,23] in detection of posterior compartment and bowel endometriosis (see **Table 1**). Other techniques that have been suggested for improved sensitivity include using a transrectal approach and/or a bowel preparation for better visualization of the bowel wall as well as instillation of extra gel in the vagina.[21] Limitations of sonographic technique, despite meticulous efforts, include anterior compartment detection of endometriosis (bladder and vesicouterine pouch detection) and detection within the middle compartment (torus uterinus and round ligaments). However, because posterior compartment endometriosis is the most frequently involved compartmental region by deep endometriosis, this modality, when performed with specialized endometriosis sonographic technique, represents an effective screening examination in this population.

MR Imaging

MR imaging of the pelvis is frequently performed for the detection of endometriosis, either as the second-line imaging examination (after US) for the detection/confirmation of endometriosis or as the initial examination in a patient for whom there is a high clinical suspicion for endometriosis. MR imaging can be performed with either a 1.5-T or 3-T magnet, using a high-resolution phased-array surface coil for improved resolution. There is no consensus regarding whether to perform the examination around the timing of the patient's menstrual cycle.[24] Fasting before the examination for 4 hours is typically recommended in order to empty the upper gastrointestinal tract so that the patient will not have material to vomit with supine positioning, with antiperistaltic administration, or after intravenous (IV) contrast administration. The bladder should be moderately full to improve detection of implants in the anterior compartment. Some practices recommend a bowel enema to clear out the colon; however, others have reported equal sensitivity and specificity without an enema.[24,25]

Patients are positioned supine on the scanner, with abdominal strapping after phased coil array

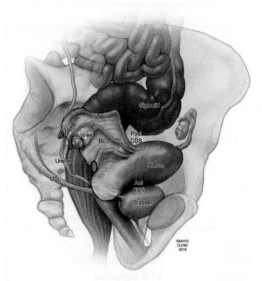

Fig. 1. The regions of the normal female pelvis. Ovarian endometriomas are found in the ovaries. Deep endometriosis can involve any region of the pelvis. For functional and clinical relevance, the pelvis can be artificially divided into the posterior, middle, and anterior compartments. The posterior compartment includes the posterior cul-de-sac (Post CDS), which comprises the uterosacral ligaments (USL), rectovaginal septum (not shown), anterior rectal wall (not shown), and sigmoid colon (Sigmoid). In the middle compartment, deep endometriosis can involve the uterine body (Uterus), fallopian tubes (FT), and uterine ligaments; here the broad ligament is shown (BL). In the anterior compartment, deep endometriosis can involve the bladder (Bladder), vesicouterine pouch/vesicovaginal pouch (depicted as the anterior cul-de-sac [Ant CDS]). SB, small bowel. (Used with permission of Mayo Foundation for Medical Education and Research, all rights reserved.)

placement. Antiperistaltic agents are generally recommended; however, the type of agent (oral agents, nonoral agents), dose, and route (intramuscular, subcutaneous, or IV) is debated; at New York University, the authors give 1 mg IV glucagon immediately before the acquisition of the 3-plane T2-weighted images (because these are the most sensitive sequences for the detection of subtle endometriosis, after which the glucagon often wears off). The administration of vaginal (gel) and rectal contrast (gel or water) is optional; the authors have the patient self-administer vaginal gel via a syringe on the table before placing the phased array coil.

For MR imaging sequences (**Table 2**), 3-plane 2-dimensional T2 turbo spin echo (TSE) -weighted images are standard for acquisition; 3-dimensional T2-weighted images are considered optional (because of their decreased contrast resolution). Half-Fourier acquisition in coronal plane single-

shot TSE images is considered standard in addition to true T2 TSE-weighted images, particularly because these allow for a larger field of view to assess for ureteral endometriosis and hydronephrosis in the kidneys. T1-weighted images without and with fat suppression are standard, because the fat suppression is useful for the detection of subtle foci of hemorrhage, which may be obscured on non–fat-saturated images. Dixon technique or conventional in- and out-of-phase T1-weighted images are useful for the differentiation of fat-containing lesions, such as dermoid cysts from endometriomas, both of which have high signal on non–fat-saturated T1-weighted images. The addition of diffusion-weighted images, susceptibility-weighted images, and postcontrast images is considered optional in the imaging for endometriosis.[25–28]

IMAGING PROTOCOLS
Imaging Findings/Pathology

The main different types of endometriotic lesions are ovarian endometriomas, superficial peritoneal implants, and DIE (see **Box 1** and **Table 2**). Ovarian endometriomas occur when ectopic endometrial tissue in the ovary hemorrhages, forms a hematoma, and is enveloped by ovarian parenchyma.[29] On gross pathology, endometriomas have thick fibrotic walls, associated with dense fibrotic adhesions with internal contents containing thick chronic blood products (thus the common pathologic term "chocolate cyst").[30] Superficial peritoneal implants of endometriosis are "powder burn" regions (<5 mm deep) seen on laparoscopy that are below the resolution of US or MR imaging. DIE is defined as a solid endometriotic implant more than 5 mm deep to the peritoneum.[7]

DIAGNOSTIC CRITERIA
Ultrasound

Sonographic appearance of endometriomas
Ovarian endometriomas occur when ectopic endometrial tissue in the ovary hemorrhages, forms a hematoma, and is enveloped by ovarian parenchyma (**Box 2**). An ovarian endometrioma has different imaging appearances on US, with the classic appearance being a cyst containing homogeneous uniform low-level echoes with increased posterior through transmission (**Fig. 4**). This finding has been described in as many as 95% of endometriomas and only 19% of nonendometriomas.[31] Another feature is the presence of peripheral echogenic foci (thought to reflect cholesterol deposits) seen in up to 36% of endometriomas versus only 6% of nonendometriomas.[31] Endometriomas tend

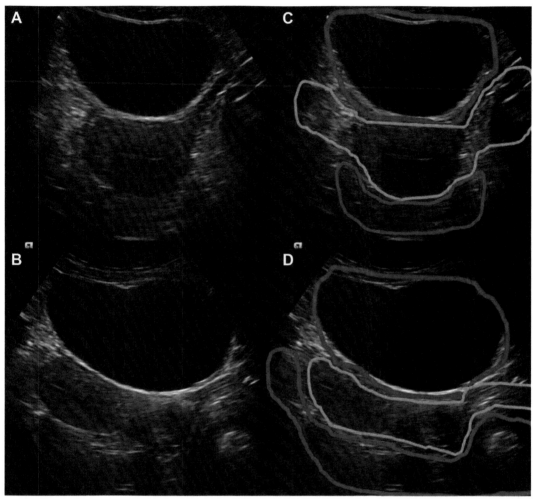

Fig. 2. Normal pelvic compartments on transabdominal pelvic sonogram. Transabdominal sonographic images of a normal pelvis in transverse (*A*) and long (*B*). Corresponding images in the same planes in transverse (*C*) and long, (*D*) with color coding of the 3 compartments (blue = anterior compartment; orange = middle compartment; and red = posterior compartment).

to be multilocular (in up to 50%) and bilateral (up to 50%)[31] (**Fig. 5**). However, endometriomas may have a variable appearance because of the range of appearance of the internal blood products within them, which can cause fluid-fluid levels, echogenic regions, or a solid appearance.[32] In these cases, additional evaluation with MR imaging may be warranted to better evaluate and to exclude malignancy.

The primary differential diagnosis of an endometrioma is a hemorrhagic cyst, which is a common cause of pelvic pain (thought to occur from hemorrhage into a corpus luteum cyst or follicular cyst). On US, a hemorrhagic cyst classically has internal reticular strands with retractile clot; the combination of such features is associated with a likelihood ratio greater than 67.[31] However, these features

may not be seen, and instead, homogeneous low-level echoes mimicking that of an endometrioma may be present. Hemorrhagic cysts are unlikely to have the peripheral echogenic foci occasionally seen in endometriomas, and they are less likely to be bilateral or multifocal. Sonographic follow-up demonstrating resolution at 6 to 12 weeks is diagnostic of a hemorrhagic cyst.

Another differential diagnosis of an endometrioma is an ovarian epithelial neoplasm, which may contain low-level internal homogeneous echoes similar to an endometrioma. This imaging appearance was seen in up to 6% of ovarian serous cystadenomas in the study by Patel and colleagues[31] and in up to 20% of mucinous cystadenomas in the study by Van Holsbeke.[33] To better evaluate for the presence of malignancy

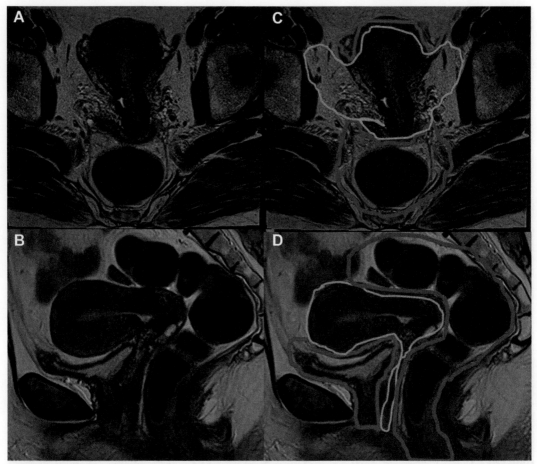

Fig. 3. Normal pelvic compartments on the female pelvis MR. Normal axial (*A*) and sagittal (*B*) T2-weighted images of the pelvis are shown. Corresponding images in the same planes of axial (*C*) sagittal (*D*) with color coding of the 3 compartments (blue = anterior compartment, orange = middle compartment, and red = posterior compartment).

(cystadenocarcinomas) in these cases, careful interrogation of the cyst should be performed to assess for internal solid components, such as papillary projections, mural nodules, and thickened septations. Ultimately, MR imaging can be performed in equivocal cases.

Sonographic appearance of hematosalpinx

Endometriosis involves the fallopian tubes up to 6% of the time in endometriosis, and external adhesions from pelvic endometriosis may also obstruct the fallopian tubes (up to 26% of the time).[34] On US, hematosalpinx appears as an extraovarian tubular structure with low-level internal echoes. A "cog-wheel" appearance of the longitudinal folds can be seen when the tube is imaged in cross-section.[35] The presence of a hematosalpinx may be the only sign on imaging of endometriosis in the pelvis.[36]

The differential diagnosis of a hematosalpinx includes pelvic inflammatory disease (PID) or fallopian tube malignancies. Pyosalpinx of PID can be differentiated clinically by the presence of extreme tenderness on examination as well as the clinical signs of infection (fever, white count). On imaging, hyperemia surrounding the fallopian tube with fatty proliferation/edema in the adjacent fat suggests a pyosalpinx. Fallopian tube carcinoma presents sonographically with solid, vascular internal nodules within the fallopian tube and tends to occur in an older demographic group.[32]

Sonographic appearance of deep infiltrating endometriosis

Deep endometriosis on sonography is subtle and presents as hypoechoic nodular or infiltrating regions in classic locations in the pelvis (in the posterior compartment, uterosacral ligaments,

---

Box 1
Specialized endometriosis ultrasound protocol

1. Before the ultrasound, a targeted physical examination should be performed by the physician (radiologist or gynecologist) reporting fixation of uterus, cervical/vaginal tenderness, visible endometriosis implants.

2. Standard ultrasound Transabdominal/Transvaginal pelvic examination (as described by the Practice Parameter of the AIUM). This includes measuring in 2 tangential planes and documenting the following: (1) the uterus (including uterine size, shape, and orientation; the endometrium; the myometrium; and the cervix); (2) the adnexa (ovaries and fallopian tubes); and (3) the cul-de-sac (including attempts to evaluate bowel posterior to the uterus).

   a. This is considered "Step 1" of the ultrasound evaluation, looking for signs of adenomyosis or ovarian endometriomas.

3. Targeted compartmental sonographic evaluation as described by the IDEA group, evaluating the anterior, middle, and posterior compartments. For this component of the evaluation (steps 2–4 of the evaluation), the following are required:

   a. Step 2 is the evaluation of transvaginal "soft markers" (ie, site-specific tenderness and ovarian mobility).

   b. Step 3 is the evaluation of the pouch of Douglas using the ultrasound "sliding sign."

   c. Step 4 is the assessment for deep infiltrating endometriosis nodules in the anterior and posterior compartments.

4. Optional: Tenderness guided transvaginal sonography:

   A. Evaluation of the cul-de-sac, bowel wall, and rectovaginal septum while gently palpating with the probe to elicit the areas of tenderness.

   B. This technique involves incremental evaluation of the pelvis, beginning with the ovary, moving posteriorly toward the cul-de-sac slowly, while palpating and evaluating regions of discomfort. In the medial region, the uterosacral ligaments are assessed, and the posterior cervical lip and rectovaginal septum are evaluated, along with the rectum, and the posterior cervix. The cervix should be moved slightly with the probe, while observing the movement of the cervix and uterus with the operator's hand. Fixated movement will suggest adhesions. The bowel should be observed for peristalsis (any regions without peristalsis will suggest implants in those regions).

Data from Guerriero S, Condous G, van den Bosch T, et al. Systematic approach to sonographic evaluation of the pelvis in women with suspected endometriosis, including terms, definitions and measurements: a consensus opinion from the International Deep Endometriosis Analysis (IDEA) group. Ultrasound Obstet Gynecol 2016;48(3):318-32; and Benacerraf BR, Groszmann Y. Sonography should be the first imaging examination done to evaluate patients with suspected endometriosis. J Ultrasound Med 2012;31(4):651–3.

---

rectovaginal septum, rectosigmoid, or bladder) (Fig. 6). Occasionally, the infiltrative regions of DIE may have internal hyperechoic foci or complex internal cysts.[21,37]

The differential diagnosis for DIE includes malignancy, particularly within the posterior compartment, which is a common site for peritoneal implants to distribute. To help differentiate endometriosis from malignant peritoneal disease, the history is useful (malignancy is unlikely in a young premenopausal patient without signs and symptoms of bloating or weight loss), and the presence of additional sites of endometriosis in the pelvis (ovarian endometriomas) supports the diagnosis of endometriosis.[32] However, if the lesion is large, hypervascular, and there are no other sites of disease, malignancy should be

suspected, and additional evaluation with MR is recommended.

Abdominal wall endometriosis
Abdominal wall endometriosis typically occurs at the site of prior surgery or trauma in the abdominal wall. It can occur independently of the presence of endometriosis elsewhere in the body and is thought to occur secondary to direct implantation of endometrial cells into the abdominal wall during surgery.[37] This phenomenon has an incidence of between 0.3% and 15% after cesarean section.[22] On sonography, these typically palpable nodules have hypoechoic echotexture, irregular borders, and increased vascularity, with or without internal cysts (Fig. 7). Typically, patients present with cyclical pain in the nodule, corresponding to the

Table 2
Endometriosis MR protocol at 3 T

Sequence	Plane	Slice Thickness, mm	Field of View, cm	Matrix	Repetition Time (ms)	Echo Time (ms)	No. Averages	B Value (s/mm²)	Contrast Delay
Patient self-administers 3 × 12-cc syringes; vaginal contrast (US gel)									
Tru FISP Scout	T1/T2	3 plane Cor/Sag/Ax	7-8	40	192 × 144	700	1.13	1		
Inject IV glucagon, do T2 sequences immediately after injection									
T2 TSE	T2	Sag	4	30–35 (adjust to body habitus)	512 × 256	4870	102	2		
HASTE	T2	Cor	5		320 × 256	Infinite	93	1		
T2 TSE	T2	Ax	4		448 × 291	5110	99	2		
Diffusion	T2	Ax	6		160 × 120	6600	70	2	b0, b50, b100, b400, b800	
In/out	T1	Ax	5		256 × 232	168	1.1/2.2 (3T)	1		
Pre-VIBE	T1	Sag	2.5		256 × 205	3	1.22	1		
Pre-VIBE	T1	Ax	3		256 × 179	2.6	1.05	1		
Post-VIBE	T1	Sag/Ax	2.5		256 × 205	3	1.22	1		30, 60, 180 s

The example given is for Siemens 3T Magnetom VIDA (Erlangen, Germany).
Abbreviations: Ax, axial; Cor, coronal; Sag, sagittal.

Diagnostic criteria for endometriosis on ultrasound and MR imaging

US:

Endometrioma:

- Cyst with homogeneous internal low-level echoes
- Cyst with peripheral echogenic foci
- Multilocular (with above features)
- Bilateral (with above features)

Hematosalpinx:

- Extraovarian tubular structure with internal low-level echoes
- Extraovarian tubular structure with incomplete septations ("cog-wheel" appearance)

Deep infiltrating endometriosis

- Hypoechoic nodular regions ± internal hyperechoic foci or complex cystic areas
- Infiltrating hypoechoic tissue ± internal hyperchoic foci or complex cystic areas

MR imaging:

Endometrioma:

- Cyst with uniformly high signal on T1-weighted image (T1WI), with corresponding uniformly low signal on T2-weighted image (T2WI; "shading sign" of Togashi)
- Cyst with peripheral T2 dark spot

Hematosalpinx:

- Extraovarian tubular structure with internal high signal on T1WI ± low signal on T2WI
- Extraovarian tubular structure with incomplete septations with high signal on T1WI

Deep infiltrating endometriosis

- Ill-defined nodular regions, low signal on T2W1 (usually *without* high signal on T1WI, but may occasionally have foci of internal high signal on T1WI)
- Infiltrating retractile regions, low signal on T2WI (usually *without* high signal on T1WI, but may occasionally have foci of internal high signal on T1WI)

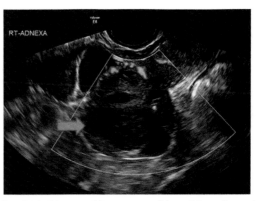

Fig. 4. A 31-year-old woman with pelvic pain and infertility. Transvaginal sonogram in the region of the right adnexa demonstrates a right ovarian cyst containing uniform low-level echoes (*arrow*) with increased posterior through transmission, and no internal vascularity, consistent with an ovarian endometrioma.

pain within the palpable abnormality suggests the diagnosis of an endometrioma. MR may be helpful for presurgical planning, because both smooth muscle tumors and abdominal wall endometriomas are surgically resected; however, the approach is different (there is a tissue-sparing conservative approach for endometriomas, vs the need for wide negative margins for desmoid tumors).

MR
MR Appearance of Endometriomas

The MR appearance of endometriomas is classically described as uniformly high signal on T1-weighted images with uniform low signal on T2-weighted images, a phenomenon termed "shading" by Togashi and colleagues[38] in 1991 (**Fig. 8**). Of 354 pathologically confirmed lesions, the overall diagnostic sensitivity, specificity, and accuracy of the shading sign for differentiating endometriomas from other gynecologic lesions were 90%, 98%, and 96%, respectively.[38] Since that time, Corwin and colleagues[39] evaluated a dataset of 74 lesions and found that the T2 shading sign of Togashi had a sensitivity, specificity, and positive predictive value of 93%, 45%, and 72%. Corwin and colleagues[39] postulated that the difference in specificity between the 2 studies (in terms of the T2 shading sign) may be a reflection of the different echo time (TE) of the T2-weighted imaging sequences. The Togashi paper had an average TE of 60 to 80 milliseconds, but the Corwin paper had an average TE of 95 milliseconds, thus making the study by Corwin and colleagues[39] more sensitive to a small amount of blood products, but less specific. The Corwin paper

stimulation of the endometrial glands during the menstrual cycle.

The differential for the sonographic finding of an irregular palpable mass in the abdominal wall is broad and includes smooth muscle tumors of the anterior abdominal wall (desmoid tumors and fibrous tumors). Typically, the presence of cyclical

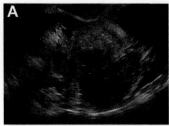 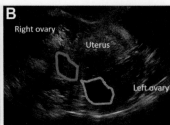

Fig. 5. A 41-year-old woman with pelvic pain with US showing "kissing ovaries." Transvaginal sonogram in an oblique plane through the pelvis (A) demonstrates posterior displacement of both ovaries behind the uterus. The right ovary (labeled in B) contains an endometrioma (blue), which contacts the left ovary, which also has an endometrioma (orange). This configuration is termed "kissing ovaries" and is consistent with endometriosis.

proposed a new "T2 dark spot sign," defined as discrete, markedly hypointense foci within the cyst on T2-weighted images with or without T2 shading, which had a sensitivity of 36%, specificity of 93%, and positive predictive value of 89% for the diagnosis of endometrioma as opposed to a hemorrhagic cyst (Fig. 9).

As described above under the Ultrasound section, the primary differential diagnosis of an endometrioma is a hemorrhagic cyst. Use of the aforementioned T2 shading sign and T2 dark spot sign is associated with a good sensitivity and excellent specificity for the diagnosis of an endometrioma. Other diagnostic considerations include a mature cystic teratoma/dermoid cyst. On MR imaging, a mature cystic teratoma will be high signal on T1-weighted images *without* fat saturation (similar to an endometrioma), but unlike an endometrioma, the cystic teratoma will follow the signal of bulk fat on every sequence. Thus, on a T1-weighted frequency selective fat-saturation sequence, the mature cystic teratoma will be low in signal, whereas an endometrioma will have high signal.

MR Appearance of Hematosalpinx

Thirty percent of women with endometriosis have tubal involvement at the time of operative exploration.[36,40] On MR imaging, hematosalpinx manifests as a distended tubular structure adjacent to the ovary demonstrating internal high signal on T1-weighted images (40% of distended tubes in endometriosis have hyperintense contents).[41] If a

hematosalpinx is seen in isolation, it is suggestive of endometriosis.[41,42] However, in up to 60% of patients with endometriosis with a dilated fallopian tube seen at the time of surgery, imaging does not show internal high signal on T1-weighted images.[41] In addition, it is atypical to see T2 shading within the lumen of the distended fallopian tube even when there is high signal on T1-weighted images.[42] T2 shading is not seen because of the fact that the endometriotic implants are mostly along the surface of the tube and not within the lumen of the tube, such that the chronic bleeding within the implants leads to adhesions along the tubal surface, but not within the lumen.

The differential diagnosis of a hematosalpinx on MR imaging is the same as that described above under hematosalpinx on US and again includes PID or fallopian tube malignancies. Pyosalpinx of PID can be differentiated by the clinical signs of infection (fever, white count). On MR imaging, hyperemia surrounding the fallopian tube with stranding in the adjacent fat would suggest a pyosalpinx. Fallopian tube carcinoma demonstrates solid, enhancing internal nodules within the fallopian tube and tends to occur in an older demographic group.[32]

MR Appearance of Deep Infiltrating Endometriosis

DIE is defined as a solid endometriotic implant more than 5 mm deep to the peritoneum. Typical locations include the rectovaginal septum,

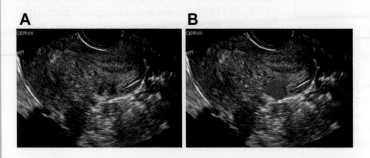

Fig. 6. A 31-year-old woman with rectovaginal endometriotic implant. Transvaginal sonogram in the sagittal plane centered on the cervix is shown in (A), with the rectovaginal implant (of the same image) demonstrated, shaded in red in (B).

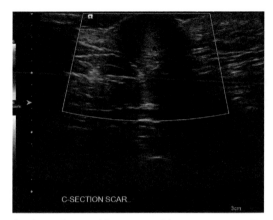

Fig. 7. A 40-year-old woman with a cesarean section scar endometrioma. A 40-year-old woman with cyclical pain of the anterior abdominal wall and a history of prior cesarean section. Axial transabdominal sonogram demonstrates a hypoechoic to slightly isoechoic mass of the anterior abdominal wall with low-level internal vascularity. This mass was excised and was consistent with endometriosis.

uterosacral ligaments, rectosigmoid colon, uterine body, round ligaments, bladder, and vagina. DIE has a varied imaging appearance on MR imaging, typically demonstrating low signal on T1-weighted images with corresponding low signal on T2-weighted images, with a spiculated, fibrotic appearance. Preoperative imaging has traditionally been performed with TVUS, which has an excellent sensitivity and specificity for detection of ovarian endometriomas, but a limited sensitivity for detection of DIE,[43] and has a high operator variability. Older studies with MR imaging demonstrated limited accuracy in detection of endometriosis; however, with advanced MR imaging techniques and increased awareness by radiologists of this entity, along with the superior reproducibility of MR imaging scans (as opposed to transvaginal sonography), newer studies have demonstrated a high interobserver agreement for MR imaging in detection of deep endometriosis.[26,44–46]

Table 1 describes the frequency of involvement of each region in the pelvis by

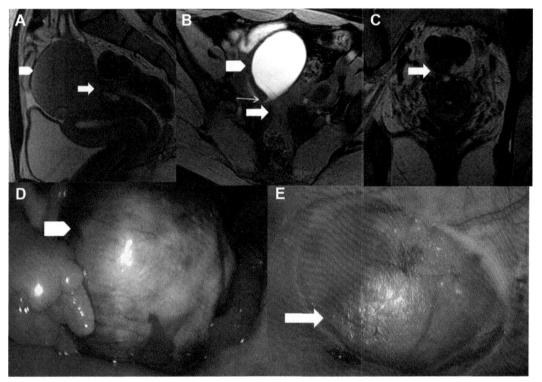

Fig. 8. A 30-year-old woman with tricompartmental deep endometriosis. A 30-year-old G0 woman with 2 years' constant right pelvic pain and deep dyspareunia. Sagittal T2 (*A*) and axial T1-weighted with fat saturation (*B*) and coronal T2 (*C*). MR imaging shows fibrotic tethering of large right endometrioma (*arrowhead* in A, B, and D) and rectosigmoid colon (*regular arrow* in A, B, and C) deep infiltrative endometriosis to the posterior uterine body with punctate T1 hyperintense endometriotic implants on the uterine serosa (*thin arrow*). Intraoperative correlation shows the right ovarian endometrioma (*arrowhead* in D) and the endometriosis bulging into the rectal lumen (*arrow* in E).

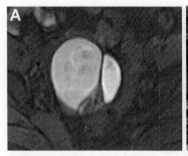
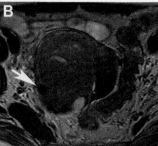

Fig. 9. T2 dark spot sign. A 35-year-old woman with axial T1- (*A*) weighted and axial T2- (*B*) weighted images through the pelvis showing a uniformly high signal (on T1-weighted images, *A*) right ovarian cyst, which demonstrates both uniform loss of signal on T2-weighted images, consistent with shading as well as a more focal T2 dark spot (*arrow* in *B*), consistent with an ovarian endometrioma.

endometriosis. The uterosacral ligaments are the most commonly involved region of DIE and can be seen as thickened regions of low signal on T2-weighted images. The rectosigmoid colon is the most commonly involved intestinal segment (see **Fig. 8**). This area of the colon needs to be carefully evaluated for length and depth of invasion by DIE. If the muscularis propria is involved (seen on imaging as luminal invasion), then patients may benefit from segmental or partial (saline-lift procedure) resection of the involved segment of bowel, and a colorectal surgeon should be consulted preoperatively with appropriate consent obtained from the patient. Bladder involvement typically presents with dysuria and less commonly with cyclical hematuria. On MR imaging, bladder involvement by endometriosis presents with a focus of low signal on T2-weighted images, often with internal high signal on T2-weighted images, corresponding to ectopic endometrial glands (**Fig. 10**). T1-weighted imaging is variable, occasionally demonstrating foci of high signal.[42] The round ligaments may be involved by endometriosis, with prevalence of disease involvement of up to 14%[13–15] (**Fig. 11**). The appearance of round ligament involvement on MR imaging is T2 hypointense thickening or nodularity with enhancement postcontrast.

Abdominal wall endometriosis can occur in patients because of direct implantation of endometrial glands and stroma during cesarean section or laparoscopic intervention, with the reported incidence after cesarean section as high as 0.3% and 15%.[22] Seventy percent of patients with abdominal wall endometriomas have cyclical pain associated with the patient's menstrual cycle; however, the pain may be constant. On MR imaging, these masses demonstrate variable signal on T1-weighted images (sometimes high signal on T1-weighted images is seen, but often not), with typically low signal on T2-weighted images, with or without internal foci of high signal on T2-weighted images. These regions will demonstrate progressive enhancement postcontrast. The presence of internal foci of high signal on T2-weighted images is nearly pathognomonic. The differential diagnosis of a spiculated enhancing mass in the anterior abdominal wall includes smooth muscle tumors of the anterior abdominal wall (desmoid tumors and fibrous tumors). The imaging features (internal foci of high signal on T1, low signal on T2, internal cystic foci) combined with the typical symptoms of cyclical pain allow the diagnosis of an abdominal wall endometrioma to be made preoperatively most of the time.

DIFFERENTIAL DIAGNOSIS
Pearls/Pitfalls/Variants

Pearls

- T1 bright adnexal lesions may be endometriomas, look for the associated (see **Box 2**):
  - T2 shading sign of ovarian endometrioma
  - T2 dark spot sign of ovarian endometrioma
- Hematosalpinx is specific for endometriosis

Complications/pitfalls

- Rupture
- Infection
- Malignant transformation
- Intraluminal (rectal) invasion
- Missing subtle disease
- Undercalling frozen pelvis
- Peritoneal carcinomatosis of another primary
- Crohn disease
- Decidualized endometriosis of pregnancy

Variants

- Abdominal wall endometriosis
- Perineal endometriosis
- Ureteral endometriosis
- Diaphragmatic endometriosis
- Appendiceal endometriosis
- Invasive endometriosis of the posterior uterine wall

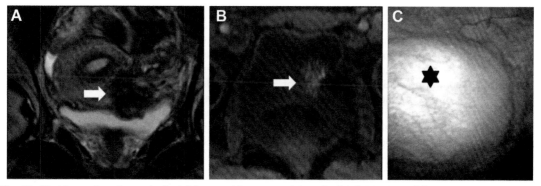

Fig. 10. Bladder wall endometriosis. A 36-year-old woman with cyclical pelvic pain and frequent urinary tract infections. Coronal T2- (*A*) and axial T1-weighted MR imaging with fat saturation (*B*) shows bladder invasive endometriosis with T1 and T2 hyperintense glandular foci (*arrow* in *A* and *B*). Image (*C*) during cystoscopy demonstrates a submucosal bladder lesion (*star*) with pathology demonstrating deep endometriosis of the bladder wall.

WHAT THE REFERRING PHYSICIAN NEEDS TO KNOW

- Endometriosis is a common gynecologic condition (estimated 10% prevalence in women of reproductive age).[4]

- Endometriosis does not have pathognomonic-associated symptoms or biomarkers. Most patients who are sent for imaging present with chronic pelvic pain or infertility.[47]

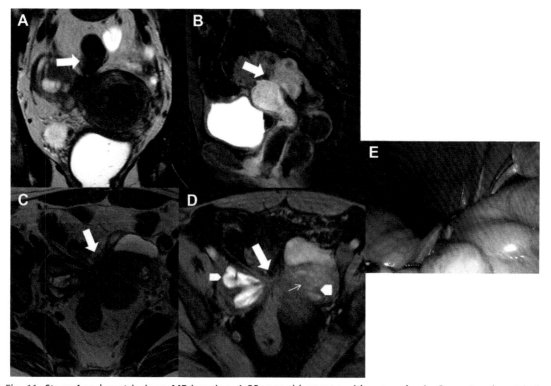

Fig. 11. Stage 4 endometriosis on MR imaging. A 38-year-old woman with menorrhagia. Stage 4 endometriosis with "kissing ovaries" morphology and obliteration of the posterior cul-de-sac by bowel invasive endometriosis. Coronal (*A*) and axial (*C*) T2-weighted MR images show the hypointense fibrotic retraction of both ovaries and the rectum to the posterior uterus (*arrow* in *C*). Thickening of the right round ligament is also seen just anterior to the right ovary (*C, D*). Postcontrast T1-weighted images with fat saturation (*B*) show invasion of the rectum by the endometriosis (*arrow* in *A* and *B*). Axial T1-weighted imaging with fat saturation (*D*) shows bilateral T1 hyperintense hemorrhagic ovarian endometriomas and ovarian (*white arrowhead*) and serosal implants (*thin arrow*). Intraoperative image (*E*) shows obliteration of the posterior cul-de-sac by the extensive deep endometriosis.

- Endometriosis is classified intraoperatively in the 3 following ways: (1) a superficial peritoneal lesion (occult on imaging), (2) an ovarian endometrioma, or (3) deep endometriosis (endometriotic lesions extending >5 mm below the peritoneum). Knowledge of the extent of involvement of endometriosis in the pelvis is useful in determining appropriate therapy.[18]
- Unless trained, many general radiologists do not notice regions of deep endometriosis on pelvic MR imaging. If radiologists can detect this disease, it helps clinicians to appropriately consider care options/fertility options for the patient.
- Describing endometriosis in terms of its compartment of involvement (anterior, middle, and posterior) helps the operative surgeon know the degree of dissection required and the operative approach.
- US and MR imaging may underestimate disease extent of endometriosis. If there is 3-compartmental involvement on imaging, it will likely correspond to a "frozen pelvis" for the operative surgeon (ie, multiple adhesions between organs and/or bowel).

DISCLOSURE

No financial disclosures.

REFERENCES

1. Giudice LC. Clinical practice. Endometriosis. N Engl J Med 2010;362(25):2389–98.
2. Chatman DL, Ward AB. Endometriosis in adolescents. J Reprod Med 1982;27(3):156–60.
3. Sangi-Haghpeykar H, Poindexter AN 3rd. Epidemiology of endometriosis among parous women. Obstet Gynecol 1995;85(6):983–92.
4. Bazot M, Bharwani N, Huchon C, et al. European Society of Urogenital Radiology (ESUR) guidelines: MR imaging of pelvic endometriosis. Eur Radiol 2017; 27(7):2765–75.
5. Cheng YM, Wang ST, Chou CY. Serum CA-125 in preoperative patients at high risk for endometriosis. Obstet Gynecol 2002;99(3):375–80.
6. Menakaya UA, Rombauts L, Johnson NP. Diagnostic laparoscopy in pre-surgical planning for higher stage endometriosis: is it still relevant? Aust N Z J Obstet Gynaecol 2016;56(5):518–22.
7. De Cicco C, Corona R, Schonman R, et al. Bowel resection for deep endometriosis: a systematic review. BJOG 2011;118(3):285–91.
8. Schenken RS. Endometriosis classification for infertility. Acta Obstet Gynecol Scand Suppl 1994;159: 41–4.
9. Schenken RS. Familial endometriosis. J Soc Gynecol Investig 2003;10(3):123.
10. Schenken RS. Delayed diagnosis of endometriosis. Fertil Steril 2006;86(5):1305–6 [discussion: 1317].
11. Practice Committee of the American Society for Reproductive Medicine. Treatment of pelvic pain associated with endometriosis: a committee opinion. Fertil Steril 2014;101(4):927–35.
12. de Ziegler D, Borghese B, Chapron C. Endometriosis and infertility: pathophysiology and management. Lancet 2010;376(9742):730–8.
13. Chamie LP, Blasbalg R, Pereira RM, et al. Findings of pelvic endometriosis at transvaginal US, MR imaging, and laparoscopy. Radiographics 2011; 31(4):E77–100.
14. Chapron C, Fauconnier A, Vieira M, et al. Anatomical distribution of deeply infiltrating endometriosis: surgical implications and proposition for a classification. Hum Reprod 2003;18(1):157–61.
15. Gui B, Valentini AL, Ninivaggi V, et al. Deep pelvic endometriosis: don't forget round ligaments. Review of anatomy, clinical characteristics, and MR imaging features. Abdom Imaging 2014;39(3):622–32.
16. Foti PV, Farina R, Palmucci S, et al. Endometriosis: clinical features, MR imaging findings and pathologic correlation. Insights Imaging 2018;9(2): 149–72.
17. Chamie LP, Pereira RM, Zanatta A, et al. Transvaginal US after bowel preparation for deeply infiltrating endometriosis: protocol, imaging appearances, and laparoscopic correlation. Radiographics 2010;30(5): 1235–49.
18. Coutinho A Jr, Bittencourt LK, Pires CE, et al. MR imaging in deep pelvic endometriosis: a pictorial essay. Radiographics 2011;31(2):549–67.
19. American Institute of Ultrasound in Medicine (AIUM), American College of Radiology (ACR), American College of Obstetricians and Gynecologists (ACOG), Society for Pediatric Radiology (SPR), Society of Radiologists in Ultrasound (SRU). AIUM practice guideline for the performance of ultrasound of the female pelvis. J Ultrasound Med 2014;33(6): 1122–30.
20. Guerriero S, Condous G, van den Bosch T, et al. Systematic approach to sonographic evaluation of the pelvis in women with suspected endometriosis, including terms, definitions and measurements: a consensus opinion from the International Deep Endometriosis Analysis (IDEA) group. Ultrasound Obstet Gynecol 2016;48(3):318–32.
21. Benacerraf BR, Groszmann Y. Sonography should be the first imaging examination done to evaluate patients with suspected endometriosis. J Ultrasound Med 2012;31(4):651–3.
22. Bazot M, Lafont C, Rouzier R, et al. Diagnostic accuracy of physical examination, transvaginal sonography, rectal endoscopic sonography, and magnetic

resonance imaging to diagnose deep infiltrating endometriosis. Fertil Steril 2009;92(6):1825–33.

23. Chamie LP, Blasbalg R, Goncalves MO, et al. Accuracy of magnetic resonance imaging for diagnosis and preoperative assessment of deeply infiltrating endometriosis. Int J Gynaecol Obstet 2009;106(3):198–201.

24. Bazot M, Darai E. Diagnosis of deep endometriosis: clinical examination, ultrasonography, magnetic resonance imaging, and other techniques. Fertil Steril 2017;108(6):886–94.

25. Manganaro L, Vittori G, Vinci V, et al. Beyond laparoscopy: 3-T magnetic resonance imaging in the evaluation of posterior cul-de-sac obliteration. Magn Reson Imaging 2012;30(10):1432–8.

26. Bazot M, Darai E, Hourani R, et al. Deep pelvic endometriosis: MR imaging for diagnosis and prediction of extension of disease. Radiology 2004;232(2):379–89.

27. Bazot M, Gasner A, Ballester M, et al. Value of thin-section oblique axial T2-weighted magnetic resonance images to assess uterosacral ligament endometriosis. Hum Reprod 2011;26(2):346–53.

28. Bazot M, Gasner A, Lafont C, et al. Deep pelvic endometriosis: limited additional diagnostic value of postcontrast in comparison with conventional MR images. Eur J Radiol 2011;80(3):e331–9.

29. Brosens IA, Puttemans PJ, Deprest J. The endoscopic localization of endometrial implants in the ovarian chocolate cyst. Fertil Steril 1994;61(6):1034–8.

30. Woodward PJ, Sohaey R, Mezzetti TP Jr. Endometriosis: radiologic-pathologic correlation. Radiographics 2001;21(1):193–216 [questionnaire: 288–94].

31. Patel MD, Feldstein VA, Chen DC, et al. Endometriomas: diagnostic performance of US. Radiology 1999;210(3):739–45.

32. Jones LP, Morgan MA, Chauhan A. The sonographic spectrum of pelvic endometriosis: pearls, pitfalls, and mimics. Ultrasound Q 2019;35(4):355–75.

33. Van Holsbeke C, Zhang J, Van Belle V, et al. Acoustic streaming cannot discriminate reliably between endometriomas and other types of adnexal lesion: a multicenter study of 633 adnexal masses. Ultrasound Obstet Gynecol 2010;35(3):349–53.

34. Jenkins S, Olive DL, Haney AF. Endometriosis: pathogenetic implications of the anatomic distribution. Obstet Gynecol 1986;67(3):335–8.

35. Rezvani M, Shaaban AM. Fallopian tube disease in the nonpregnant patient. Radiographics 2011;31(2):527–48.

36. Gougoutas CA, Siegelman ES, Hunt J, et al. Pelvic endometriosis: various manifestations and MR imaging findings. AJR Am J Roentgenol 2000;175(2):353–8.

37. Chamie LP, Ribeiro D, Tiferes DA, et al. Atypical sites of deeply infiltrative endometriosis: clinical characteristics and imaging findings. Radiographics 2018;38(1):309–28.

38. Togashi K, Nishimura K, Kimura I, et al. Endometrial cysts: diagnosis with MR imaging. Radiology 1991;180(1):73–8.

39. Corwin MT, Gerscovich EO, Lamba R, et al. Differentiation of ovarian endometriomas from hemorrhagic cysts at MR imaging: utility of the T2 dark spot sign. Radiology 2014;271(1):126–32.

40. Kim MY, Rha SE, Oh SN, et al. MR imaging findings of hydrosalpinx: a comprehensive review. Radiographics 2009;29(2):495–507.

41. Outwater EK, Siegelman ES, Chiowanich P, et al. Dilated fallopian tubes: MR imaging characteristics. Radiology 1998;208(2):463–9.

42. Siegelman ES, Oliver ER. MR imaging of endometriosis: ten imaging pearls. Radiographics 2012;32(6):1675–91.

43. Savelli L, Manuzzi L, Pollastri P, et al. Diagnostic accuracy and potential limitations of transvaginal sonography for bladder endometriosis. Ultrasound Obstet Gynecol 2009;34(5):595–600.

44. Varol N, Maher P, Healey M, et al. Rectal surgery for endometriosis–should we be aggressive? J Am Assoc Gynecol Laparosc 2003;10(2):182–9.

45. Bazot M, Thomassin I, Hourani R, et al. Diagnostic accuracy of transvaginal sonography for deep pelvic endometriosis. Ultrasound Obstet Gynecol 2004;24(2):180–5.

46. Abbott JA, Hawe J, Clayton RD, et al. The effects and effectiveness of laparoscopic excision of endometriosis: a prospective study with 2-5 year follow-up. Hum Reprod 2003;18(9):1922–7.

47. Agarwal SK, Chapron C, Giudice LC, et al. Clinical diagnosis of endometriosis: a call to action. Am J Obstet Gynecol 2019;220(4):354.e1-12.

48. Guerriero S, Ajossa S, Minguez JA, et al. Accuracy of transvaginal ultrasound for diagnosis of deep endometriosis in uterosacral ligaments, rectovaginal septum, vagina and bladder: systematic review and meta-analysis. Ultrasound Obstet Gynecol 2015;46(5):534–45.

49. Nisenblat V, Bossuyt PM, Farquhar C, et al. Imaging modalities for the non-invasive diagnosis of endometriosis. Cochrane Database Syst Rev 2016;(2):CD009591.

50. Scardapane A, Lorusso F, Bettocchi S, et al. Deep pelvic endometriosis: accuracy of pelvic MRI completed by MR colonography. Radiol Med 2013;118(2):323–38.

51. Valentini AL, Gui B, Micco M, et al. How to improve MRI accuracy in detecting deep infiltrating colorectal endometriosis: MRI findings vs. laparoscopy and histopathology. Radiol Med 2014;119(5):291–7.

Magnetic Resonance Imaging of the Female Pelvic Floor
Anatomy Overview, Indications, and Imaging Protocols

Rania Farouk El Sayed, MD, PhD

KEYWORDS

- Pelvic floor anatomy • MR imaging anatomy of pelvic floor muscles • MR imaging of pelvic floor
- Indications for MR imaging of pelvic floor dysfunctions
- Indications and imaging protocols of pelvic floor dysfunctions

KEY POINTS

- The "classic 3-compartment approach," "active and passive conceptual approach," and the "multi-layered system approach" are established different approaches for description of pelvic floor anatomy.
- The "functional 3-part pelvic supporting systems approach," a new, more function-based classification of pelvic floor support system, is discussed in detail.
- Indications, patients' preparation, and hardware requirements for MR imaging of pelvic floor dysfunction and MR-defecography are included.
- The MR imaging protocols define the most important prerequisites for a diagnostic MR examination according to the concordance of experts from European Society of Urogenital Radiology, European Society of Gastrointestinal and Abdominal Radiology, and Society of Abdominal Radiology societies.

INTRODUCTION

Pelvic floor disorders are often complex with symptoms ranging from vague low back pain to major fecal incontinence and urinary incontinence.

Symptoms are divided arbitrarily into different areas: urinary disorders, fecal disorders, sexual dysfunction, and pelvic discomfort, although symptoms of all types often coexist in the same individual.[1]

When a patient presents for evaluation, she may be unaware that many of her symptoms may be related to pelvic floor dysfunction (PFD). The clinician should elicit a comprehensive history encompassing all pertinent areas. Obtaining a comprehensive history is a particular challenge in reconstructive pelvic surgery, in which anatomic aberrations are often striking, but understanding the symptoms related to them is inadequate. The reoperation rate after initial pelvic floor surgery is reported to be approximately 29%.[2] The commonness of the need for reoperation indicates that better treatments are necessary; however, clinicians specialized in this field affirmed that such improvement will be possible only if research clarifies the causative mechanisms and the reasons that surgery fails.[3]

Magnetic resonance (MR) imaging has been effectively used to evaluate PFD, with very good reported sensitivity, specificity, and positive predictive value. The modality relies on (a) static sequences with a high spatial resolution to delineate the passive and active elements of the pelvic organ support system and (b) fast imaging

Cairo University MRI Pelvic Floor Center of Excellency and Research Lab Unit, Department of Radiology, Cairo University Hospitals, Kasr El Ainy Street, Cairo 11956, Egypt
E-mail address: rania729.re@gmail.com

Radiol Clin N Am 58 (2020) 291–303
https://doi.org/10.1016/j.rcl.2019.11.005
0033-8389/20/© 2019 Elsevier Inc. All rights reserved.

dynamic (cine) sequences during straining and evacuation to detect functional abnormalities.[4] This article reviews in detail the basic essential anatomic information the radiologist needs to know to become competently capable not only of writing a full report based on solid scientific information but also of providing state-of-the art care for patients who present for MR imaging for PFD.[5,6] Full competence means that the radiologist will know the steps for taking a full relevant medical history,[7] can confidently determine which radiologic studies to order to allow for a detailed diagnostic report, to know the mandatory steps for patient preparation, and to assemble the MR imaging findings in a schematic to best meet the needs of the urologist, gynecologist, and proctologist who will treat the patients.

Overview of Pelvic Floor Normal Anatomy

There are several approaches for functional description of pelvic floor (Fig. 1):

A. Classic 3-compartment approach
- The pelvic floor is divided into the following 3 major compartments:
  Anterior: Includes urinary bladder, urethra, and urethral support system
  Middle: Includes vagina (anterior and posterior wall) and uterocervical support
  Posterior: Contains rectum and supporting structure
- Patients with abnormalities in 1 compartment often have disorders in another[8]
B. Active and passive conceptual approach
- Pelvic floor components are divided into passive and active structures
  o Passive structures

- Pelvic bones
- Supportive connective tissue
  o Active structures
- Pelvic floor muscles
- This classification cannot precisely explain pathogenesis of various dysfunctions.[8]
C. Multilayered system approach
- Considers passive and active components of pelvic floor as an integrated multilayer system[8,9] organized from cranial to caudal into the following:
  o First layer: Endopelvic fascia
  o Second layer: Pelvic diaphragm
  o Third layer: Urogenital diaphragm
  o Fourth layer: Perineum
D. Functional 3-part pelvic supporting systems approach (Fig. 2)
- The components of this functional approach are described in full detail in the later discussion, "Static MR Images" of the pelvic floor examination.
- It is a new, more function-based classification of pelvic floor support system.[5]
- This approach is based on fact that each passive and active structural component of the pelvic floor plays a role in urinary and fecal continence, preventing pelvic organ prolapse. In this approach, all structures that contribute to the same function are grouped under 1 system.
  o Urethral support system
- Structures that maintain urinary continence:
  - Urethral support ligaments
  - Level III endopelvic fascia
  - Puborectalis muscle
  o Vaginal support system:

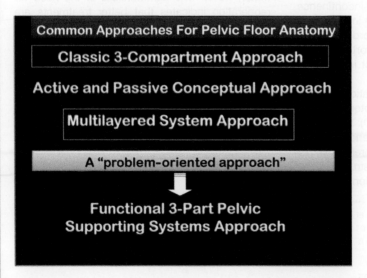

Fig. 1. Four approaches describing the anatomy of the pelvic floor.

Common Approaches For Pelvic Floor Anatomy

Classic 3-Compartment Approach

Active and Passive Conceptual Approach

Multilayered System Approach

A "problem-oriented approach"

Functional 3-Part Pelvic Supporting Systems Approach

- Supporting elements that prevent prolapse:
  - Level I and II endopelvic fascial
  - Iliococcygeus muscle
  - Anal sphincter complex:
    - Anal sphincter muscles together with other supporting elements maintain fecal continence

Multilayered System Approach

Essential anatomic and functional information to understand the concept of the "Multilayered system approach" includes the following:

Supportive connective tissue

Supportive connective tissue is a complex network of connective tissue, and variations occur between the main components according to the type of the supportive structures[5]:

A. Ligaments:
  - Form a well-defined layer composed of specialized aggregation of connective tissue and have well-organized fibrous collagen

  - Include arcus tendineus levator ani (ATLA) and arcus tendineus fascia pelvis ligaments, which are dense, obliquely oriented linear pure connective tissue structures at the pelvic sidewall

B. Endopelvic fascia:
  - Forms a diffuse layer that consists of less well-defined connective tissue
  - Has a functional correlation, whereby it envelops pelvic organs, including parametrium and paracolpium, giving support to the uterus and upper vagina, respectively[8,10]

Layers of pelvic support

(a) First layer: Endopelvic fascia
  - Parametria includes broad, cardinal, and uterosacral ligaments
  - Paracolpium refers to connective tissue that attaches vagina to pelvic walls (**Fig. 3**)
    - Anteriorly, pubocervical fascia and ligaments extend from the posterior surface of the pubis to the cervix, giving support to the bladder
    - Posteriorly, rectovaginal fascia inserts into the perineal body, levator plate, and

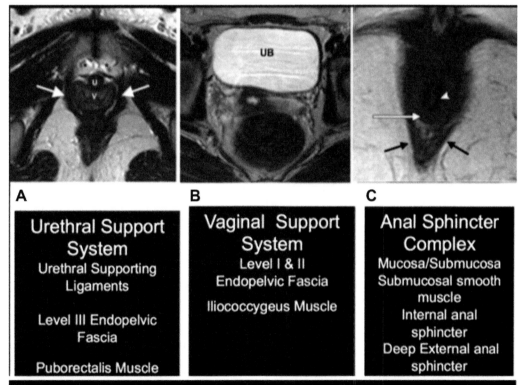

A

Urethral Support System
Urethral Supporting Ligaments

Level III Endopelvic Fascia

Puborectalis Muscle

B

Vaginal Support System
Level I & II
Endopelvic Fascia

Iliococcygeus Muscle

C

Anal Sphincter Complex
Mucosa/Submucosa
Submucosal smooth muscle
Internal anal sphincter
Deep External anal sphincter

Functional 3-Part Pelvic Supporting Systems Approach

Fig. 2. The Functional 3-Part pelvic support system approach and the components of each system. (*A*) Urethral support system. (*B*) Vaginal support system. (*C*) The anal sphincter complex. Arrow points to internal anal sphincter. Arrowhead points to submucosal smooth muscle. U, urethra; V, vagina; UB, urinary bladder.

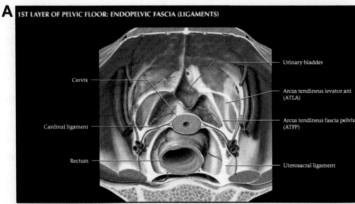

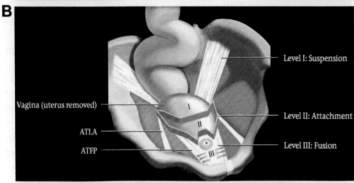

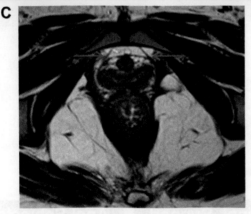

Fig. 3. (A) Overview of the pelvis shows the fascia with the bladder, cervix, and rectum cut away. Endopelvic fascia is a continuous adventitial layer, covering the pelvic diaphragm and viscera. It is a complex network of connective tissue composed of collagen, fibroblasts, elastin, smooth muscle cells, and neurovascular bundles. Ligaments are a more well-defined aggregate of connective tissue. (B) The type of support the vagina receives at each level (uterus removed). In level I (suspension), the paracolpium suspends the vagina from the lateral pelvic walls. Fibers of level I extend both vertically and posteriorly toward the sacrum. In level II (attachment), the vagina is attached to the arcus tendineus fasciae pelvis and the superior fascia of levator ani. In level III (fusion), the vagina, near the introitus, is fused laterally to the levator ani. (C) Axial oblique T2WI TSE MR image shows the arcus tendineus fascia pelvis (ATFP) (arrows) on either side of the symphysis pubis. (From [(El Sayed RF . Overview of the Pelvic Floor. In: Shaaban AM, Editor. Diagnostic Imaging: Gynecology 2nd Edition. Philadelphia: Elsevier-Amirsys; 2015. 8/2 -8/28 ; with permission.)

uterosacral ligament. It support the rectum and forms a restraining layer that prevents the rectum from protruding forward, blocking formation of a rectocele (Fig. 3A)
- Levels of vaginal support
  Pubocervical fascia is divided into 3 levels (Fig. 3B, C)
  - *Level I (suspension)*
    - Upper portion of the vagina adjacent to the cervix (cephalic 2 to 3 cm of the vagina)
    - Suspended from above by relatively long connective tissue fibers of the upper paracolpium
    - Functional significance: it provides upper vaginal support
- *Level II (attachment)*
  - Is a midportion of the vagina
  - The paracolpium becomes shorter at this level
  - Attaches the vaginal wall more directly to arcus tendineus fascia pelvis
  - Stretches the vagina transversely between the bladder and rectum
- *Level III (Fusion)*
  - Corresponds to the region of the vagina that extends from the introitus to 2 to 3 cm above the hymenal ring

o Near introitus, the vagina is fused laterally to levator ani
o Posteriorly, attaches to perineal body
o Anteriorly, blends with the urethra
o At this level, there is no intervening paracolpium between the vagina and the adjacent structures, as opposed to levels I and II

(b) Second layer: Pelvic diaphragm
- *Definition*: Formed by coccygeus and levator ani muscles and acts as a shelf to support pelvic organs (**Fig. 4**)
- Coccygeus muscle
  o Forms the posterior part of the pelvic diaphragm
  o Arises from the tip of the ischial spine along the posterior margin of the internal obturator muscle, inserts into the lateral side of the coccyx and lowest part of the sacrum
  o The coccygeus muscle is not part of the levator ani, having a different function and origin
- Levator ani muscle
  o Components
    The levator ani is divided anatomically into 3 components and is differentiated according to origin and direction of fiber bundles[11–14] (**Fig. 4A**)
    Puborectalis muscle
    - Arises from the superior and inferior pubic rami
    - Unites with contralateral puborectalis muscle, posterior to the rectum, forming a sling
    - Does not insert onto any skeletal structure
    Pubococcygeus muscle (**Fig. 4B**)
    - Arises from the back of the pubic bone and the anterior part of the obturator fascia
    - Inserts into the lateral aspect of the coccyx
    Iliococcygeus muscle
    - Arises from the fascia overlying obturator internus
    - Inserts into the lateral aspect of the coccyx, overlapping with fibers of pubococcygeus muscle in a staggered arrangement
  o Functional correlation of levator ani muscle
    ■ Puborectalis muscle:
      - Urethral pressure
        o Puborectalis muscle aids in maintaining urethral pressure
        o Some of its anteromedial fibers attach to the vagina and may assist

in direct elevation and support of the urethrovesical neck, thus affecting urethral pressure and continence
- Pelvic organ support
  o Direct support for rectum
  o Indirect support to vagina, bladder, and urethra by drawing these structures ventrally toward the pubic bone
  o Traction force contributes to more acute anorectal angle (and thus the anal canal is closed). Posterior curve to the vagina and horizontal levator plate
- Anal continence
  o Constant tone causes anterior displacement of the anal canal, resulting in an acute anorectal angle
  o Acute angulation resists fecal outflow and is essential in maintaining rectal continence
  o Under physiologic conditions, this angle can be altered either to augment continence or to assist defecation
  o To facilitate defecation, the puborectalis is relaxed, and brief Valsalva maneuver augments pelvic floor descent
  o To defer defecation, the puborectalis contracts, causing the rectum to become more perpendicular to the anal canal, which elevates the pelvic floor and lengthens the anal canal[5,14]
    ■ Iliococcygeus muscle
      - Stretches in a horizontal plane from the rectal hiatus to the coccygeus muscle, where the upper one-third of the vagina and cervix lie upon it
        o This horizontal part assists in development and maintenance of the vaginal axis
        o This muscle is active at rest and contracts further during rectus abdominis contraction to maintain proper vaginal axis
      - Levator plate
        o Is the main part of the levator ani muscle seen on the sagittal MR images
        o Is formed by fusion of the right and left iliococcygeus muscle slings in midline
        o Forms a horizontal shelf that supports pelvic organs in normal asymptomatic volunteers

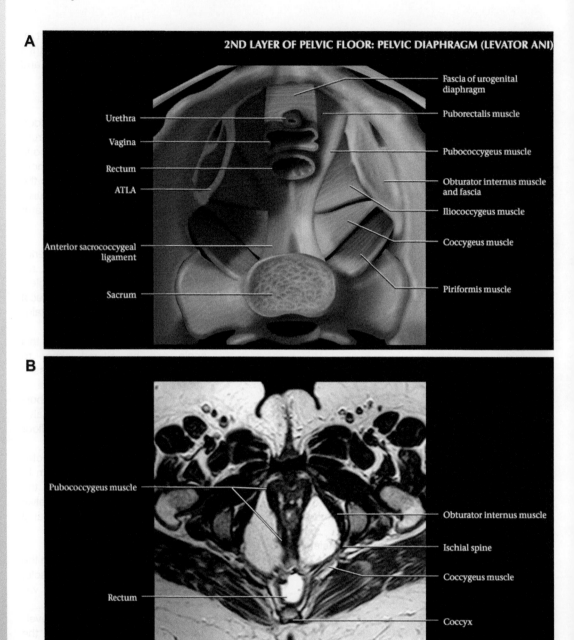

Fig. 4. (*A*) Superior view of the pelvic floor. The puborectalis, pubococcygeus, and iliococcygeus muscles form the levator ani. The obturator internus is covered by a fascial layer, which forms a thick band, the ATLA. This is a crucial area of attachment for the levator ani. The levator ani muscle with the coccygeal muscles forms the pelvic diaphragm (floor). The piriformis muscle contributes to the posterior wall. (*B*) Axial oblique T2WI MR image shows the pelvic floor and parts of the levator ani. The pubococcygeus muscle passes posteriorly. It has a bony attachment that is different from the puborectalis, which forms a sling around the anorectal junction with no bony attachment. (*From* [(El Sayed RF . Overview of the Pelvic Floor. In: Shaaban AM, Editor. Diagnostic Imaging: Gynecology 2nd Edition. Philadelphia: Elsevier-Amirsys; 2015. 8/2 -8/28 ; with permission.)

○ Is evaluated during evacuation, straining, and withholding in the sagittal plane

○ Contracts by a combination of squeeze and inward lift

○ Movement reflects multicomponent action of levator ani, where the puborectalis provides inward squeeze and iliococcygeus provides upward lift[5,15]

(c) Third layer: urogenital diaphragm

- Location and description
  ○ The cavity of pelvis is divided by the pelvic diaphragm into the main pelvic cavity above, and perineum below (**Fig. 5**).
  ○ The urogenital diaphragm is a fibromuscular layer directly below the pelvic diaphragm also known as the deep perineal pouch
  ○ Classically, the urogenital diaphragm is described as a trilaminar structure, which includes deep to superficial[5]
    ▪ The superior fascial layer of urogenital diaphragm is formed by the deep fascia of the pelvic floor
    ▪ The deep transverse perineal muscles are sandwiched between the superior and inferior fascia
    ▪ The inferior fascial layer of urogenital diaphragm forms the perineal membrane
  ○ Perineal body
    ▪ Is a fascial condensation posterior to the vagina
    ▪ Is an insertion site of the perineal muscle and external anal sphincter

(d) Fourth layer: Perineum

- Location and description
  ○ The perineum is the superficial soft tissues below pelvic diaphragm.
  ○ It is a diamond-shaped area bounded anteriorly by the symphysis pubis, posteriorly by the tip of the coccyx, and laterally by the ischial tuberosities (**Fig. 6**).
- Divisions
  ○ The perineum is divided by an arbitrary line between the ischial tuberosities into the urogenital triangle anteriorly, containing the urethra, the vagina, the perineal membrane, and the external genital muscles and the anal triangle posteriorly[5,14,16] (**Fig. 6A**)
  ○ Most superficial layers of the perineum is the external genital muscles and includes the superficial transverse perineal, bulbospongiosus, and ischiocavernosus muscles (see **Fig. 6B**)

Pelvic floor muscle and endopelvic fascial interaction

- Normal
  ○ Muscles give active support to pelvic floor, whereas ligaments give passive support to hold the pelvic organs in place
  ○ When the levator ani muscle (**Fig. 7**) functions properly, the following occurs:
    ▪ The pelvic floor is closed
    ▪ The ligaments and fasciae are under no tension
    ▪ The fasciae simply act to stabilize the pelvic organs in their position above the levator ani muscle[5,14,16]
- Abnormal
  ○ When pelvic muscles relax or are damaged, ligaments are put under strain
  ○ Pelvic organs lie between high abdominal pressure and low atmospheric pressure
  ○ In this situation, pelvic organs must be held in place by ligaments
  ○ Ligaments can sustain these loads for short periods
  ○ If damaged pelvic floor muscles cannot close levator hiatus, connective tissues must support pelvic organs for extended periods
  ○ Connective tissue will eventually fail to hold the vagina and other pelvic organs in place[5,14,16]

MR Imaging of Pelvic Floor

Indications for MR imaging of PFD

- According to the recently published consensus paper of European Society of Urogenital Radiology and European Society of Gastrointestinal and Abdominal Radiology recommendations, the indications of MR imaging in each compartment are listed in **Box 1** in descending order from those that scored the highest number of agreement among both the group members and the literature review. The indications for MR imaging of the pelvic floor that scored the highest number of agreement among the group members and the literature review are rectal outlet obstruction (92% agreed on), rectocele (92%), recurrent pelvic organ prolapse (POP; 85%), enterocele (85%), and dyssynergic defecation (anismus) (85%).[17]

Patients' preparation and hardware requirements

- All patients undergo cleansing rectal enema (using warm water) the night before MR imaging

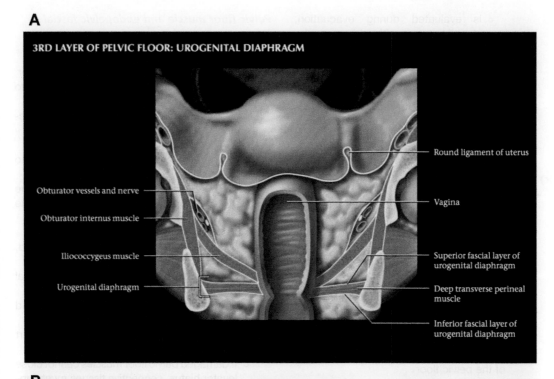

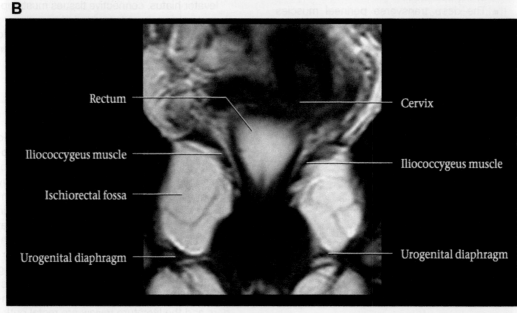

Fig. 5. (*A*) Coronal graphic of the pelvic floor shows the urogenital diaphragm. It is the fibromuscular layer directly below the pelvic diaphragm (levator ani muscles). It is a trilaminar structure with the deep transverse perineal muscle sandwiched between superior and inferior fascial layers. It is part of the perineum, which is located below the levator ani and includes the external genitalia. (*B*) Coronal T2WI MR at the level of the urogenital (UG) diaphragm shows its location below the pelvic diaphragm. The UG diaphragm is part of the perineum. (*From* [(El Sayed RF. Overview of the Pelvic Floor. In: Shaaban AM, Editor. Diagnostic Imaging: Gynecology 2nd Edition. Philadelphia: Elsevier-Amirsys; 2015. 8/2 -8/28 ; with permission.)

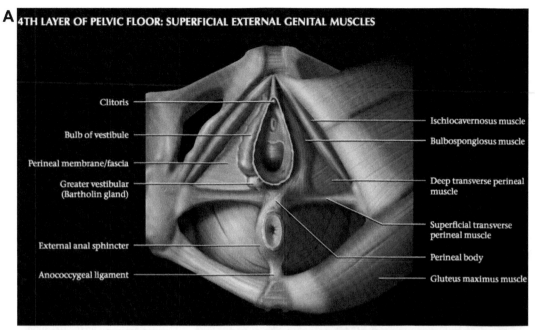

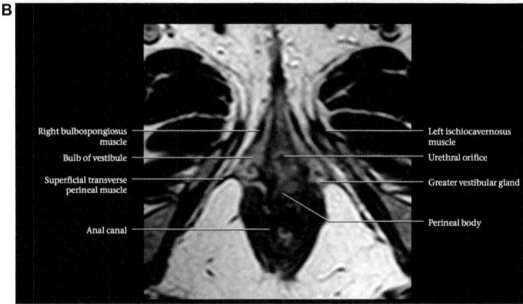

Fig. 6. (A) The external genital muscle is located anteriorly in the urogenital triangle, whereas the anal sphincter complex and perineal body are in the anal triangle. The perineal body is a thickened, midline condensation of fibrous tissue at the midpoint of a line joining the ischial tuberosities. At this point, several important muscles converge and are attached: The external anal sphincter, paired bulbospongiosus muscles, paired superficial transverse perineal muscles, and fibers of the levator ani. (B) Axial oblique T2WI MR image in a woman at the level of the superficial external genital muscle shows the extension of the bulbospongiosus muscle. (From [(El Sayed RF . Overview of the Pelvic Floor. In: Shaaban AM, Editor. Diagnostic Imaging: Gynecology 2nd Edition. Philadelphia: Elsevier-Amirsys; 2015. 8/2 -8/28]; with permission.)

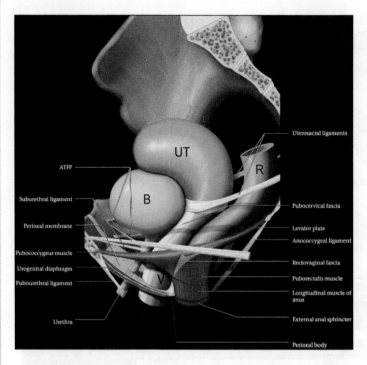

Labels on figure:
Uterosacral ligaments
UT
ATFP
R
Suburethral ligament
B
Perineal membrane
Pubocervical fascia
Pubococcygeus muscle
Levator plate
Urogenital diaphragm
Anococcygeal ligament
Pubourethral ligament
Rectovaginal fascia
V
Puborectalis muscle
Longitudinal muscle of anus
Urethra
External anal sphincter
Perineal body

Fig. 7. Graphic of the pelvis illustrates the multilayered system approach that considers the passive and active components of pelvic floor as an integrated multilayer system. From cranial to caudal, the pelvic support system consists of endopelvic fascia, pelvic diaphragm, perineum, and the external genital muscles. The muscles (levator ani) give active support to the pelvic floor, whereas the ligaments give passive support holding organs in place. When the levator ani is functioning properly, the pelvic floor is closed and the ligaments and fasciae are under no tension. When the musculature is damaged and cannot close the levator hiatus, ligaments are put under strain and will eventually fail, resulting in pelvic organ prolapse. B, bladder; UT, uterus; R, rectum. (*From* [(El Sayed RF. Overview of the Pelvic Floor. In: Shaaban AM, Editor. Diagnostic Imaging: Gynecology 2nd Edition. Philadelphia: Elsevier-Amirsys; 2015. 8/2–8/28; with permission.)

- MR protocol requires no oral or intravenous administration of contrast agents
- Full patients' history of pelvic floor disorder should be taken before scanning
- The bladder should be moderately filled; therefore, voiding 2 hours before the examination is recommended
- Ultrasound gel (90 to 120 mL) is placed into the rectum
- The patient is examined in the supine position with the knees elevated (eg, on a pillow with firm consistency) because this was found to facilitate straining and evacuation
- A pad is placed under the patient to add more comfort to the patient when evacuating the rectum and to avoid contamination of the MR table
- Patient training
  ○ The patient is informed that the evacuation phase is crucial for a complete diagnostic study
  ○ The radiologist should explain that this phase is important because POP is often only evident when abdominal pressure increases, and this is best achieved during evacuation of the rectum
- Hardware requirements: The patient should be examined at least in a 1.5-T MR imaging

unit with a phased array coil, because this is the most agreed-upon field strength
- The coil should be centered low on the pelvis to ensure complete visualization of prolapsed organs
- The recommended patient preparation is summarized in **Box 2**[17,18]

MR imaging protocol
Static MR imaging sequences According to the concordance of experts, high-resolution T2-weighted images (T2WI) (eg, turbo spin echo; fast spin echo) in 3 planes are recommended for static images.[17,19,20]

Dynamic (kinematic) MR imaging sequences
- Dynamic refers to the kinematic part of the study, imaging during evacuation "MR imaging defecography," and "dynamic cine MR" imaging in the 3 orthogonal planes during different grades of staining.[4,18]
- Steady state (eg, fast imaging with steady-state precession [FISP], gradient-recalled acquisition in the steady state [GRASS], fast field echo [FFE]) or balanced state free precession sequence (eg, true fast imaging with steady-state precession [trueFISP], fast imaging employing steady-state acquisition [FIESTA], balanced fast field echo [B-FFE]) in the sagittal plane is recommended for evacuation.

Box 1

Most common indications for MR imaging of pelvic floor dysfunction[a]

Indications

Anterior compartment

Stress urinary incontinence

Recurrence after surgical POP repair

Middle compartment

Recurrence after surgical POP repair

Enterocele/peritoneocele POP

Posterior compartment

Outlet obstruction

Rectocele

Anismus

Fecal incontinence

Recurrence after surgical POP repair

Rectal intussusception

Nonspecific compartment

Pelvic pain/perineal pain

Descending perineal syndrome

[a] The indications of MR imaging in each compartment are listed in descending order from those that scored the highest number of agreement among both the group members and the literature review.

Data from [El Sayed RF, Alt CD, Maccioni F, Meissnitzer M, Masselli G, Manganaro L, Vinci V, Weishaupt D. Magnetic resonance imaging of pelvic floor dysfunction - joint recommendations of the ESUR and ESGAR Pelvic Floor Working Group. On Behalf of ESUR and ESGAR Pelvic Floor Working Group . European Radiology,2017; 27(5):2067–2085. DOI 10.1007/s00330-016-4471-7].

Box 2

Checklist for the recommended patients' preparation and MR imaging protocols

A. Patient's preparation

- Acquire equipment: preferably a 1.5-T magnet and phased array coil
- Take patient's history of pelvic floor disorder
- Ask the patient to void 2 hours before the examination
- Train the patient on how to perform squeezing, straining, and evacuation
- Use a diaper for protection
- Do rectal filling with ultrasonic gel
- Examine the patient in the supine position with elevated knees on a high pillow

B. MR imaging protocol

1. Recommended static sequences

   T2-weighted TSE, FSE, RARE in sagittal, transverse, and coronal plane

2. Recommended dynamic SSFP or BSFP sequences in sagittal plane

   Straining phase

   Evacuation phase

   Squeezing phase

BSFP, balanced state free precession; FSE, fast spin echo; RARE, rapid acquisition with relaxation enhancement; SSFP, steady-state free precession; TSE, turbo spin echo.

Data from [El Sayed RF, Alt CD, Maccioni F, Meissnitzer M, Masselli G, Manganaro L, Vinci V, Weishaupt D. Magnetic resonance imaging of pelvic floor dysfunction - joint recommendations of the ESUR and ESGAR Pelvic Floor Working Group. On Behalf of ESUR and ESGAR Pelvic Floor Working Group . European Radiology,2017; 27(5):2067–2085. DOI 10.1007/s00330-016-4471-7].

- The dynamic sequence should not exceed 20 seconds each, because breath holding is required.
- MR imaging during evacuation is mandatory, because certain abnormalities and the full extent of POP are only visible during evacuation.
- The evacuation sequence should be repeated until the rectum is emptied to exclude rectal intussusception (total time duration around 2–3 minutes).
- If no evacuation of the rectal content at all or a delayed evacuation time (>30 seconds to evacuate two-thirds of the rectal content) is present, anismus should be considered.
- Because the performance of adequate pelvic stress during the dynamic sequences is important in order to assess the full extent of PFD, quality control of the study is essential.
  o The study can only be considered diagnostic if a clear movement of the abdominal wall is seen during squeezing and straining.
- The MR imaging protocols[17,18] are summarized in **Box 2**.
- **Fig. 8** illustrates the recommended imaging sequences and the patient maneuvers.

DISCLOSURE

The author has nothing to disclose.

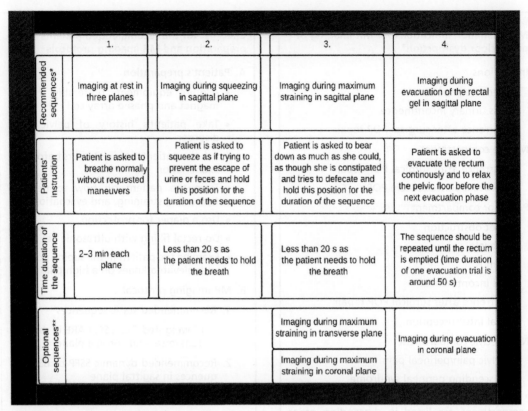

	1.	2.	3.	4.
Recommended sequences*	Imaging at rest in three planes	Imaging during squeezing in sagittal plane	Imaging during maximum straining in sagittal plane	Imaging during evacuation of the rectal gel in sagittal plane
Patients' instruction	Patient is asked to breathe normally without requested maneuvers	Patient is asked to squeeze as if trying to prevent the escape of urine or feces and hold this position for the duration of the sequence	Patient is asked to bear down as much as she could, as though she is constipated and tries to defecate and hold this position for the duration of the sequence	Patient is asked to evacuate the rectum continously and to relax the pelvic floor before the next evacuation phase
Time duration of the sequence	2–3 min each plane	Less than 20 s as the patient needs to hold the breath	Less than 20 s as the patient needs to hold the breath	The sequence should be repeated until the rectum is emptied (time duration of one evacuation trial is around 50 s)
Optional sequences**			Imaging during maximum straining in transverse plane / Imaging during maximum straining in coronal plane	Imaging during evacuation in coronal plane

Fig. 8. Schedule of the recommended imaging sequences, the instructions given to the patient, and the time duration per sequence. *, 100% agreement of expert opinion and level of evidence 2. **, Level of evidence 2 without expert consensus (3/8).

REFERENCES

1. Maglinte DD, Kelvin FM, Fitzgerald K, et al. Association of compartment defects in pelvic floor dysfunction. AJR Am J Roentgenol 1999;172(2): 439–44.
2. Seynaeve R, Billiet I, Vossaert P, et al. MR imaging of the pelvic floor. JBR-BTR 2006;89(4):182–9.
3. DeLancey JO. The hidden epidemic of pelvic floor dysfunction: achievable goals for improved prevention and treatment. Am J Obstet Gynecol 2005;192: 1488–95.
4. El Sayed RF, Mashed SE, Farag A, et al. Pelvic floor dysfunction: assessment with combined analysis of static and dynamic MR imaging findings. Radiology 2008;248:518–30.
5. El Sayed RF. Overview of the pelvic floor. In: Shaaban AM, editor. Diagnostic imaging: gynecology. 2nd edition. Philadelphia: Elsevier-Amirsys; 2015. p. 8/2–8/28.
6. El Sayed RF. The urogynecological side of pelvic floor MRI: the clinician's needs and the radiologist's role. Abdom Imaging 2013;38(5):912–29.
7. Beco J, Mouchel J. Perineology: a new area. Urogynaecol Int J 2003;17:79–86.
8. DeLancey JOL. Functional anatomy of the pelvic floor. In: Bartram CI, DeLancey JOL, editors. Imaging pelvic floor disorders. Medical Radiology (Diagnostic Imaging). Berlin, Heidelberg: Springer; 2003. p. 27–38.
9. DeLancey JO. The anatomy of pelvic floor. Curr Opin Obstet Gynecol 1994;6:313–6.
10. Petros P. Reconstructive pelvic floor surgery according to the integral theory. In: Petros P, editor. The female pelvic floor: function, dysfunction and management according to the integral theory. 2nd edtion. Berlin: Springer; 2007.
11. Fröhlich B, Hötzinger H, Fritsch H. Tomographical anatomy of the pelvis, pelvic floor, and related structures. Clin Anat 1997;10(4):223–30.
12. Strohbehn K, Ellis JH, Strohbehn JA, et al. Magnetic resonance imaging of the levator ani with anatomic correlation. Obstet Gynecol 1996;87(2):277–85.
13. Strohbehn K. Normal pelvic floor anatomy. Obstet Gynecol Clin North Am 1998;25:683–705.
14. Klutke CG, Siegel CL. Functional female pelvic anatomy. Urol Clin North Am 1995;22(3):487–98.
15. Singh K, Reid WM, Berger LA. Magnetic resonance imaging of normal levator ani anatomy and function. Obstet Gynecol 2002;99(3):433–8.

16. DeLancey JO. Functional anatomy of the pelvic floor. In: Bartram CI, DeLancey JO, Halligan S, et al, editors. Imaging pelvic floor disorders. New York: Springer; 2003. p. 27–38.

17. El Sayed RF, Alt CD, Maccioni F, et al. Magnetic resonance imaging of pelvic floor dysfunction–joint recommendations of the ESUR and ESGAR Pelvic Floor Working Group. On Behalf of ESUR and ESGAR Pelvic Floor Working Group. Eur Radiol 2017; 27(5):2067–85.

18. El Sayed RF. Pelvic floor imaging. In: Shaaban AM, editor. Diagnostic imaging: gynecology. 2nd edition. Philadelphia: Elsevier-Amirsys; 2015. p. 8/ 30–8/39.

19. Lienemann A, Sprenger D, Janssen U, et al. Assessment of pelvic organ descent by use of functional cine-MRI: which reference line should be used? Neurourol Urodyn 2004;23: 33–7.

20. Woodfield CA, Hampton BS, Sung V, et al. Magnetic resonance imaging of pelvic organ prolapse: comparing pubococcygeal and midpubic lines with clinical staging. Int Urogynecol J Pelvic Floor Dysfunct 2009;20:695–701.

Integrated MR Analytical Approach and Reporting of Pelvic Floor Dysfunction
Current Implications and New Horizons

Rania Farouk El Sayed, MD, PhD

KEYWORDS

- MR imaging of obstructed defecation • Dyskinetic puborectalis • Anal sphincter achalasia
- Solitary rectal ulcer syndrome • Functional 3-part pelvic floor supporting systems
- Combined analysis of dynamic and static MR imaging • Perineology
- 3-D modeling MR imaging of endopelvic fascia

KEY POINTS

- A diagnostic MR examination of pelvic floor should include MR defecography, dynamic cine MR imaging during straining, and static MR images.
- MR defecography is dedicated for detection and grading of pelvic organ prolapse and structural and functional abnormality of the evacuation process.
- Dynamic cine MR imaging at maximum straining identifies pelvic floor laxity and quantifies the degree of muscle weakness.
- Static MR images are assessed for detection and classification of structural abnormalities.
- The integrated MR analytical approach converts static and dynamic MR imaging from 2 separate types of images into an integrated system identifying specific defect in each patient.

INTRODUCTION

Many clinicians asserted that the optimal approach to treatment of PFD must be individualized for each patient on the basis of both the symptom complex and the specific anatomical and structural abnormalities. Recently, a new MR imaging analytical approach was devised that integrates data provided by both dynamic (cine) and static MR images, to define the predominant defects of the pelvic support system making it possible to pinpoint the underlying defects in each patient to the clinicians and consequently guides them to tailor treatment to the needs of each patient. This approach provides the necessary scientific evidence on which best clinical practice can be based. The first section of this article, explains why this approach was developed and how to apply it. In addition, to make it easy for radiologists to use this approach and to increase surgeons' comprehension of the overall findings, a "Data-Reporting System" was created in which all imaging findings are presented in a structured schematic MR imaging reporting template from a purely functional point of view to enhance the radiologists' interaction with clinicians and bridges the gap between radiology and surgery.

The second section emphasis on what the referring physician needs to know and their requirements to decide on the treatment plan. This section details the vital role of the radiologist in crafting and establishing new aiding tools for the clinician to use in planning reconstructive surgery. "Functional 3-Part Pelvic Supporting Systems Approach"; "Integrated MR Analytical Approach"; "Data-Reporting System"; "Three-axis perineal

Cairo University MRI Pelvic Floor Center of Excellency and Research Lab Unit, Department of Radiology, Cairo University Hospitals, Kasr El Ainy Street, Cairo 11956, Egypt
E-mail address: rania729.re@gmail.com

Radiol Clin N Am 58 (2020) 305–327
https://doi.org/10.1016/j.rcl.2019.11.007
0033-8389/20/© 2019 Elsevier Inc. All rights reserved.

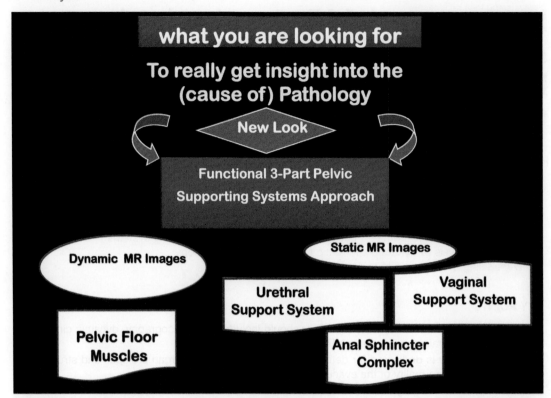

Fig. 1. The chart illustrates the link between the newly adapted 3-part pelvic support system approach and the MR imaging sequences.

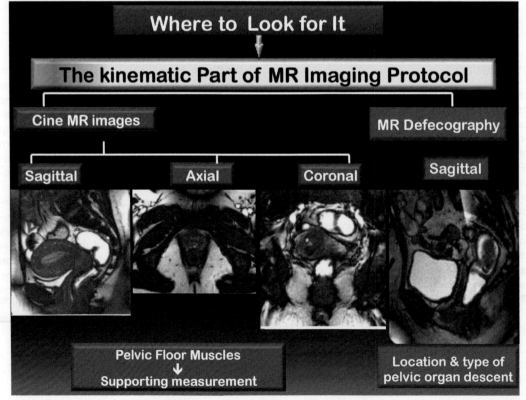

Fig. 2. Chart summarizing the essential kinematic (dynamic cine and MR defecography) imaging protocols for a diagnostic MRI study of patients with PFD.

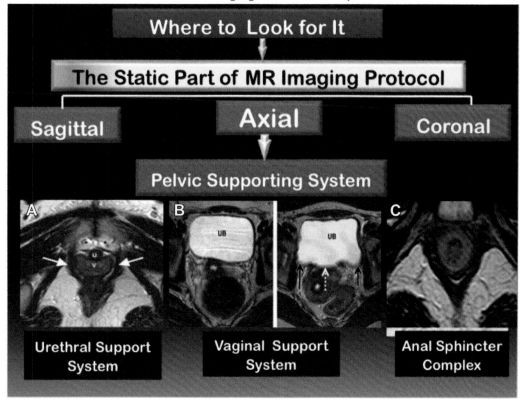

Fig. 3. For assessment of the 3-part pelvic supporting system, the radiologist should look for the underlying pathology in the static axial MR images. (A) Axial T2 weighed (T2WI) MR image of the urethral support system. Arrows point to the puborectalis muscle and asterisks indicates the space of Retzius. (B) Axial T2WI MR image of the vaginal support system. Black arrows point to the lateral endopelvic fascial defects and dashed white arrow points to the central endopelvic fascial defect. (C) Axial balanced fast field echo (BFFE) MR image shows the normal anal sphincter complex. U, urethra; UB; urinary bladder; V, vagina.

Box 1
Checklist for the recommended MR imaging reporting scheme

A. Measurements

1. Basic measurements for all compartments

   • Determine PCL.

   • Determine organ-specific reference points.

   • Measure the descent of reference points below the PCL.

2. Measurements for posterior compartment

   Measure the bulging of the anterior rectal wall during maximum straining phase and evacuation phase.

   Measure the ARA at rest, squeezing phase, straining phase and evacuation phase.

B. Reporting

1. Basic reporting for all compartments

   • Report values above the PCL as negative and below as positive.

   • Report pelvic organ mobility.

2. Reporting for anterior compartment

   • Report loss of urine at straining phase.

   • Report urethral mobility at straining phase.

3. Reporting for middle compartment

   • Report uterine descent.

- Report the content of a present enterocele.

4. Reporting for posterior compartment

- Report presence of a rectal intussusception.
- Evaluate time-effective rectal evacuation.
- Point out the change of ARA.

C. *Grading*

1. Anterior compartment

- Use the rule-of-3 grading for cystocele.
- Report cystocele as pathologic starting from °II.

2. Middle compartment

- Use the rule-of-3 grading for uterine prolapse and enteroceles.
- Report POP as pathologic starting from °II.

3. Posterior compartment

- Use the rule-of-2 grading for rectoceles.
- Report a rectocele as pathologic starting from °II.
- Use the grading for ARJ starting at 3 cm below the PCL.

Data from [El Sayed RF, Alt CD, Maccioni F, Meissnitzer M, Masselli G, Manganaro L, Vinci V, Weishaupt D. Magnetic resonance imaging of pelvic floor dysfunction - joint recommendations of the ESUR and ESGAR Pelvic Floor Working Group. On Behalf of ESUR and ESGAR Pelvic Floor Working Group . European Radiology,2017; 27(5):2067–2085. 10. 1007/s00330-016-4471-7].

evaluation (TAPE) Approach"; "Individualized, defect- specific treatment Approach"; "3-D modeling of the predominant pelvic supporting system defect" are the rising stars of the upcoming new horizon in the diagnosis of the complex disorders of the pelvic floor, reducing the risk of surgical failure, dysfunction recurrence, and re-operation.

MR IMAGING REPORT

In order to achieve an MR imaging report that is critical in decision-making for patient management and /or operative choice, it is of paramount importance to the radiologist to understand clearly the aim of each MR sequences acquired and what to report in each set of the MR images obtained. In other words the radiologist should know "what to look for" and "where to look for it". (**Fig. 1**) illustrate this concept in details. (**Figs. 2** and **3**) provide charts summarizing the essential Kinematic and static imaging protocols for a diagnostic MRI study. In addition the charts specify in which set of the acquired MR images each of the Functional 3-part pelvic supporting system can be assessed.

A clear consensus was reached that the assessment of a MR study of the pelvic floor should include:

- Analysis of the MR Defecography for detection and grading of pelvic organ prolapse

and functional abnormality of the evacuation process.
- Assessment of the Dynamic cine MR images at maximum straining to identify pelvic floor laxity and quantifies the degree of muscle weakness.
- Analysis of static MR images for detection and classification of structural abnormalities.
- Both dynamic and static MR imaging findings as well as the results of the metric measurements should be reported in a structured MR reporting scheme1 (**Box 1**).

Analysis of MR Defecography

Dynamic MR imaging examination of pelvic floor are reported in a standardized scheme in all patients of pelvic floor dysfunction, whether the patient's main complaint is related to one or multiple compartment or whether the patients is being referred from urogynecology and/or coloproctology.

Measurements during evacuation recognize and grade the extent of POP, in addition to any structural or functional abnormalities of the evacuation process in obstructed defecation (**Fig. 4**).

Basic measurements for all compartments

- The pubococcygeal line (PCL), drawn on sagittal plane from the inferior aspect of the

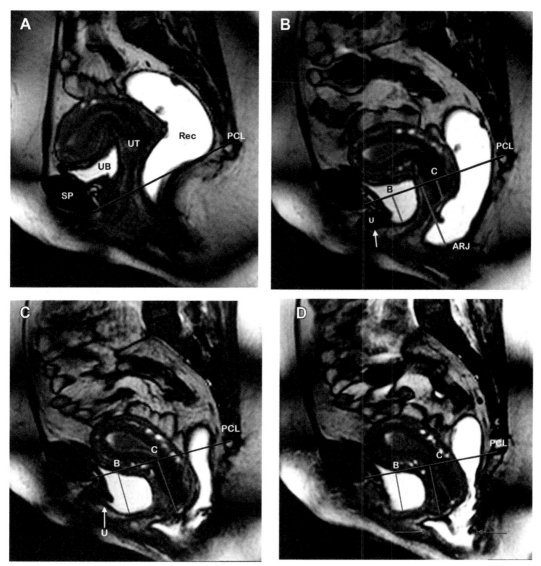

Fig. 4. MR defecography, basic measurements for all compartments. (*A*) Dynamic balanced fast field echo (BFFE) sequence in the midsagittal plane at rest shows how to plot the basic measurements of POP. The PCL, drawn on sagittal plane from the inferior aspect of the pubic symphysis to the last coccygeal joint. (*B*) Dynamic BFFE during maximum straining shows the movement of the organs compared with their location at rest. The distance from each reference point is measured perpendicularly to the PCL. In this case there is abnormal descent of the bladder, uterus and anorectal junction below the PCL. (*C, D*) MR imaging during evacuation (MR defecography) is mandatory, because certain abnormalities and the full extent of POP are visible only during evacuation. In this case, image (*C, D*) during evacuation compared with the maximum staining image (*B*) it is obvious that there is increase of the degree of the pelvic organ descent, development of new pathologies, like the loss of urine and opacification of the urethra (*white arrow* in *C*) in addition to detection of the masked intussusception, which was detected only during excavation (*red arrows* in *D*). ARJ, anorectal junction; B, bladder base; C, cervix; PCL, pubococcygeal line; PS, pubic symphysis; Rec, rectum; U, urethra; UB, urinary bladder; UT, uterus.

pubic symphysis to the last coccygeal joint, is recommended as reference line to measure POP.[1]

- After defining the PCL, the distance from each reference point is measured perpendicularly to the PCL during evacuation.

- In the anterior compartment, the organ-specific reference point is the most inferior aspect of the bladder base.
- In the middle compartment, the reference point is the anterior cervical lip (most distal edge of the cervix) or the vaginal vault after hysterectomy.
- In the posterior compartment, the reference point is the anorectal junction (ARJ).
- Measured values above the reference line have a minus sign and values below a plus sign.[2,3]

- Stress urinary incontinence (SUI) is recorded when loss of urine through the urethra is visualized at maximum straining. The absence of urine loss during MR imaging, however, does not preclude the patient experiencing symptoms.[1]

Grading of pelvic organ prolapse in anterior and middle compartments

Anterior compartments

- It has been reported that the pelvic floor may descend and widen up to 2 cm during abdominal pressure. Consequently, the pelvic organs follow the movement of the pelvic floor inferiorly but without protrusion through their respective hiatuses.
- The rule of 3 is the recommended grading system in the anterior and middle compartments starting at 1 cm below the PCL[4,5] (see **Box 1**).
- Urethrocele
  - Urethrocele is the prolapse of the female urethra into the vagina.
  - It often occurs with cystoceles; in this case, the term used is *cystourethrocele*.[6–8]
- Cystocele
  - The bladder base, in particular, may descend up to 1 cm below the PCL during straining in continent women and should not be stated as a cystocele.[9]
  - Grading of cystocele
    - Grade 0: up to +1 cm below PCL
    - Grade 1: +1 to +3 cm below PCL
    - Grade 2: +3 to +6 cm below PCL
    - Grade 3: greater than + 6 cm below PCL

Middle compartments

- True prolapse is complete organ eversion; however, the term is commonly used to generically describe any degree of pelvic organ descent.[10–12]

Classification

- Anterior vaginal wall prolapse[13,14]
  - Cystocele
  - Uterine prolapse
- Posterior vaginal wall prolapse[15]
  - Enterocele

  - Rectocele
- Vaginal vault prolapse
  - Vaginal opacification with sterile lubricating gel to enhance visualization of the vaginal apex is strongly advised, if not mandatory.[16]
- Peritoniocele
  - A peritoneocele is a protrusion of the peritoneum between the rectum and vagina that does not contain any abdominal viscera.
  - If a peritoniocele is present, the report should include the content of the peritoneal sac, because clinical examination alone may have shortcomings in identifying the content.[17–19]

Grades of pelvic organ prolapse

- Grade 0: above PCL
- Grade 1; mild: descent less than 3 cm below PCL
- Grade 2; moderate: descent 3 cm to 6 cm below PCL
- Grade 3; severe: descent greater than 6 cm below PCL
- Grade 4: cases of complete uterine prolapse[14]

Posterior compartment

Constipation and obstructed defecation

Definitions and general considerations

- Constipation describes a symptom, not clinical a sign, and is particularly subjective, meaning different things to different people.
- There is considerable individual variation in defining constipation:
  - Some patients concentrate on bowel frequency.
  - Others are more concerned about ease of defecation and stool size/consistency.
- Satisfactory definition of constipation must include both infrequent defecation and difficult evacuation.
  - Infrequent defecation
    - Usually defined as less than 3 bowel movements per week
    - Most likely associated with slow transit time
  - Difficult evacuation
    - Straining at stool is considered abnormal if it occurs for greater than 25% of time spent in lavatory
    - Indicates obstructed defecation
  - Chronic constipation
    - Very common
    - Estimated that 1 in 5 healthy, middle-aged adults have symptoms suggesting functional constipation

Obstructed defecation Outlet obstruction is due either to structural or functional underlying pathology.[20–22]

Structural pathology

1. Rectocele
   - A rectocele is diagnosed as an anterior rectal wall bulge and it is measured during maximum straining and evacuation.
   - Typically, a line drawn through the anterior wall of the anal canal is extended upward, and a rectal bulge of greater than 2 cm anterior to this line is described as a rectocele.
   - Due to the different classification of the pathology in the posterior compartment, it has different grading systems from the anterior and middle compartments.[19]
   - The rule of 2 is recommended for grading the anterior rectal wall bulge in rectoceles (see **Box 1**).
     - Grading
       - Grade 0: no outpouching
       - Grade 1: outpouching up to 2 cm
       - Grade 2: outpouching between 2 cm and 4 cm
       - Grade 3: outpouching greater than 4 cm.[23,24]
     - Anterior rectal wall bulge should be reported as pathological if it is grade II and higher, because grade I rectocele can be observed in approximately 78% to 99% of parous women.
2. Descending perineum syndrome (pelvic floor descent)
   - Defined as descent of ARJ greater than 3 cm below the PCL (see **Fig. 4**B)
   - ARJ is defined by posterior impression of puborectalis muscle at most cranial extent of anal canal.
   - Usually generalized process with associated abnormal descent of middle and anterior pelvic floor compartments
   - Often seen in combination with perineal ballooning, rectocele, intussusception, and impaired evacuation
     - Grading
       - Grade I: between 3 cm and 5 cm below the PCL
       - Grade II: with at least 5 cm[5,25]
3. Intussusception and rectal prolapse
   - Rectal prolapse is a circumferential full-thickness intussusception of the rectal wall with protrusion beyond the anal verge.
   - Intussusception (internal rectal prolapse) is full-thickness prolapse of rectum (see **Fig. 4**D) that does not protrude through the anus; it could be either
     a. Intrarectal intussusceptions that are confined to rectal ampulla
     b. Intra-anal intussusception that extends into anal canal
   - Precautions during MR imaging defecography
     - Intussusception occurs only when rectum collapses during evacuation; therefore, the end of evacuation phase is important to identify intussusception (see **Fig. 4**D).
     - Small intussusceptions of the rectal wall are considered normal findings during defecation, observed in approximately 80% of healthy subjects.[5,26]

Functional pathology

1. Dyskinetic puborectalis
   - Also called *spastic pelvic floor syndrome* or *anismus*
   - Defined as involuntary contraction of the puborectalis muscle with failure to relax, which prevents normal rectal evacuation.

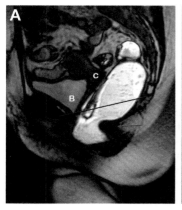
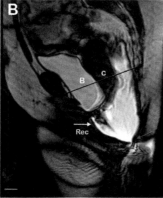

Fig. 5. MR defecography, functional outlet obstruction. (*A*) Paradoxic contraction of puborectalis during defecation (*red arrow*) and relaxed anal sphincter. (*B*) Nonrelaxing or spastic anal sphincter evident by anal canal diameter measuring less than 15 mm (*red arrows*). Note total obliteration of the posterior ARA indicating relaxed puborectalis. There is also grade 3 anterior rectocele. B, bladder; C, cervix; Rec, rectum.

- Not an uncommon cause of obstructed defecation and frequently overlooked at imaging
- Highly likely that many surgical failures occur in patients treated for rectocele because underlying anismus was not recognized
- Diagnostic criteria
  - Normal anorectal angle (ARA)
    - The ARA is the angle enclosed between a line plotted along the posterior rectal wall and the second line is plotted along the central axis of the anal canal on sagittal plane at rest, squeezing and maximum straining.
    - The change of the ARA during evacuation compared with rest expresses the functioning of the puborectal muscle; in particular, the ARA should sharpen during squeezing and should become more obtuse during straining and evacuation.
    - It is recommended to report that the ARA showed the normal changes at different maneuvers rather than the absolute value of the ARA angle, because the literature presents a widespread of normal reference values.
  - MR findings in spastic pelvic floor syndrome
    - Failure of ARA to open
    - Persistent or exaggerated puborectal impression on posterior aspect of ARJ
    - Lack of descent of pelvic floor during defecation
    - Long interval between opening of anal canal and start of defecation
    - Most pertinent finding for diagnosis of anismus is prolonged and incomplete evacuation; using 120 mL of rectal contrast, evacuation times of more than 30 seconds accurately predict this functional disorder (Fig. 5A).[5,25,27,28]
2. Spastic anal sphincter contraction
- Also known as spasmodic contraction of anal sphincter or anal sphincter achalasia
- Under normal circumstances, expansion of rectum or rectosigmoid causes internal anal sphincter (IAS) reflex relaxation.
- Patients usually present with painless constipation associated with dry stools.
- Resting anal pressure is significantly higher than normal on manometry.
- MR findings
  - Anal canal is not open with dilatation of rectum.
  - Resting dilated rectum or even giant rectum

  - MR defecography is mandatory to show rate of evacuation (see Fig. 5B).
  - Static MR should show normal anal sphincter muscle complex to exclude IAS hypertrophy.[20]

Structural and functional pathology

Solitary rectal ulcer syndrome
- Well-recognized diagnosis that describes a combination of rectal prolapse and functional pelvic floor abnormality
- MR findings
  - Usually the imaging findings in these patients are a combination of rectal prolapse and puborectalis dyskinesia.
- Pathogenesis: incompletely understood
  - Prolapsed rectal mucosa is forced downward due to pressures generated during defecation and is compressed by force of paradoxic puborectalis contraction, leading to mucosal ischemia and ulceration secondary to repeated straining.
  - Proctoscopy usually reveals rectal inflammation and ulceration and is accompanied by specific histopathological changes within prolapsing mucosa.[5]

Analysis of Dynamic Cine MR Images at Maximum Straining

- Analysis of the dynamic MR images is dedicated to supportive measurements.
  - These are 5 measurements of supporting structures measured in the 3 orthogonal plane (Fig. 6).
  - They are all considered to reflect the status and the weakness of the levator ani.
  - They have proved of value in identification of pelvic floor laxity and quantification of the degree of weakness. They also are useful for follow-up assessment.

Dynamic Sagittal Cine MR images

H-line
  - Measured from inferior aspect of pubic symphysis to ARJ
  - Length of H-line: 5.8 cm
M-line
  - Drawn as perpendicular line from PCL to posterior aspect of H-line
  - Length of M-line: 1.3 cm $\pm$ 0.5 SD
Levator plate angle
  - Levator plate angle (LPA) is drawn between axis of levator plate and PCL.
  - LPA: 11.7° $\pm$ 4.8 SD

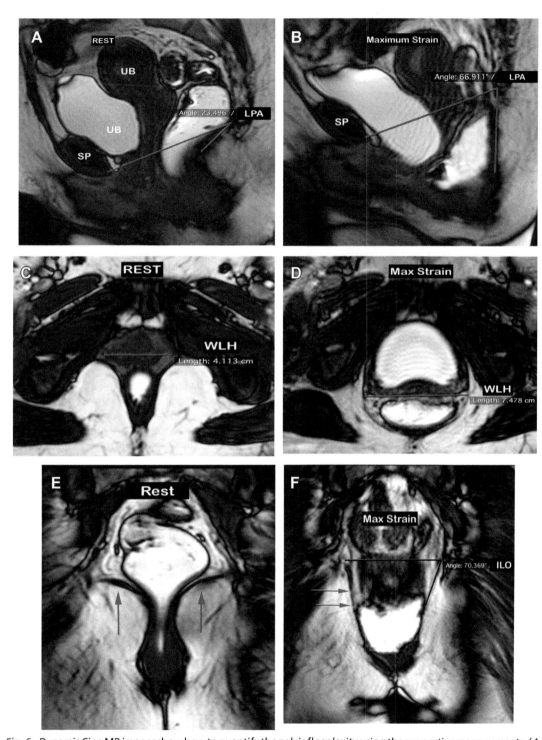

Fig. 6. Dynamic Cine MR images show how to quantify the pelvic floor laxity using the supportive measurements. (*A, B*) Dynamic BFFE MR image of patient with obstructed defection in the mid-sagittal plane at rest (*A*) during maximum straining (*B*) (*A*) shows how to plot the LPA which is enclosed between the levator plate muscle and the PCL. (*B*) Shows marked weakness of the levator plate indicated by LPA measuring 66.9°. (*C, D*) Axial BFFE MR images at rest (*C*), during maximum straining (*D*). (*C*) Shows the level where the WLH is measured at the most inferior point of symphysis pubis. The width of the levator hiatus is enclosed between the puborectalis muscle sling. (*D*) The WLH measures 7.5 cm indicating muscle weakness; the transverse diameter of the muscle reflects the extent of its ballooning and weakness during straining. (*E, F*) Coronal BFFE MR images, at rest (*E*), during maximum straining

Dynamic Axial Cine MR images

- o Width of levator hiatus (WLH)
    - ▪ Measured on axial image at most inferior point of symphysis pubis during maximum straining
    - ▪ Distance enclosed between puborectalis muscle slings
    - ▪ WLH rarely exceeds 4.5 cm ± 0.7 SD in women with intact pelvic floor.

Dynamic Coronal Cine MR images

Iliococcygeus angle (ILCA)
- o Measured on coronal posterior image at level of anal canal during maximum straining
- o Angle defined by line plotted along iliococcygeus muscle sling and transverse plane of pelvis
- o Mean of ILCA is reported to be 33.4° ± 8.2 SD in women with intact pelvic floor.

Table 1 gives an overview of the published reference values for quantitative MR measurements of the pelvic floor.

Analysis of the Static MR Images

- It is important to establish the new era of the added value of the static MR image analysis after adapting the new functional 3-part pelvic supporting systems approach, on which the new insight of the defect-specific approach of patient management was established.[9,15]
- Analysis of static images is based on thorough examination of the pelvic organ supporting elements and characterizations of the defects in each of its components: the urethral supporting system, the vaginal supporting system, and the anal sphincter complex.

Urethral Supporting System

Scrutiny of the urethral support system involves imaging of the 1) urethral ligaments, 2) endopelvic fascia (level III fascial support), and 3) the puborectalis muscle[9] (Fig. 7).

Urethral ligaments
MR imaging of normal urethral ligaments
- o Meticulous cadaveric dissection identified *ventral and dorsal* urethral ligaments on axial T2-weighted turbo spin-echo sequences. The MR imaging findings in volunteers correlated with the MR imaging and gross anatomic findings in cadavers.[9,29]

    The ventral urethral ligaments include
    - ▪ The pubourethral (PUL) ligaments, which were found to consist of a group of 3 distinct but related ligaments: proximal PUL (PPUL), intermediate PUL (IPUL), and distal PUL (DPUL). All have a similar anteroposterior orientation running from the ventral urethral surface to the pubic bone. Functionally, the most important is the PPUL, which contributes to suspension of anterior urethral region and appears to counteract opening of posterior vesicourethral angle during stress. The DPUL supports and fixes the distal urethra.
    - ▪ The periurethral ligament and paraurethral ligaments that link the proximal urethra to puborectal sling [29,30]

    Dorsal Urethral ligament:
    - ▪ A sling-like ligament, the suburethral ligament, was identified along the dorsal aspect of the urethra. It runs posterior to urethra and has a distinct plane of cleavage from the anterior vaginal wall. It extends anterolaterally to pelvic sidewalls forming a suburethral sling. To the best of the author's knowledge, this ligament has not been previously reported.[29]
- o The PPUL, periurethral, paraurethral, and suburethral ligaments had visibility scores of 3 (moderately visible) or 4 (easily visible) on MR imaging in 47%, 65%, 47%, and 53% of volunteers, respectively.[29]

(F). (E) Shows how to the plot the iliococcygeus angle, it is measured between one of the iliococcygeus muscle slings (*red arrows* in E) and the transverse plane of the pelvis in posterior coronal images at the level of the anal canal. The ILCA reflects the degree of descent and movement of the muscle. (F) Shows the abnormal elongation of the iliococcygeus muscle slings during maximum straining (*double red arrows*). The iliococcygeus muscle should move downward during straining with no excessive caudal descent or elongation. The dynamic cine MR images of this patient in the 3 orthogonal planes during maximum straining show gross evidences of marked pelvic floor muscle weakness. BFFE, Balanced Fast Field Echo; ILO, Iliococcygeous; LPA, Levator Plate Angle; Max, maximum; PCL, pubococcygeal line; SP, symphysis pubis; UB, urinary bladder; WLH, width of levator hiatus.

MR imaging of urethral ligaments abnormalities

- On images obtained in the axial plane, abnormalities are classified as follows:
  - Distortion, when internal architectural changes with waviness of the ligaments are seen
  - Defects, defined by discontinuity of the ligament with visualization of the torn parts [30–32]

Level III endopelvic fascial support

MR imaging of normal level III Fascia

- On static axial T2 weighted MR images, level III fascia supports mid urethra and maintains the following relationships:
  - a) Central positioning of mid urethra
  - b) Small, symmetric-appearing space of Retzius
  - c) Preserved H-shaped vagina
- Functionally, level III fascia provides urethral support and has special importance to urinary continence because the endopelvic fascia at this level is better developed than at more superior levels; therefore, level III provides better support for vesical neck than higher levels. Loss of this normal support at vesical neck may result in SUI.

MR imaging of level III fascial defect

- Level III fascial defect is assessed at the level of urethra and bladder neck.
- The defect is recognizable by the drooping mustache sign, which is caused by the fat in the prevesical space against the bilateral sagging of the detached lower third of the anterior vaginal wall from the arcus tendineus fascia pelvis.[29]

Puborectalis muscle

MRI of the puborectalis muscle

- On the static axial T2 weighted MR images the puborectalis is seen as a sling encasing urethra, vagina, and rectum. It has no attachment to bladder neck but its anterior portion lies in close proximity to mid and lower urethra
- Functionally it is hypothesized that weakness of puborectalis contributes to problems with urinary continence

MRI of puborectal muscle defect

- Muscle defect is recognizable by disruption of the normal symmetrical appearance of the muscle sling or of its attachment to the symphysis pubis

Vaginal Supporting System

Vaginal supporting structures include: 1) Level I and II endopelvic fascia and 2) the iliococcygeus muscle **(Fig. 8)**.[33–35]

Table 1 Overview of the published reference values for quantitative MR measurements of the pelvic floor	
Parameters	**Reference Value ± SD**
Anterior compartment according to PCL	
Bladder base position at rest	−2.3 ± 0.46 cm
Bladder base position during straining	0.81 ± 1.11 cm
Middle compartment according to PCL	
Anterior cervical lip position at rest	4.31 ± 0.78 cm
Anterior cervical lip position during straining	−0.79 ± 1.65 cm
Posterior compartment	
Anterior bulge of the rectal wall during straining (rectocele)	2.6 ± 0.6 cm
ARJ at rest	≤3 cm below the PCL
ARJ during squeezing	Elevation of ARJ
ARJ during straining	2.99 ± 1.03 cm
ARA at rest	85°–95°
ARA during squeezing	71° sharpening of 10°–15°
ARA during straining or defecation	103° 15°–25° more obtuse
Measurements for quantification of the pelvic floor laxity	
H-line during straining	5.8 ± 0.5 cm
M-line during straining	1.3 ± 0.5 cm
LPA during straining	11.7 ± 4.8°
ILCA at rest	20.9 ± 3.5°
ILCA during straining	33.4 ± 8.2°
Transverse diameter of levator hiatus at rest	3.3 ± 0.4 cm
Transverse diameter of levator hiatus during straining	4.5 ± 0.7 cm

Data from [El Sayed RF, Alt CD, Maccioni F, Meissnitzer M, Masselli G, Manganaro L, Vinci V, Weishaupt D. Magnetic resonance imaging of pelvic floor dysfunction - joint recommendations of the ESUR and ESGAR Pelvic Floor Working Group. On Behalf of ESUR and ESGAR Pelvic Floor Working Group. European Radiology,2017; 27(5):2067–2085. 10.1007/s00330-016-4471-7].

Level I and II endopelvic fascia

MRI of normal level I and II Fascia

- On static axial T2 weighted MR images, level I landmark is at the level of the funds of the

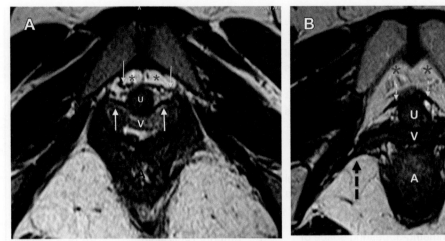

Fig. 7. Static MR image of normal and abnormal urethral supporting system. (*A*) Axial T2-weighted MR image of a woman with a normal urethral support system shows the suburethral ligament (*white arrows*), periurethral ligament (*yellow arrows*), small symmetric Retzius space (*asterisks*) and the normal insertion of the puborectalis muscle on to the posterior pubic symphysis, some anteromedial fibers attach to the vagina and help support the urethrovesical neck. (*B*) Axial T2-weighted MR image in a woman with SUI and history of childbirth perineal tear and forceps delivery, the MR image shows complex multiple urethral supporting system injuries that include bilateral detachment of the suburethral ligament. The ligament on the right side is subluxed backward (*white arrow*) and the periurethral ligament (*yellow arrows*). Also note the abnormal configuration of the Retzius space (drooping mustache) (*asterisks*), with loss of the H-shaped vagina (V), indicating disruption of level III endopelvic fascia. The most severe injury detected is the bilateral detachment of the puborectalis muscle slings from the pubic bone (*black dashed arrow*). It is important to report all of these findings, because it would affect treatment planning. A, anal canal; U, Urethra; V, vagina.

bladder. Level II corresponds to the middle portion of vagina, and is assessed at the bladder base.

- Normally attached lateral vaginal support results in straight posterior wall of urinary bladder.

MRI of Level I and II fascial defect
- Paravaginal defect:
  - In the axial plane, a paravaginal defect in the fascia is visualized as sagging of the fluid-filled posterior urinary bladder wall, caused by the detachment of the vaginal supporting fascia from the lateral pelvic wall, known as the saddlebags sign.
- Central defect
  - A central defect is indicated by sagging of the central part of the urinary bladder posterior wall.

Iliococcygeus muscle
MRI of the Iliococcygeus muscle
- On static coronal T2 weighted MR images, normally attached iliococcygeus muscle has dome-shaped appearance at rest with upward convexity. With straining, muscle becomes horizontal with basin-shaped configuration.
- Functionally, it is hypothesized that weakness of iliococcygeus muscle contributes to vaginal prolapse.

MRI of Iliococcygeus muscle defect
- In the coronal plane, the iliococcygeus muscle is assessed for loss of the normal symmetrical appearance of its muscle slings or defect and/or disruption of its attachment to the obturator internus muscle.[35]

Anal Sphincter Complex
MR imaging of normal anal sphincter complex
- On axial T2-weighted balanced fast field echo (BFFE) images, the consecutive layers of the anal sphincter from the lumen outward include (**Fig. 9A**)
  - The innermost high signal intensity layer (the combined mucosa and submucosa)
  - The low signal intensity layer (the submucosal smooth muscle)
  - The IAS (of homogenous intermediate to high signal intensity)
  - The deep external anal sphincter (EAS) (of low signal to intermediate signal intensity)
- IAS
  - Composed of smooth muscle fibers
  - It measures 2-mm to 3-mm thickness with progressive increase in thickness with advancing age
  - Functional correlation

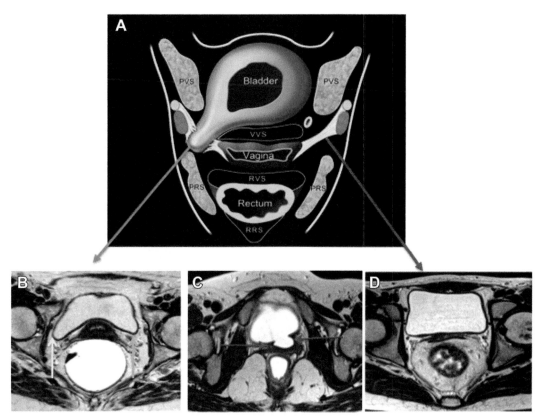

Fig. 8. Static MR image of normal and abnormal vaginal support system. (A) In this graphic, there is right-sided endopelvic fascial detachment causing a paravaginal defect. Because of the defective support mechanism, there is sagging of the right posterolateral wall of the urinary bladder (blue arrow) to fill the resulting defect. On the left side, however, the vagina is suspended between the 2 ATFP ligaments by lateral fascial extensions. These lateral extensions fuse with the pubocervical fascia superiorly and the rectovaginal fascia inferiorly. Pelvic organs are separated from each other by spaces that allow organs to move independently from each other. RRS, retrorectal space; PRS, pararectal space or ischiorectal fossa; PVS, paravesical space; VVS, vesicovaginal space; RVS, rectovaginal space. (B) Axial T2-weighted MR image obtained in a woman with POP shows the consequences of ATFP detachment with sagging of the posterior vaginal wall (saddlebags sign) (green arrow). It is asymmetric with the larger defect on the right (yellow arrow). The degree of sagging of the bladder wall corresponds to the size of the fascial defect. This may help determine the appropriate surgical approach: surgical repair of fascia, if the defect is small, versus use of mesh, if the defect is large. (C) Axial T2-weighted MR image obtained in a woman with POP shows bulging of the central part of the posterior urinary bladder wall. The red arrows point to the site of defect, which results in this type of bulge. In a central defect, the lateral attachment of the fascia to the ATFP is intact with stretching and redundancy of the central pubocervical fascia. Because a central defect is not due to fascial tear but rather fascial stretching, the bladder wall bulging usually is small compared with paravaginal defects. (D) Axial T2-weighted MR image shows normal level II endopelvic fasciae, the landmark to define level II is the midvagina at the level of the bladder base. It is important to emphasize that although injury of urethral ligaments can be visualized in some cases, the fascia is not; however, the integrity of the fascia can be inferred by the appearance of surrounding organs. The posterior bladder wall is seen as a straight line, indicating that level II endopelvic fascia is intact as indicated by the red arrow in A. ATFP, arcus tendineus fascia pelvis. ([A] From El Sayed RF. Overview of middle compartment. In: Shaaban AM, editor. Diagnostic Imaging: Gynecology, 2nd edition. Elsevier, Amirsys; 2015. p. 8/68–8/79; with permission.)

- Maintains anal sphincter resting tone (contributes up to 85% of maximal anal resting pressure)
- Intersphincteric space
  - Intersphincteric space is a thin, fat-containing space between the IAS and outer striated muscles.
  - It contains longitudinal smooth muscle layer
- EAS

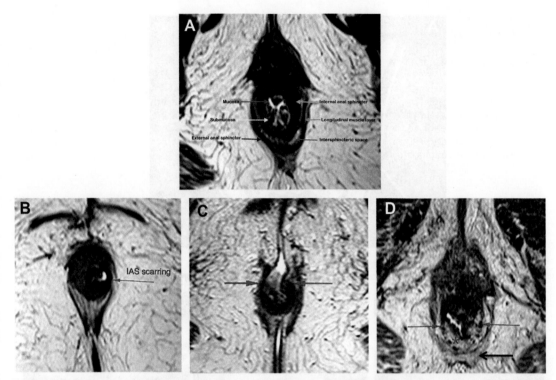

Fig. 9. Static MR image of normal and pattern of injury of the anal sphincter complex (ASC). (A) The ASC shows 4 layers of different signal intensity. The mucosa is the thin, folded inner layer of high signal intensity. The submucosa is of low signal intensity and has a folded internal contour and smooth outer contour. The internal anal sphincter (IAS) appears as a homogeneous isointense to hyperintense (relative to the striated muscle) smooth circular band surrounding the anal canal. The longitudinal smooth muscle layer and the fatty component of the intersphincteric space are more prominent at the distal part of the deep EAS (DEAS). (B–D) are all axial oblique T2-weighted MR images in 3 different patients presenting with fecal incontinence each patient has different site, side, and type of anal sphincter complex injury (B) shows thinning and low signal intensity of the left lateral aspect of the IAS, indicating fibrosis and scarring. (C) Shows discontinuity of the DEAS and IAS muscles ring (red arrows). A muscle defect should be described according to clock face; this is an anterior defect extending from the 10 o'clock to 2 o'clock positions. (D) MR image of a complex case of anal sphincter muscle injury from inner to outer; there is extensive atrophy of the of IAS posteriorly (red arrows) compared with its anterior aspect. Loss of muscle is more on the right side, with subsequent shift of the lumen posterior and to the right. Wide intersphincteric space (asterisk) with thinning of the longitudinal smooth muscle plus fatty degeneration of the DEAS (black arrow).

- Cylindrical striated muscle layer under voluntary control
- Predominantly composed of slow-twitch muscle fibers, capable of prolonged contraction
- The EAS measures 2.7 cm in height (shorter anteriorly in women, approximately 1.5 cm).
- Nerve supply: inferior rectal branch of pudendal nerve (S2, S3) and perineal branch of S4
- Functional correlation
  - Contributes 15% to 20% of resting anal tone
  - Voluntary control of sphincter complex
  - Major role in continence control, such as during intra-abdominal pressure or to defer defecation[36]

MR imaging of anal sphincter injury
- Lesions of the anal sphincter are classified according to 1) the muscle injured and 2) the type of lesion (see Figs. 9B–D):
  - According to the muscle injured:
    - The internal anal sphincter
    - The external anal sphincter
  - According to lesion types:
    - A sphincteric defect is defined as discontinuity of the muscle ring.
    - Scarring is defined as a low signal intensity deformation of the normal pattern of the muscle layer.[37,38]
    - Fragmentation and fraying of the muscle fiber this is usually seen in motor car injury, explosion or falling in sitting position.

WHAT THE REFERRING PHYSICIAN NEEDS TO KNOW

Magnitude of Pelvic Floor Dysfunction, Current Treatment, and Reported Recurrence Rate

The most prevalent forms of dysfunction are urinary incontinence, POP, and anal incontinence, all of which affect women 3 times to 7 times more often than men, at an estimated incidence of 23.7% of women in the United States.[39] Approximately 10% to 20% of these patients are symptomatic, and, by the age of 70 years, an estimated 1 in 10 undergoes pelvic floor surgical repair. It also is expected that there will be an increased demand for imaging this population.

Although multiple factors predispose for PFD, the precise pathologic mechanism is poorly understood, and treatment often is started regardless of the specific anatomic lesion involved. This situation was reflected in a study by Olsen and colleagues,[40] who reported that 29% of the procedures performed for incontinence and prolapse were reoperations, suggesting the need for advances in the treatment of these disorders. Clinicians[35,40,41] stated, however, that such advancement in treatment plans could be achieved based only on advanced imaging either in resolution and/or image interpretation and analysis.

Clinician's Requirements for Treatment Advancement

- Several clinicians who specialize in the field of PFD have stated that a "wide variety of surgical procedures have been used, with several based on weak scientific evidence."[42] Other studies[32,35] reported that PFD, such as SUI, results from specific damage to muscles, fascial structures, and nerves of the pelvic floor. Hence, it is required to define the damage occurring in each element of the continence mechanisms, to be able to precisely select treatment plans that are based on the abnormality found in individual patients. They emphasized on the value of switching from the current empirical treatment approach, which is based on a symptom complex that assigns a woman who says she has urine leakage to treatment of SUI to a therapeutic model that investigates and is based on the specific neuromuscular and fascial defect that results in the symptom complex.
- What had long been missing was a tool for accurately defining the anatomic and structural abnormalities in each patient.

NEW HORIZONS AND RADIOLOGIST'S ROLE

Recent advancements in imaging of the anatomic structures with MRI has allowed superior soft tissue resolution and consequently provided a more realistic glimpse of the structural relationships in vivo.[43,44] Based on this imaging advancements several new concepts in imaging, analysis, interpretation, and reporting MRI of pelvic floor had evolved.

Correlation Between Static and Dynamic MR Images

- The terms, *individualized*, *defect-specific treatment approach*, and *combined analysis of static and dynamic MR images*, have been adopted in the author's institutional Cairo University MRI Pelvic Floor Center of Excellency and Research Lab based on original research work, which documented the presence of specific defect in each individual patient, even if 2 patients present with the same symptoms.[15]
- The basis of this approach is simultaneous analysis of findings obtained from static and dynamic MR images of the same patient with correlation with the data obtained to determine whether a particular anatomic defect in the pelvic supporting system detected on static images is associated with a specific dysfunction on dynamic images. The most marked type of defect is reported as the predominant defect **Fig. 10**
- The author recently developed correlative analytical approach that converts static and dynamic MR imaging from 2 separate types of images into an integrated system that can more precisely identify the underlying anatomic defect responsible for symptoms in individual patients with PFD, even allowing differentiation of the underlying anatomic defect when any 2 patients have the same symptoms. This type of information, when reported by a radiologist to a clinician, allows clinicians to contemplate a holistic view of the pelvic floor and gives insight into the diagnosis of these complex disorders.[45]
- To make it easy for radiologists to use this approach and to increase surgeons' comprehension of the overall findings, an MR imaging reporting template is shown in (**Fig. 11**). In this template, all MR findings are presented in a schematic form that synthesizes data for ease of use by clinicians from several different

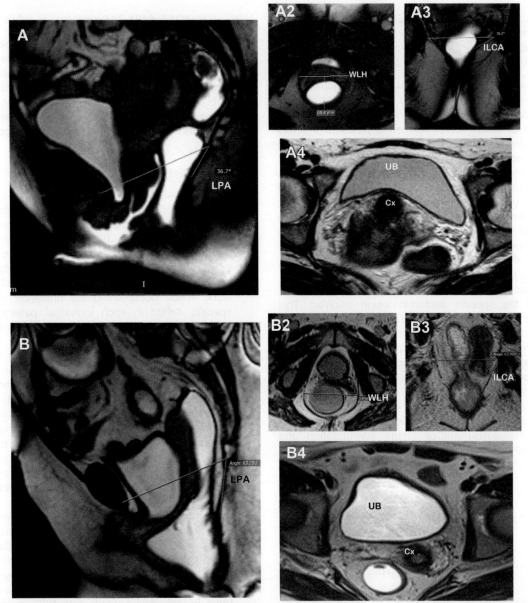

Fig. 10. Correlative analytic approach and how to apply it. (*A*) and (*B*) are dynamic MR images of 2 different patients during evacuation, both patients their MR images show 3 compartments POP but of different grades. (*A*) Shows grade I cystocele, uterine descent and abnormal Ano-rectal junction descent (ARJD). (*B*) shows grade II cystocele, uterine descent, moderate rectocele and abnormal ARJD. The clinicians can diagnose most of these findings if not all of them. How to apply the correlative approach: the radiologist should start with the dynamic cine MR image in the three orthogonal planes to evaluate the degree of pelvic floor muscle weakness. Images A, A2, A3 show mild degree of pelvic floor muscle weakness indicated by the LPA measuring 36.7°, WLH 5.9 cm, and ILCA angle of 26.3° respectively. The radiologist should then assess the static image (A4); which shows bilateral level I endopelvic fascial defect larger on the left side indicated by the deeper sagging of the UB wall on the left side compared to its right side. The final step is correlation between the dynamic and the static MR findings, which reveals that the POP is due to the large fascial defects in (A4) compared with the moderate sagging of the levator plate in (A). This patient is candidate for surgical fascial repair. Applying the same steps for reporting the MR images of the second patient (*B*) reveals the LPA of 63.2°, WLH measures 8.59 cm in (B1), and ILCA of 63.9 degree in (B3). The corresponding axial T2-weighted image (B4) at level II endopelvic fascia reveals almost intact fascia reflected by the straight posterior UB wall. In this patient despite that the MR images showed the same POP as the first patient; however, correlation between dynamic and static MR findings shows that the more advanced degree of muscle weakness compared with the fascial status indicates that muscle weakness is the main factor responsible for POP. Physiotherapy in such case is mandatory, not surgical repair of the fascia. Cx, cervix; ILCA, Iliococcygeus angle; LPA, levator plate angle; POP, pelvic organ prolapse; UB, urinary bladder; WLH, width of levator hiatus.

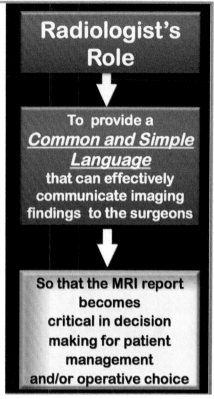

MR Reports

MR Defecography

> ➤ The sagittal plane revealed the following POP
> ➤ The Evacuation phase revealed ARDs

Dynamic MRI to assess Pelvic Floor Muscle Weakness

> ➤ Sagittal plane : Levator Plate Angle LPA
> ➤ Axial plane : Width of Levator Hiatus WLH
> ➤ Coronal plane : Iliococcygeus Angle ILCOA

Static MRI Sequences for Pelvic Support

> ➤ Urethral and Vaginal supporting system
> ➤ The Anal Sphincter Complex ASC
> ➤ Pelvic Floor Muscle PFM

OPINION: -

MRI defecography phase revealed:

- • Pelvic organ prolapse in 3 compartments
- • Descending perineal syndrome

Dynamic cine MR images in three orthogonal planes :

- • Advanced pelvic floor muscle weakness

Static MR Images revealed:

- • Diminished muscle bulk of the deep EAS.

Correlation between static and dynamic MRI

- • The predominant defect: Muscle weakness

Radiologist's Role

To provide a *Common and Simple Language* that can effectively communicate imaging findings to the surgeons

So that the MRI report becomes critical in decision making for patient management and/or operative choice

Fig. 11. A guide to radiologists on how to report the MR imaging findings systematically and comprehensively on both the static and dynamic images, using a recently developed integrated MR imaging analytical approach from a purely functional point of view that could enhance radiologists' interaction with clinicians and bridges the gap between radiology and surgery, consequently both of them can share the management decisions in each patient. ARDs, ano rectal junction descent; EAS, external anal sphincter; POP, pelvic organ prolapse.

subspecialties. A diagnostic algorithm (**Fig. 12**) can be used to help tailor imaging according to the patient's symptoms and the clinical findings.[45]

Three-axis Perineal Evaluation

Beco and Mouchel[46] have defined a 3-axis perineal evaluation (TAPE) approach, which they call *perineology* (**Fig. 13**).

Concept

The investigators recommended TAPE in the assessment of a patient presenting with PFD, even if the main symptom is apparently related to 1 of the 3 pelvic compartments. This is because, anatomically, each organ system in the pelvic floor—urinary, genital, and intestinal—traverses the pelvis and exits through its own orifice. Thus, these systems are intricately related in function and structural support, which is why, among patients with PFD, 95% have abnormalities in all the 3 pelvic compartments, even if a

patient is presenting with symptoms that involve only 1 compartment.[46] Therefore, disorders of each of these components should be evaluated in light of their impact on the function of the surrounding structures and the functional anatomy of the pelvic floor. Hence, the investigators believed that physicians treating women with PFD should adopt a global approach, taking into consideration all the 3 pelvic compartments, and must clearly understand the anatomy of the pelvis and the associated urinary, genital, and anorectal abnormalities. This calls for noninvasive preoperative and postoperative imaging methods that can depict the 3 pelvic compartments simultaneously. MR imaging is ideal for this purpose.[45]

Aim

The aim of perineology is anatomic restoration with respect to biomechanics and physiology, so that each defect must be corrected without inducing trouble on other levels, which is why

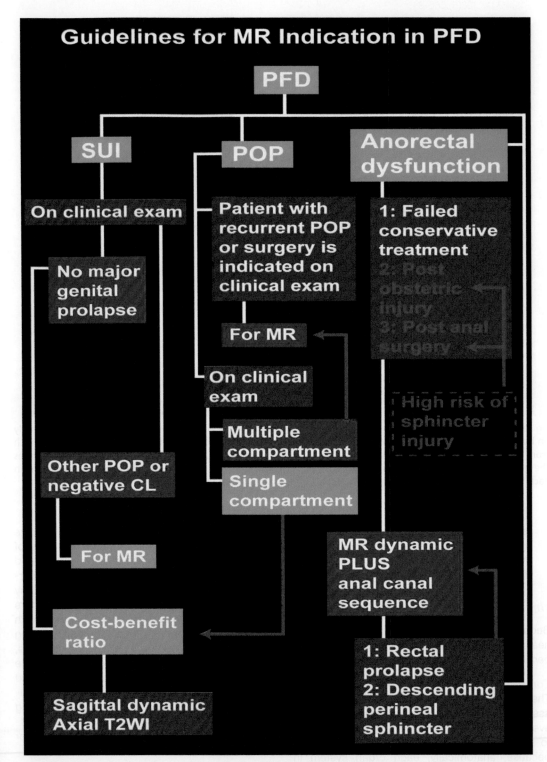

Fig. 12. This diagnostic algorithm can be used as a guideline to help tailor imaging according to a patient's symptoms and the clinical findings. The radiologist should be aware that defects in multiple compartments are present in 90% of patients with PFD. It is essential to consider all 3 pelvic compartments as an integrated unit. (*From* El Sayed RF. Multicompartmental imaging. In: Shaaban AM, editor. Diagnostic Imaging: Gynecology, 2nd edition. Elsevier, Amirsys; 2015. p. 8/88–8/101; with permission.)

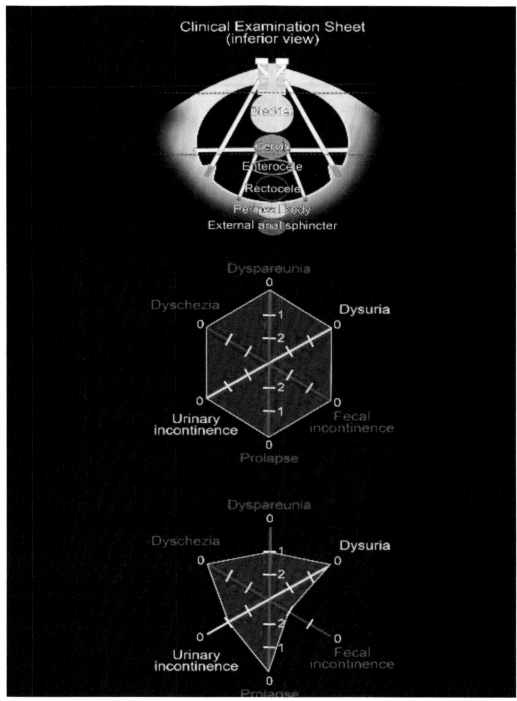

Fig. 13. (Top) This clinical examination sheet can be used to record examination findings. Each structure is assessed and noted, with the degree of POP recorded. (Middle) The TAPE is a plot to graphically represent the functional state of the perineum. Each of the 3 axes reflects a spectrum of related perineal pathologies. The gynecologic axis is in red, encompassing dyspareunia and prolapse. The urologic axis is in yellow, representing dysuria and urinary incontinence. The coloproctologic axis is in pink, reflecting dyschezia and fecal incontinence. For each axis, there are 3 levels of severity: 0 = not present, 1 = mild, and 2 = severe. (Bottom) This TAPE is of a patient with problems on all 3 axes: mild dyspareunia, severe fecal incontinence, and mild urinary incontinence. Knowing the physical examination findings and patient symptoms helps the radiologist tailor the MR examination and address the specific complaint. (From El Sayed RF. Multicompartmental imaging. In: Shaaban AM, editor. Diagnostic Imaging: Gynecology, 2nd edition. Elsevier, Amirsys; 2015. p. 8/88–8/101; with permission.)

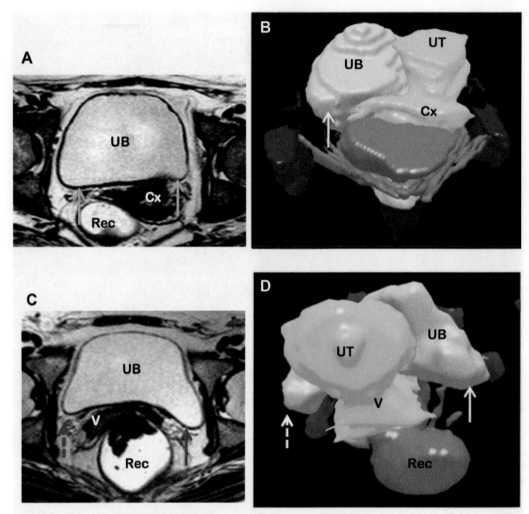

Fig. 14. 3D- Modeling of the predominant pelvic supporting system defect. (*A*) Static axial T2WI of a normal healthy volunteer with no pelvic floor dysfunction shows straight posterior urinary bladder wall indicating normal level I endopelvic fascia (*green arrows*). (*B*) The corresponding 3-D reconstruction post imaging processing using manual segmentation of sequential source images, shows that the intact fascia is reflected on the urinary bladder posterior wall (*white arrow*) in the 3D model same as in the 2D MR image. (*C*) Static Axial T2W MR image of female patient with POP shows sagging of the posterior urinary bladder wall, to fill the gap caused by detachment of the pubocervical fascia from the lateral pelvic wall (*red arrows*). (*D*) Is the corresponding 3-D modeling of the MR image effectively portraying the sagging urinary bladder (*white arrows*). Introducing the 3D- advanced post imaging processing modeling in our institution and research lab and its outcome has impressively enhanced the preoperative interpretation of the fascial defect by the surgeons. For example in this case the size of the defects on the right side (*dashed arrows* in C and D) are identical if compared to the larger defect on the left side solid (*arrows* in C and D) provide the surgeons with vivid information about the structural damage that will need to be repaired during the operation. To our knowledge applying this 3D modeling specifically on pelvic supporting endopelvic fascia has not been reported before. Cx, cervix; Rec, rectum; UB, urinary bladder; UT, uterus; V, vagina.

this approach is the result of the fusion between the disciplines of urogynecology and coloproctology. Combining TAPE with the author's recently developed integrated MR analytical approach puts a complete assessment of the patient, both clinically and radiologically, within reach of both radiologists and clinicians.[46]

Three-dimensional Modeling MR Imaging of the Functional 3-part Pelvic Supporting Systems

Concept

MR imaging is the imaging gold standard in PFD. Reducing rate of recurrence depend on accurate preoperative assessment. Despite the importance of MR imaging, surgeons may find difficulties in the interpretation of the MR images, especially in complex cases.

This raises the concept of 3-D postprocessing of MR images to perform a complementary 3-D model, which could be easily read by the surgeons.

Apart from the well-established role of 3-D surface rendering in maxillofacial reconstructive surgeries, in recent years, the conception of 3-D models has been gaining space as a promising aiding diagnostic modality in the preoperative planning in other new specialties ,for example, as perianal lesions, but this is an option yet little explored in the treatment of anal fistulas.[47,48]

Hypotheses

In the author's pelvic floor research laboratory, the author hypothesized that introducing 3-D modeling MR imaging would enhance preoperative interpretation of the predominant pelvic supporting system defect by the surgeons.

The 3D model was achieved by 3D reconstruction advanced post imaging processing technology named "manual segmentation" of huge number of sequential source images. Axial T2 weighted MR imaging sequence was used as the source images for segmentation. After manual segmentation, surface rendering is applied to obtain the final 3D model, which demonstrates each anatomical structure in a different colour.

Objectives

The generated (engineered) model gave a better orientation to complex cases (**Fig. 14**) and was utilized by the surgeons in the author's institute as a road map for pelvic floor reconstructive surgery planning, even more challenging the 3-D model was taken advantage of during surgery.

Summary

Although multiple factors predispose for PFD, the precise pathologic mechanism is poorly understood, and treatment often is started regardless of the specific anatomic lesion involved, possibly due to lack of understanding of normal anatomy and physiology of the pelvic floor, lack of solid data on selection criteria for the various surgical techniques, and sparsity of data on the outcome of different procedures.

All diagnostic modalities, including physical examination and standard MR imaging assessment, are directed toward 2 basic goals: detecting if prolapse of a specific organ is present and determining the degree of prolapse.

The author of this article believes, as do others, that as new modalities of evaluation emerge, anatomic concepts of form and function change.

With changing concepts, it is necessary to reexamine and redefine the underlying anatomy, which requires a functional classification system based on scientific evidence. On the basis of the new 3-part pelvic support system classification,[4] a correlative analytical approach was created that can pinpoint each patient's structural and anatomic defects, providing better data for treatment planning.

In conclusion, the functional 3-part pelvic supporting systems approach; integrated MR analytical approach; TAPE approach; individualized, defect-specific treatment approach; and 3-D modeling of the predominant pelvic supporting system defect are the tools of the upcoming new horizon in the diagnosis of the complex disorders of the pelvic floor. They are all considered in the author's research laboratory as the rising stars for a new era of MR imaging, image analysis, diagnosis, and treatment decisions of PFD based on a concrete more realistic glimpse of the structural relationships in vivo.

Disclosure

The author has nothing to disclose.

ACKNOWLEDGMENTS

The author would like to thank Professor Dr Haney Sami Shawali head of Department of Radiology, Cairo University and Professor Dr Hatem El Azizi for their enthusiasm and efforts to establish "Cairo University MRI center of Excellency and Research Lab Unit". The author also thank Dr Mary Salah, PhD candidate, for her contribution to the 3D modeling reconstruction project.

REFERENCES

1. El Sayed RF, Alt CD, Maccioni F, et al. Magnetic resonance imaging of pelvic floor dysfunction - joint recommendations of the ESUR and ESGAR Pelvic Floor Working Group. On Behalf of ESUR and ESGAR Pelvic Floor Working Group. Eur Radiol 2017; 27(5):2067–85.

2. Morren GL, Balasingam AG, Wells JE, et al. Triphasic MRI of pelvic organ descent: sources of measurement error. Eur J Radiol 2005;54:276–83.

3. Woodfield CA, Krishnamoorthy S, Hampton BS, et al. Imaging pelvic floor disorders: trend toward comprehensive MRI. AJR Am J Roentgenol 2010; 194:1640–9.

4. Pannu HK, Kaufman SH, Geoffrey WC, et al. Dynamic MR imaging of pelvic organ prolapse: spectrum of abnormalities. Radiographics 2000;20(6): 1567–82.

5. Kelvin FM, Maglinte DD, Hornback JA, et al. Pelvic prolapse: assessment with evacuation proctography (defecography). Radiology 1992;184: 547–51.

6. El Sayed RF. Female pelvic floor dysfunction. In: Morcos SK, Thomse HS, editors. Urogenital imaging: a problem-oriented approach. Chichester (England): Wiley-Blackwell; 2009. p. 399–413.

7. Bump RC, Mattiasson A, Bo K, et al. The standardization of terminology female pelvic floor dysfunction. Am J Obstet Gynecol 1996;175:10–7.

8. Kilpatrick CC. Anterior and posterior vaginal wall prolapse (Cystoceles, Urethroceles, Enteroceles, and Rectoceles). Kenilworth (NJ): Merck and the Merck Manuals; 2017.

9. Elsayed RF. Anterior compartment Imaging. In: Shaaban AM, editor. Diagnostic imaging gynecol. 2nd editionn. Philadelphia: Amirsys Elsevier; 2015. 8/60–8/67.

10. Lienemann A, Anthuber C, Baron A, et al. Dynamic MR colpocystorectography assessing pelvic floor descent. Eur Radiol 1997;7:1309–17.

11. Lalwani N, Moshiri M, Lee JH, et al. Magnetic resonance imaging of pelvic floor dysfunction. Radiol Clin North Am 2013;51(6):1127–39.

12. Colaiacomo MD, Masselli G, Polettini E, et al. Dynamic MR imaging of the pelvic floor: a pictorial review. Radiographics 2009;35:1–42.

13. Etlik Ö, Arslan H, Odaba si H, et al. The role of the MR-fluoroscopy in the diagnosis and staging of the pelvic organ prolapse. Eur J Radiol 2005;53: 136–41.

14. Comiter CV, Vasavada SP, Barbaric ZL, et al. Grading pelvic prolapse and pelvic floor relaxation using dynamic magnetic resonance imaging. Urology 1999;54:454–7.

15. Elsayed RF. Middle compartment imaging. In: Shaaban AM, editor. Diagnostic imaging gynecol. 2nd edition. Philadelphia: Amirsys Elsevier; 2015. 8/80–8/87.

16. Halligan S, Bartram C, Hall C, et al. Enterocele revealed by simultaneous evacuation proctography and peritoneography: does "defecation block" exist? Am J Roentgenol 1996;167:461–6.

17. Cortes E, Reid WMN, Singh K, et al. Clinical examination and dynamic magnetic resonance imaging in vaginal vault prolapse. Obstet Gynecol 2004;103: 41–6.

18. Fielding JR. Practical MR imaging of female pelvic floor weakness. Radiographics 2002;22:295–304.

19. Kelvin FM, Maglinte DDT, Hale DS, et al. Female pelvic organ prolapse: a comparison of triphasic dynamic MR imaging and triphasic fluoroscopic cystocolpoproctography. AJR Am J Roentgenol 2000;174:81–8.

20. Elsayed RF. Overview of posterior compartemnt. In: Shaaban AM, editor. Diagnostic imaging gynecol. 2nd edition. Philadelphia: Amirsys Elsevier; 2015. 8/88–8/101.

21. Lowry AC, Simmang CL, Boulo P, et al. From The American Society of Colon and Rectal Surgeons, The Association of Coloproctology of Great Britain and Ireland, and the Colorectal Surgical Society of Australia. Consensus statement of definitions for anorectal physiology and rectal cancer report of the tripartite consensus conference on definitions for anorectal physiology and rectal cancer. Washington, DC, May 1, 1999.

22. Shorvon PJ, McHugh S, Diamant NE, et al. Defecography in normal volunteers: results and implications. Gut 1989;30:1737–49.

23. Kruyt RH, Delemarre JB, Doornbos J, et al. Normal anorectum: dynamic MR imaging anatomy. Radiology 1991;179:159–63.

24. Mortele KJ, Fairhurst J. Dynamic MR defecography of the posterior compartment: indications, techniques and MRI features. Eur J Radiol 2007;61: 462–72.

25. Elsayed RF. Imaging of obstructed defecation. In: Shaaban AM, editor. Diagnostic imaging gynecol. 2nd edition. Amirsys: Elsevier; 2015. 8/88–8/101.

26. Maccioni F. Functional disorders of the anorectal compartment of the pelvic floor: clinical and diagnostic value of dynamic MRI. Abdom Imaging 2013;38:930–51.

27. Elshazly WG, El Nekady AA, Hassan H. Role of dynamic magnetic resonance imaging in management of obstructed defecation case series. Int J Surg 2010;8:274–82.

28. Halligan S, Bartram CI, Park HJ, et al. Proctographic features of anismus. Radiology 1995;197:679–82.

29. El-Sayed RF, Morsy MM, el-Mashed SM, et al. Anatomy of the urethral supporting ligaments defined by dissection, histology, and MRI of female cadavers and MRI of healthy nulliparous women. AJR Am J Roentgenol 2007;189:1145–57.

30. Elsayed RF. Overview of anterior compartment. In: Shaaban AM, editor. Diagnostic imaging gynecol. 2nd edition. Philadelphia: Amirsys Elsevier; 2015. 8/40–8/58.

31. Stoker J, Rociu E, Bosch JL, et al. High-resolution endo-vaginal MR imaging in stress urinary incontinence. Eur Radiol 2003;13:2031–7.

32. DeLancey JO. Fascial and muscular abnormalities in women with urethral hypermobility and anterior vaginal wall prolapse. Am J Obstet Gynecol 2002; 187:93–8.

33. Berek JF. Incontinence, prolapse, and disorders of the pelvic floor. In: Berek JF, Adashi EY, Hillard PA,

editors. Novak gynecology, 12th edition. Baltimore (MD): Williams & Wilkins; 2007. p. 619–76.

34. Huddleston HT, Dunnihoo DR, Huddleston PM 3rd, et al. Magnetic resonance imaging of defects in DeLancey's vaginal support levels I, II, and III. Am J Obstet Gynecol 1995;172:1774–8.

35. DeLancey JO. Anatomy and biomechanics of genital prolapse. Clin Obstet Gynecol 1993;36:897–909.

36. Elsayed RF. Overview of posterior compartment. In: Shaaban AM, editor. Diagnostic imaging gynecol. 2nd edition. Philadelphia: Amirsys Elsevier; 2015. 8/88–8/101.

37. Bartram CI. Fecal incontinence. In: Bartram CI, DeLancey JOL, editors. Imaging pelvic floor disorders. Berlin: Springer; 2003.

38. Elsayed RF. Imaging of fecal incontinence. In: Shaaban AM, editor. Diagnostic imaging gynecol. 2nd edition. Philadelphia: Amirsys Elsevier; 2015. 8/88–8/101.

39. Bump RC, Norton PA. Epidemiology and natural history of pelvic floor dysfunction. Obstet Gynecol Clin North Am 1998;25:723–46.

40. Olsen AL, Smith VJ, Bergstrom JO, et al. Epidemiology of surgically managed pelvic organ prolapse and urinary incontinence. Obstet Gynecol 1997;89: 501–6.

41. Petros PEP. Reconstructive pelvic floor surgery according to the integral theory. In: Petros PEP, editor. The female pelvic floor: function, dysfunction and management according to the integral theory. 2nd edition. Berlin: Springer; 2007. p. 122–3.

42. Black N, Downs S. The effectiveness of surgery for stress incontinence in women: a systematic review. Br J Urol 1996;78:497–551.

43. El Sayed RF, Fielding JR, El Mashed S, et al. Preoperative and postoperative magnetic resonance imaging of female pelvic floor dysfunction: correlation with clinical findings. J Women's Imag 2005;7: 163–80.

44. Kaufman HS, Buller JL, Thompson JR, et al. Dynamic pelvic magnetic resonance imaging and cystocolpoproctography alter surgical management of pelvic floor disorders. Dis Colon Rectum 2001;44: 1575–84.

45. Elsayed RF. Multicompartmental imaging. In: Shaaban AM, editor. Diagnostic imaging gynecol. 2nd edition. Philadelphia: Amirsys Elsevier; 2015. 8/88–8/101.

46. Beco J, Mouchel J. Perineology: a new area. Urogynaecol Int J 2003;17:79–86.

47. Júnior ECS, Nogueirac AT, Rochad BA, et al. Three-dimensional virtual reconstruction as a tool for preoperative planning in the management of complex anorectal fistulas. J coloproctol (Rio J., Impr.) 2018;38(1):77–81.

48. Sahnan K, Adegbola SO, Tozer PJ, et al. P126 Experience of 3D modelling in perianal fistula disease and survey of international surgical interest. J Crohns Colitis 2017;11(1):140–1.

Imaging of Acute Pelvic Pain: Nonpregnant

Jeffrey Dee Olpin, MD[a],*, Loretta Strachowski, MD[b]

KEYWORDS

- Female ● Pelvic pain ● Premenopause ● Nonpregnant ● Ultrasound ● Computed tomography
- Magnetic resonance

KEY POINTS

- Pelvic pain is a common condition that affects women of all ages and is defined as acute when less than 3 months' duration.
- The differential diagnosis of acute pelvic pain in the nonpregnant woman is broad, including a variety of gynecologic and nongynecologic entities.
- Ultrasound serves as the primary imaging modality for the evaluation of acute pelvic pain in the nonpregnant woman.

INTRODUCTION

Pelvic pain is a common condition that affects women of all ages and is defined as acute when less than 3 months in duration.[1] The etiology of acute pelvic pain in women of reproductive age often poses a diagnostic dilemma because many signs and symptoms are nonspecific. In addition, the clinical presentation of each disorder can vary widely. A detailed history regarding onset, character and duration of pain, constitutional symptoms, relevant laboratory values, and gynecologic, sexual, and social history can aid in the diagnosis. In the nonpregnant woman, the differential diagnosis of acute pelvic pain is broad, including a variety of gynecologic and nongynecologic entities.[1] Imaging plays a central role in the diagnosis and behooves the radiologist to become familiar with the most common etiologies.

IMAGING PROTOCOLS

Although ultrasound, computed tomography (CT), and magnetic resonance (MR) imaging are all used in the evaluation of acute pelvic pain in nonpregnant women, the selection of imaging modality for initial evaluation should be driven by the most clinically suspected disorder[2] (**Box 1**). However,

as CT uses ionizing radiation, its use should be avoided in young women of reproductive age unless there is a clear risk-to-benefit ratio.

GYNECOLOGIC ETIOLOGIES

Multiple conditions of the female reproductive tract may account for acute pelvic pain in the nonpregnant woman of reproductive age (**Box 2**). The following is a discussion of some of the more common etiologies.

ADNEXAL DISORDERS
Functional Cysts

Ovarian follicles are estrogen-mediated cystic lesions containing an oocyte that progressively enlarges during the first half of the menstrual cycle. One or more dominant follicles eventually emerge within the ovary ranging from 17 to 28 mm in diameter.[3] At midcycle, the dominant follicle evolves into a corpus luteum that secretes hormones to prepare for implantation and support early pregnancy.[4] A follicle that fails to expel an oocyte may continue to enlarge as a follicular cyst. Although most follicular cysts are asymptomatic, rapid cystic enlargement or rupture may result in acute pelvic pain. Follicular cysts generally

a University of Utah Health Sciences Center, 30 North 1900 East #1A71, Salt Lake City, UT 84132, USA;
b University of California, San Francisco, 1001 Potrero Avenue, San Francisco, CA 94110, USA
* Corresponding author.
E-mail address: Jeffrey.olpin@hsc.utah.edu

Radiol Clin N Am 58 (2020) 329–345
https://doi.org/10.1016/j.rcl.2019.11.002

measure between 3 and 10 cm and may remain hormonally sensitive.[5] A discriminatory size of 3 cm also differentiates a physiologic corpus luteum from a corpus luteal cyst.

On ultrasound , follicular cysts are unilocular, round or oval, anechoic intraovarian lesions with posterior acoustic enhancement.[4] The inner margin is uniformly smooth and a peripheral rim of compressed ovarian parenchyma is often seen.[3,6] Follicular cysts are typically sharply marginated, unilocular, thin-walled cysts with simple internal fluid attenuation on CT. On MR, follicular cysts are isointense to simple fluid on various pulse sequences: uniformly hypointense on T1-weighted images and uniformly hyperintense on T2-weighted images.[4] The thin walls of follicular cysts are typically best appreciated on T2-weighted images, and may enhance on T1-weighted contrast-enhanced images[7] (Fig. 1).

In contrast, on ultrasound , a corpus luteum has a thick wall, smooth or crenulated inner margin,

and commonly demonstrates intense peripheral flow.[6] The highly friable nature of its luteinized walls explains the common appearance of echoes within the central cystic component (see the next section, "Hemorrhagic cysts"). Corpus luteal cysts often demonstrate smooth or crenulated thickened walls with robust enhancement on CT and MR, but should never contain any discrete enhancing solid components (Fig. 2).

Hemorrhagic Cysts

Hemorrhagic cysts result from intracystic bleeding into a follicle or corpus luteum. Although many hemorrhagic cysts are discovered incidentally, others present with severe pain due to rapid enlargement or rupture.[8] Although hemorrhagic cysts are typically smaller than 5 cm, they may exceed 10 cm in size.

On ultrasound , hemorrhagic cysts are cystic ovarian lesions containing internal fibrin strands that are often described as reticular, lacelike, fishnet, or cobweb in appearance.[6,9] Retractile clot may demonstrate straight or concave margins, the latter of which has a 100% specificity for a benign hemorrhagic cyst[10] (see Fig. 4). Peripheral vascularity is often seen on color Doppler interrogation. Acute rupture of a hemorrhagic cyst may reveal hematoma and/or hemoperitoneum within the adnexa or cul-de-sac (Fig. 3).

On CT, hemorrhagic cysts demonstrate higher attenuation than that of simple fluid, typically greater than 30 Hounsfield units. On MR, these lesions frequently demonstrate internal signal intensity higher than that of simple fluid on T1-weighted images due to the presence of internal blood products, although the signal intensity may vary depending on the chronicity of the cyst. These lesions are typically intermediate to high signal intensity on T2-weighted images.[7]

Ovarian Torsion

Ovarian torsion occurs when the ovary and accompanying support structures twist on its vascular pedicle. Predisposing risk factors include prior pelvic surgery, early pregnancy, ovulation induction medication, and intraovarian lesions in 50% to 80% of reported cases.[11,12] Lesions that tend to twist are often larger (>4–5 cm) and are much more commonly benign than those lesions due to malignancy, endometriosis, or infection, which "fix" the ovary in place.[13] However, torsion can likewise occur in prepubertal girls with normal ovaries.[11] Classic symptoms of ovarian torsion include sudden onset of sharp or stabbing pelvic pain. Less specific symptoms, such as pain-induced nausea and vomiting, are seen in 70%

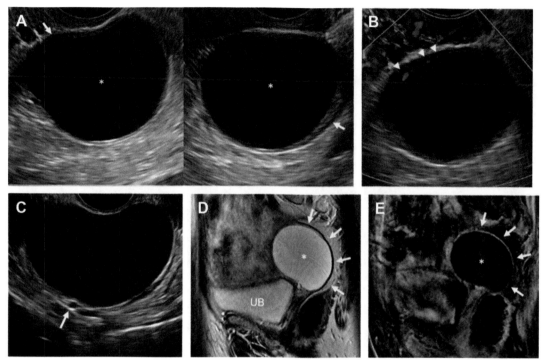

Fig. 1. Follicular cysts. (*A*) Longitudinal and transverse TVS shows a simple (unilocular, anechoic) cyst (*asterisks*) with compressed ovarian parenchyma (*arrows*) demonstrating (*B*) flow (*arrowhead*) on color Doppler. (*C*) Large simple cyst with peripheral ovarian tissue (*arrow*) on TVS. MR imaging 2 days later for unremitting pain shows high signal (*asterisks*) on T2 sagittal image (*D*) with a thin dark wall (*arrows*) that on T1+FS + C is low signal (*asterisks*) with thin uniform wall enhancement (*arrows*).

to 85% of women with torsion. The twisting of the ovarian vascular pedicle can compromise arterial, venous, and lymphatic flow to the affected ovary. As ovarian salvage rates are known to be inversely proportional to time to surgical intervention, imaging plays a critical role in prompt diagnosis.[14]

The classic ultrasound appearance of ovarian torsion is diffuse edema manifest as ovarian enlargement (5–20 cm) or increased surrounding ovarian parenchymal thickness when an intraovarian lesion is present. Other manifestations of edema include peripheralization of ovarian follicles ("string of pearls" sign) and adjacent free fluid. Additional grayscale findings of torsion include unusual ovarian location, uterine deviation/tilting and visualization of the twisted pedicle.[13,15]

Although duplex Doppler interrogation of the ovary may aid in the diagnosis of torsion, the presence or absence of flow within the ovary or twisted pedicle may play a greater role in assessing ovarian viability.[15] An absence of both arterial and venous flow is classically seen in high-grade torsion. However, arterial flow may be preserved in the setting of early or partial torsion in which only venous flow is compromised. Color Doppler evaluation may reveal a twisted or corkscrew appearance of the vascular pedicle, the so-called

"whirlpool sign"[16] (**Fig. 4**). The presence of flow within the twisted pedicle by Doppler interrogation can aid in assessing the viability of the ovary in experienced hands.[16] Most importantly, the presence of flow within the ovary does not exclude torsion and should never negate worrisome grayscale ultrasound findings when torsion is clinically suspected.[15]

CT findings of torsion mirror those seen on ultrasound, including asymmetric ovarian enlargement, hypoattenuation, hypoenhancement, unusual situs, deviation/titling of the uterus toward the ipsilateral side, and stranding of adnexal fat when ischemia is present.[13] The twisted pedicle sign may be seen on CT and is more frequently appreciated in the coronal plane[17] (**Fig. 5**).

Pelvic Inflammatory Disease

Pelvic inflammatory disease (PID) is a spectrum of infection of the upper female genital tract including endometrium, fallopian tubes, ovaries, and peritoneal cavity. PID is one of the most common causes of acute pelvic pain in sexually active women, affecting 1 million women and resulting in 275,000 hospitalizations per year.[18] The most

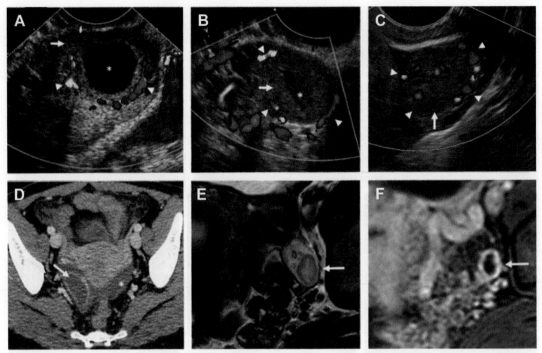

Fig. 2. Corpora lutea (CL). (*A–C*) Color Doppler TVS shows the characteristic thick wall (*arrow*) and peripheral vascularity (*arrowheads*) of CL. Centrally, the cystic component is anechoic with smooth inner margin in (*A*), has internal echoes and crenulated inner margin in (*B*), and solid appearance in (*C*). (*D*) CT of a ruptured CL with peripheral vascularity (*arrow*) and high attenuation free fluid (*asterisks*). (*E*) MR axial T2 and (*F*) T1+FS + C shows the thick wall, crenulated inner margin and robust peripheral enhancement of a CL.

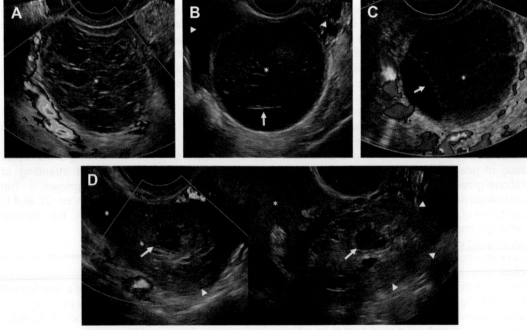

Fig. 3. Hemorrhagic cysts (HC). (*A–C*) demonstrate avascular unilocular cysts with internal reticular pattern (*asterisks*) characteristic of HC. Retractile clot (*arrow*) with straight (*B*) and concave (*C*) margins is highly specific for HC. (*D*) Transverse and longitudinal TVS of a ruptured HC (*arrow*) with adjacent hematoma (*arrowheads*) and hemoperitoneum (*asterisk*).

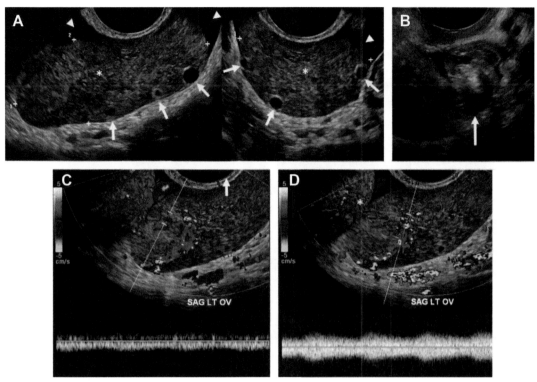

Fig. 4. Ovarian torsion, ultrasound . (A) Longitudinal and transverse TVS shows an edematous left ovary (*asterisks*) measuring 6.7 cm, peripheralization of follicles (*arrows*), and adjacent fluid (*arrowheads*). (B) An adjacent "whirlpool" sign (*arrow*) of the twisted pedicle. Color Doppler interrogation shows (C) venous and (D) arterial flow. At surgery, the left ovary was dusky and twisted 3 times, but viable.

common pathogens in PID are *Neisseria gonorrhea* and *Chlamydia trachomatis*, although polymicrobial infection is implicated in 30% to 40% of cases.[19–21] Infection typically spreads from the vagina when the cervical mucus plug is expelled during menses and spreads in ascending order to involve the uterus, tubes, and ovaries, often asymmetrically. Several discrete, often coexisting entities have been described, including cervicitis, endometritis, myometritis, salpingitis, pyosalpinx, tubo-ovarian complex (TOC), and tubo-ovarian abscess (TOA).[19]

PID should be suspected in any female individual presenting with acute pelvic pain, fever, and leukocytosis.[22] Untreated PID can eventually result in pyosalpinx and TOA, often requiring imaging-guided or surgical drainage.[20] Severe PID may result in tubal scarring with increased incidence of infertility, ectopic pregnancy, and chronic pelvic pain.[22] Although PID is considered a clinical diagnosis, imaging can greatly aid in the detection and guiding appropriate management of PID-related complications.[22]

Pelvic ultrasound is frequently normal in early PID, although affected women may complain of cervical motion tenderness with transvaginal sonography. Sonographic features of PID-induced endometritis include endometrial thickening, heterogeneity, and hypervascularity and occasionally intracavitary fluid ± echoes.[4] Increased vascularity within the myometrium may suggest endomyometritis. Echogenic fluid may develop in the pelvic cul-de-sac. Pyosalpinx may develop in the setting of salpingitis, which manifests as a thick-walled, hypervascular tubal-shaped structure between the uterus and ovary. A "cogwheel" sign may be present as thickened longitudinal folds of the fallopian tubes demonstrate a nodular appearance when seen in cross section[23] (Fig. 6). TOAs may develop in which the margins between tube and ovary are obscured, resulting in a complex, thick-walled cystic adnexal mass or tubo-ovarian complex.[5] The term TOC is used by some as distinct from TOA when an adjacent edematous ovary is inseparable from the tubal process. On ultrasound, a TOA presents as a heterogeneous, complex cystic adnexal mass ± thickened walls, fluid-debris levels, and surrounding hypervascularity without an identifiable ovary[5] (Fig. 7).

CT may be performed in women with acute pelvic pain when clinical suspicion of PID is equivocal

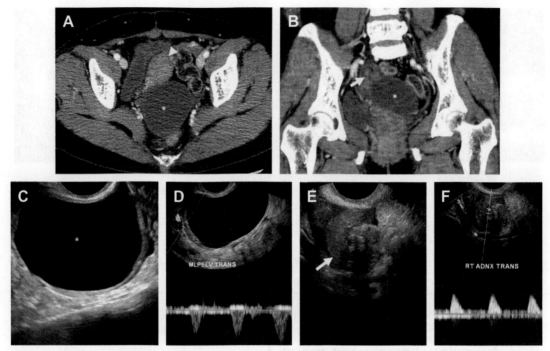

Fig. 5. Ovarian torsion, CT/ultrasound. (*A*) Axial and (*B*) coronal CT shows a large 6-cm cyst (*asterisks*) in the midline cul-de-sac, tilting of the uterus (*arrowhead*) and twisted pedicle sign (*arrow*). (*C –F*) Grayscale and Doppler TVS shows a midline simple cyst (*asterisk*) with preserved flow and right adnexal "whirlpool" sign (*arrow*).

and/or a nongynecologic condition is suspected. Although CT findings in early PID may be absent, mild pelvic edema with haziness and stranding of pelvic fat may be seen. Enhancing, thick-walled

fallopian tubes may be dilated with high attenuation fluid or layering internal debris in the setting of pyosalpinx.[4] The ovaries may be enlarged, heterogeneous, and edematous in the setting of

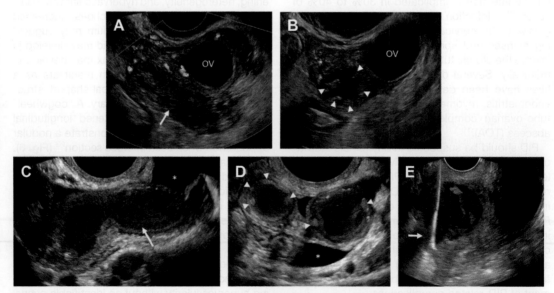

Fig. 6. Pyosalpinges. (*A*) Longitudinal and (*B*) transverse TVS shows an elongated thick-walled tubular structure with peripheral vascularity (*arrow*) next to the ovary and thickened endosalpingeal folds (*arrowheads*). (*C*) Echogenic fluid in a thick-walled tube (*arrow*), adjacent fluid (*asterisk*) and "cogwheel" sign in (*D*) axial plane. (*E*) TVS-guided aspiration and drainage (*arrow*) was performed.

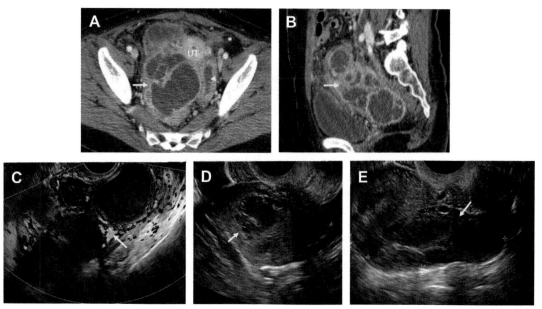

Fig. 7. TOAs. (*A*) Axial and (*B*) sagittal CT for suspected nongynecologic etiology shows a large right adnexal enhancing fluid collection (*arrows*), and smaller process on the left (*arrowhead*). Stranding (*asterisk*) is noted in adjacent fat. (*C*) Longitudinal and (*D*) transverse TVS on the right shows a multiloculated collection with internal debris and hyperemic walls (*arrows*). (*E*) Longitudinal TVS on the left shows a similar elongated collection (*arrow*). Ovaries were not identified bilaterally.

oophoritis. CT findings in the setting of advanced PID include progressive fallopian tube dilatation with complex fluid or layering internal debris in the setting of pyosalpinx.[4] Tubo-ovarian or pelvic abscesses may present as complex adnexal fluid collections, often with internal septations (see **Fig. 7**). Adjacent organ involvement may likewise be seen with mural thickening of small bowel, colon, and bladder. Patients with concomitant right upper quadrant pain may demonstrate perihepatic fluid and hepatic capsular and peritoneal enhancement from infectious perihepatitis, otherwise known as Fitz-Hugh-Curtis syndrome[21] (**Fig. 8**). MR imaging is infrequently used in suspected acute PID, but may be of benefit in the evaluation of complications from chronic PID.

Ovarian Hyperstimulation Syndrome

Ovarian hyperstimulation syndrome is a clinical syndrome resulting in bilateral ovarian enlargement with symptoms associated with extravascular fluid accumulation.[24] The condition most commonly occurs in the setting of exogenous human chorionic gonadotropin (hCG) administration, resulting in cystic enlargement of the ovaries and fluid shift from the intravascular to the third space.[24] Diffuse ovarian enlargement may present as diffuse abdominal and pelvic pain, nausea, and vomiting.[24] Marked ovarian enlargement predisposes women to ovarian torsion, which often

poses a diagnostic dilemma given an overlap in clinical and imaging features. Abdominal distention may likewise occur due to the development of ascites. Extravascular fluid accumulation may

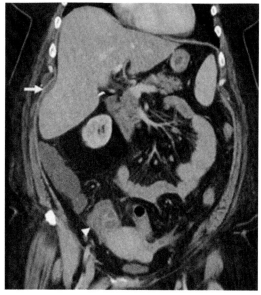

Fig. 8. Fitz-Hugh-Curtis (FHC) syndrome. TOAs in the right adnexa (*arrowhead*) in a woman with clinical PID, right pelvic and right upper quadrant pain. Perihepatic fluid and capsular enhancement (*arrow*) is diagnostic for FHC syndrome.

result in life-threatening hypovolemic shock or even death in rare instances.[8]

On ultrasound , bilateral symmetric ovarian enlargement is typically seen, often exceeding 12 cm in diameter. Multiple cysts of varying size can be seen, often demonstrating the classic "spoke-wheel appearance."[25] Ascites, pleural effusions, and pericardial effusions may occur due to capillary leak (**Fig. 9**).

Ovarian Vein Thrombophlebitis

Ovarian vein thrombophlebitis is a relatively rare condition that occurs primarily in the postpartum setting.[26] However, the condition can occur in the setting of other disease processes, such as malignancy, PID, inflammatory bowel disease, sepsis, or recent abdominal or pelvic surgery. Ovarian vein thrombosis involves the right ovarian vein in 70% to 90% of cases, likely due to a longer length and less competent valves compared with the left. Ovarian vein thrombosis generally presents clinically as pelvic pain, fever, and right-sided abdominal mass.[27]

Ultrasound is often inconclusive for ovarian vein thrombophlebitis due to body habitus and overlying bowel gas with a reported sensitivity of 55% and specificity of 41%.[28] CT is widely considered the initial imaging modality of choice for suspected ovarian vein thrombophlebitis.[29] CT findings include a hypodense filling defect and enlargement of the vein[30] (**Fig. 10**). MR angiography is considered the gold standard in the evaluation of suspected ovarian vein thrombophlebitis with a sensitivity and specificity of 92%.[29] However, MR has significant disadvantages, including limited availability, relatively high expense, and lengthy examination time.

UTERINE DISORDERS
Intrauterine Contraceptive Device Malpositioning

Intrauterine device (IUD) utilization has significantly increased over the past several decades as an attractive alternative for reversible, temporary contraception. As such, IUD-associated complications of displacement, myometrial penetration, and perforation resulting in acute pelvic pain are on the rise. Predisposing factors for malpositioning include structural uterine abnormalities, such as fibroids, an excessively anteverted or retroverted uterus, and inherently small endometrial cavity.[31]

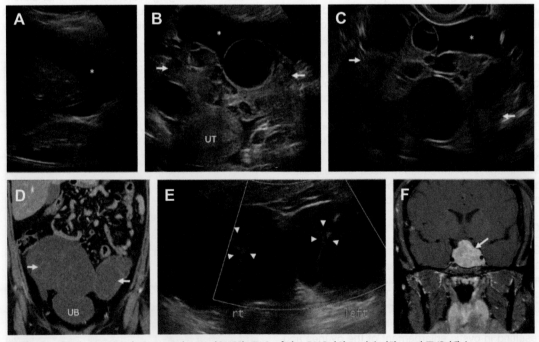

Fig. 9. Ovarian hyperstimulation syndrome (OHSS). TAS of the RUQ (A), pelvis (B), and TVS (C) in a woman on ovulation induction medication shows ascites (*asterisks*) in the Morrison pouch and pelvis, with marked ovarian enlargement (>10 cm) containing numerous cysts (*arrows*). (D) Coronal CT shows marked bilateral ovarian enlargement (*arrows*). TAS (E) shows intervening vascularized ovarian tissue (*arrowhead*) between large cysts creating a "spoke-wheel" appearance. New-onset galactorrhea prompted brain MR imaging (F), which revealed a pituitary macroadenoma (*arrow*) as the etiology of spontaneous OHSS.

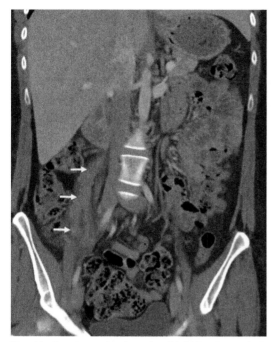

Fig. 10. Ovarian vein thrombophlebitis. Coronal CT shows a markedly dilated right ovarian vein filled with thrombus (*arrows*) with adjacent inflammatory fat stranding.

On ultrasound , the echogenic stem of the device should be oriented along the long axis of the endometrial cavity and the 2 horizontal arms transversely oriented within the fundal portion of the endometrium.[5] Three-dimensional (3D) ultrasound can provide a composite view of the IUD device within the endometrial cavity on a single coronal image, and is now considered the standard of care in the assessment of IUD positioning in routine clinical practice[32] (**Fig. 11**). A conventional radiograph of the pelvis is generally performed to assess for the presence of an intraperitoneal IUD if the device cannot be visualized within the pelvis on either transabdominal ultrasound (TAS) or transvaginal ultrasound (TVS). CT and MR play little roles in the assessment of suspected IUD malpositioning, although clinically occult device malpositioning may be incidentally detected (**Fig. 12**).

Leiomyoma Degeneration, Prolapse, and Torsion

Leiomyomas or fibroids are very common benign smooth-muscle, estrogen-dependent tumors of the uterus with an estimated prevalence of 20% in women older than 30 years.[33] Fibroids are commonly categorized as intramural, subserosal, or submucosal according to anatomic location in

order of prevalence.[4] Fibroids undergo degeneration if they outgrow their blood supply. Although most degenerating fibroids are asymptomatic, fibroid degeneration can result in acute pelvic pain and/or vaginal bleeding in up to 30% of cases.[4]

Submucosal fibroids that are pedunculated may prolapse through the cervix or into the vagina resulting in acute, laborlike pain often accompanied by bleeding. Complications of prolapsed fibroids include torsion, necrosis, and superimposed infection.[34] Although prolapsed fibroids are most commonly a clinical diagnosis, imaging is often useful for surgical planning to evaluate the site of stalk attachment within the uterine cavity.[34] Likewise, pedunculated subserosal fibroids with a sufficiently long vascular pedicle may rotate around its own axis. Although uncommon, torsion of a fibroid may result in hemorrhagic infarction and life-threatening peritonitis if left untreated.[35]

Ultrasound is the most commonly used imaging modality in suspected fibroid degeneration. In general, most fibroids become progressively heterogeneous as degeneration occurs; however, areas of increased echogenicity or anechoic cystic spaces ± internal debris and thick septations may be seen.[4] Degenerating fibroids are generally hypovascular or avascular compared with background myometrium with color Doppler interrogation (**Fig. 13**). CT and MR can be used to more definitively characterize fibroid degeneration. Gadolinium-enhanced MR sequences can be particularly useful if uterine artery embolization is being considered as a therapeutic option, as fibroids that demonstrate little to no enhancement will not respond well to embolization treatment.

On ultrasound , a prolapsed submucosal fibroid appears as a heterogeneously hypoechoic mass either within or through the endocervical canal and occasionally expanding the vagina. Color Doppler interrogation often reveals the site of attachment of the vascular pedicle within the uterine cavity; however, when inconclusive, CT and MR may be helpful for confirmation of the diagnosis and surgical planning. The appearance of a bulky mass on a long stalk protruding through the endocervix has been coined the "broccoli" sign on sagittal MR and reformatted CT images[34] (**Fig. 14**). Ultrasound findings of subserosal fibroid torsion include the characteristic corkscrew or "whirlpool" pattern on color Doppler ultrasound .[29] A pedunculated subserosal fibroid that is hypovascular on ultrasound or nonenhancing or minimally enhancing and CT or MR should raise the suspicion of torsion in the setting of acute pelvic pain (**Fig. 15**).

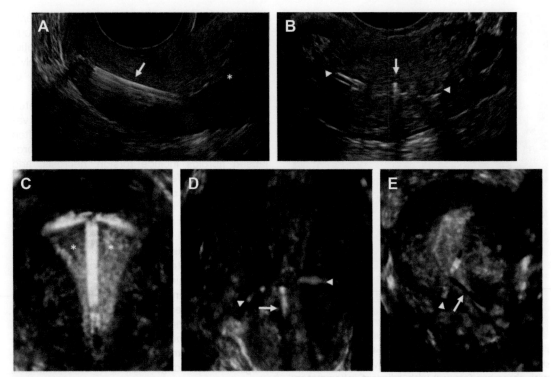

Fig. 11. Malpositioned IUDs on ultrasound . (*A*) Longitudinal, (*B*) transverse, and (*D*) 3D TVS shows a retroverted uterus with long arm (*arrows*) of an IUD low in the endocervical canal and short horizontal arms (*arrowheads*) penetrating the cervical stroma. (*C*) Three-dimensional reconstruction shows an appropriately positioned IUD within the echogenic endometrium (*asterisks*). (*E*) Mirena IUD with hypoechoic long arm (*arrow*) in lower uterine segment and right horizontal arm (*arrowhead*) penetrating the myometrium.

NONGYNECOLOGIC DISORDERS

A number of nongynecologic disorders of the gastrointestinal and urinary tract (**Box 3**) also may account for acute pelvic pain in the reproductive age woman and should always be considered, especially if a gynecologic abnormality is not identified on ultrasound. In particular, findings of appendicitis, diverticulitis, ureteral stones at the ureterovesicular junction (UVJ), and cystitis may

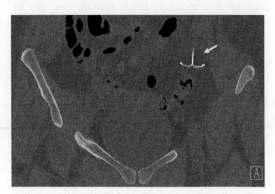

Fig. 12. Malpositioned IUD on CT. T-shaped copper IUD (*arrow*) in the left hemipelvis in a young woman on CT obtained for suspected urolithiasis.

be diagnosed on pelvic sonography and are further discussed later in this article.

Appendicitis

Appendicitis is the result of appendiceal inflammation due to luminal obstruction and superimposed infection. Although appendicitis is very prevalent, the diagnosis can be difficult to establish in women of reproductive age because of significant clinical overlap with gynecologic disorders. The diagnosis of appendicitis always must be considered in this patient population that presents with acute right-sided pelvic pain.

In the subset of women with persistent right lower quadrant pain and a normal gynecologic ultrasound, a limited ultrasound of the right lower quadrant should be performed. Sonographic -evaluation of the right lower quadrant is typically performed using a high-resolution 9 to 18 MHz linear transducer with graded compression at the site of maximum pain/ tenderness. Sonographic findings of acute appendicitis include a noncompressible, blind-ending, non-peristalsing, thick-walled tubular structure, often larger than 6 to 7 mm in diameter[36] (**Fig. 16**). A sonographic McBurney sign with point tenderness over

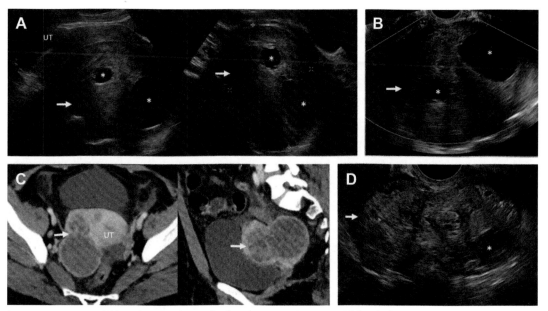

Fig. 13. Degenerated fibroids. (*A*) Longitudinal and transverse TAS and (*B*) color Doppler TVS shows a large subserosal fibroid (*arrows*) in the cul-de-sac with areas of cystic change (*asterisks*) with minimal flow. (*C*) Axial and sagittal CT and (*D*) TVS shows a right-sided, bilobed subserosal fibroid (*arrows*) with hypoattenuation, hypoenhancement, marked heterogeneity and early cystic change (*asterisks*).

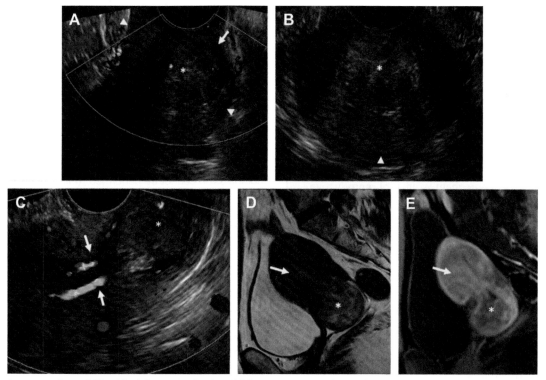

Fig. 14. Prolapsed fibroids. (*A*) Longitudinal and (*B*) transverse TVS shows the anterior and posterior cervical lips (*arrowheads*) splayed by a submucosal fibroid (*asterisk*) in the endocervical canal extending into the vagina (*arrow*). (*C*) Color TVS shows the vascular pedicle (*arrow*) of a prolapsed fibroid (*asterisk*) in the endocervix. Treatment planning MR image shows the fibroid (*asterisks*) bulging into the vagina ("broccoli" sign) on (*D*) sagittal T2 and (*E*) T1+FS + C with a clear anterior fundal attachment (*arrows*).

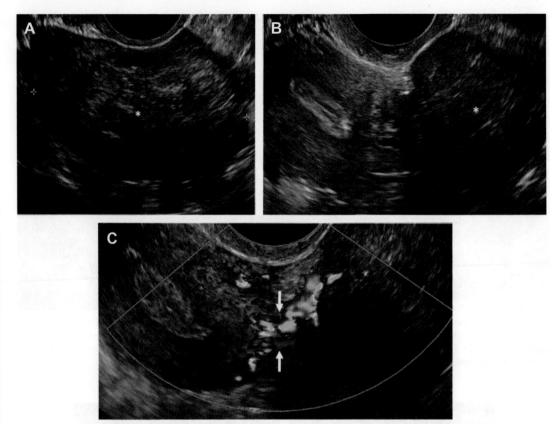

Fig. 15. Fibroid torsion. (*A*) Longitudinal and (*B*) transverse TVS shows a subserosal myoma (*asterisks*). (*C*) Probe pressure elicited tenderness and demonstrates the narrow vascular attachment with color Doppler (*arrow*).

the appendix can greatly aid in establishing the diagnosis. A shadowing, echogenic appendicolith may likewise confirm the diagnosis. Transabdominal visualization of the appendix is not always feasible,

Box 3
Nongynecologic etiologies of acute pelvic pain in the nonpregnant woman of reproductive age
Gastrointestinal
Appendicitis
Diverticulitis
Inflammatory bowel disease[a]
Enterocolitis[a]
Ischemic bowel[a]
Epiploic appendagitis[a]
Urinary Tract
Urolithiasis
Cystitis
[a] Not covered in this article as addressed in radiology literature elsewhere.

particularly in patients with a high body mass index or shadowing bowel gas. The sonographic findings of acute appendicitis may be visualized in the right adnexal region on TVS in experienced hands if the appendix is in the vicinity of the ultrasound probe.[37] The transvaginal manifestations of acute appendicitis are the same as TAS, although graded compression cannot be performed[5] (**Fig. 17**). CT or MR may be performed to confirm a suspected diagnosis of acute appendicitis in nonpregnant women, or when the ultrasound results are equivocal.

Diverticulitis

Acute diverticulitis is an intramural and pericolonic infectious or inflammatory process resulting from perforation of colonic diverticula. Patients with acute diverticulitis typically present with fever, nausea, leukocytosis, and colicky pain within the left lower quadrant. Diverticulitis is often clinically indistinguishable from other gynecologic disorders in women of reproductive age with acute left lower quadrant pain.

On ultrasound , colonic diverticula may be seen as small, round outpouchings from the colon. The wall of a normal diverticulum is too thin

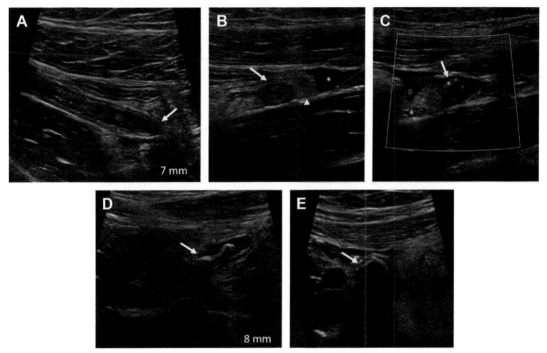

Fig. 16. Acute appendicitis, TAS. (*A*) Longitudinal, (*B*) transverse, and (*C*) color Doppler TAS shows a thickened blind-ending structure with bowel wall signature, hyperemia (*arrows*), inflamed periappendiceal fat (*arrowhead*) and adjacent fluid (*asterisk*). (*D*) Longitudinal and (*E*) transverse TAS shows a thickened appendix containing an appendicolith (*arrows*).

to be visualized on routine sonography. However, an inflamed diverticulum may demonstrate a thick hypoechoic rim reflecting underlying wall thickening (**Fig. 18**). Increased echogenicity of the pericolonic fat may likewise be seen in the setting of pericolonic inflammation. Segmental thickening of the adjacent pericolonic wall has likewise been described. CT is often used to confirm the diagnosis of acute diverticulitis in nonpregnant women if the ultrasound results are equivocal.

Urolithiasis

Urolithiasis refers to the presence of calculi anywhere along the course of the urinary tract. Renal colic accounts for a large proportion of emergency department visits for acute flank and pelvic pain

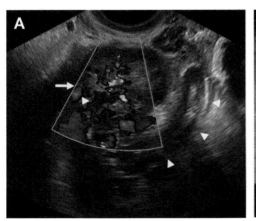
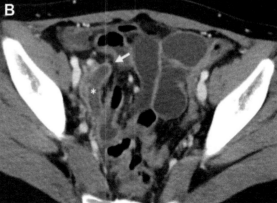

Fig. 17. Acute appendicitis, TVS. (*A*) TVS of the right adnexa to evaluate for ovarian torsion shows a nonedematous ovary (*arrow*) but reveals a tubular blind-ending structure with bowel wall signature (*arrowheads*). (*B*) CT confirms a fluid-filled, dilated appendix (*asterisk*) with stranding of periappendiceal fat adjacent to the tip of the appendix (*arrows*).

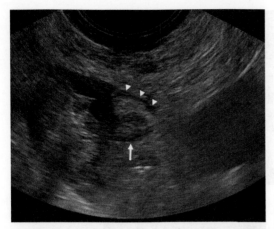

Fig. 18. Diverticulitis on TVS. TVS shows a prominent diverticulum (*arrow*) arising from the sigmoid colon with adjacent recruited inflamed fat and free fluid (*arrowheads*). Patient was focally tender with TVS.

with an estimated prevalence between 4% and 20% in economically developed countries.[38] The clinical diagnosis of upper urinary tract stones is generally straightforward, with stones at the ureteropelvic junction (UPJ) resulting in flank pain, fever, and dysuria. However, stones in the distal ureter or ureterovesical junction (UVJ) typically result in suprapubic discomfort and pain radiating to the groin and genitals, often resulting in significant clinical overlap with other gynecologic conditions.

Noncontrast CT is generally performed for suspected urolithiasis in adults. However, in the woman of reproductive age, ultrasound is commonly used to avoid ionizing radiation. Ureteral calculi present as echogenic foci with sharp posterior acoustic shadowing on grayscale imaging and may be more apparent with harmonic imaging. Color Doppler interrogation may demonstrate the so-called twinkling artifact, a focus of alternating colors behind a rough, reflective object such as a calculus. The presence of ipsilateral ureterovesical jets on color Doppler does not reliably exclude partial obstruction of a ureteral stone, although dynamic changes may be helpful in experienced hands[39] (Fig. 19). For stones larger than 5 mm, ultrasound has a reported sensitivity of 96% and a specificity of nearly 100%.[40]

Cystitis

Cystitis refers to nonspecific inflammation of the bladder and is roughly 10 times more common in women, largely due to the protective effect of a longer urethra in men and antibacterial properties of prostatic fluid.[41] Acute cystitis is generally due to bacterial infection, generally from *Escherichia coli* or *Candida* infection in immunosuppressed or diabetic patients.

Although the diagnosis of acute cystitis is often clinically established by physical examination and urinalysis, imaging may play a role in women with acute pelvic pain of suspected gynecologic origin. In general, the imaging diagnosis of cystitis may be difficult to establish on any imaging

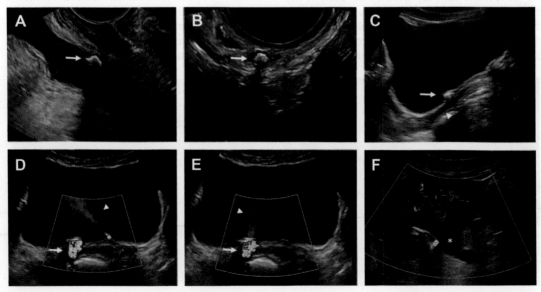

Fig. 19. UVJ stone. (*A*) Longitudinal and (*B*) transverse TVS shows a curvilinear echogenic shadowing stone (*arrows*) at the right UVJ. (*C*) TAS show the typical location of a UVJ stone (*arrow*) in the longitudinal plane within a mildly dilated ureter (*arrowhead*). (*D, E*) Doppler shows twinkling artifact (*arrow*) from the stone and ureteral jets (*arrowheads*) from both sides, although moderate obstructive right hydronephrosis (*asterisk*) is seen (*F*).

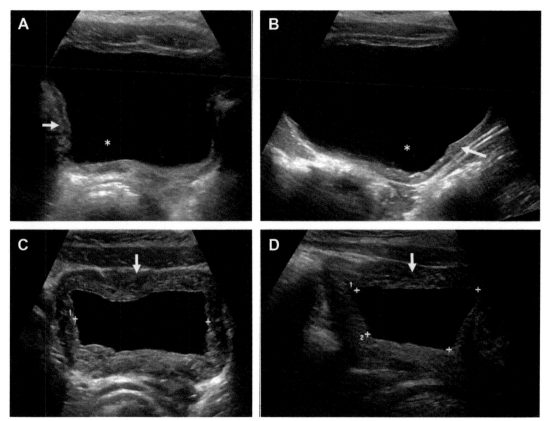

Fig. 20. Acute cystitis. Transverse and longitudinal prevoid (*A, B*) and postvoid (*C, D*) TAS of the urinary bladder shows intraluminal echoes (*asterisks*) and diffuse wall thickening (*arrows*).

modality if the bladder is underdistended or decompressed. Sonographic features of acute cystitis include intraluminal echoes, diffuse bladder wall thickening (>3 mm if distended and >5 mm if nondistended), and decreased bladder wall echogenicity[42] (**Fig. 20**). CT findings of cystitis include diffuse bladder wall changes of thickening, decreased attenuation and hyperemia, and infiltration of the perivesical fat. Bladder wall gas may be seen in the setting of emphysematous cystitis.

SUMMARY

Acute pelvic pain is commonly encountered in women of all ages. The prompt determination of pregnancy status using serum hCG is warranted in any woman capable of conceiving. If the serum hCG is negative, a thorough clinical history and physical examination are essential in triaging gynecologic versus nongynecologic etiologies to determine first-line imaging modality: pelvic ultrasound for suspected gynecologic etiologies, appendicitis, and urinary tract pathology; MR when ultrasound is nondiagnostic or inconclusive; and CT for suspected nongynecologic conditions.

A solid familiarity with the differential diagnosis of both gynecologic and nongynecologic etiologies is essential to establish the correct diagnosis and expedite appropriate clinical management. In the absence of sonographic findings, the patient with acute pelvic pain should be reassured of the very low likelihood of significant pathology.

DISCLOSURE

The authors have nothing to disclose.

REFERENCES

1. Kruszka PS, Kruszka SJ. Evaluation of acute pelvic pain in women. Am Fam Physician 2010;82(2): 141–7.
2. Bhosale PR, Javitt MC, Atri M, et al. ACR Appropriateness Criteria(R) acute pelvic pain in the reproductive age group. Ultrasound Q 2016;32(2): 108–15.
3. Levine D, Brown DL, Andreotti RF, et al. Management of asymptomatic ovarian and other adnexal cysts imaged at US: Society of Radiologists in Ultrasound Consensus Conference Statement. Radiology 2010;256(3):943–54.

4. Potter AW, Chandrasekhar CA. US and CT evaluation of acute pelvic pain of gynecologic origin in nonpregnant premenopausal patients. Radiographics 2008;28(6):1645–59.

5. Amirbekian S, Hooley RJ. Ultrasound evaluation of pelvic pain. Radiol Clin North Am 2014;52(6):1215–35.

6. Andreotti RF, Timmerman D, Benacerraf BR, et al. Ovarian-adnexal reporting lexicon for ultrasound: a white paper of the ACR ovarian-adnexal reporting and data system committee. J Am Coll Radiol 2018;15(10):1415–29.

7. Jeong YY, Outwater EK, Kang HK. Imaging evaluation of ovarian masses. Radiographics 2000;20(5):1445–70.

8. Bennett GL, Harvey WB, Slywotzky CM, et al. CT of the acute abdomen: gynecologic etiologies. Abdom Imaging 2003;28(3):416–32.

9. Laing FC, Allison SJ. US of the ovary and adnexa: to worry or not to worry? Radiographics 2012;32(6):1621–39 [discussion: 40–2].

10. Patel MD, Feldstein VA, Filly RA. The likelihood ratio of sonographic findings for the diagnosis of hemorrhagic ovarian cysts. J Ultrasound Med 2005;24(5):607–14 [quiz: 15].

11. Stark JE, Siegel MJ. Ovarian torsion in prepubertal and pubertal girls: sonographic findings. AJR Am J Roentgenol 1994;163(6):1479–82.

12. Rha SE, Byun JY, Jung SE, et al. CT and MR imaging features of adnexal torsion. Radiographics 2002;22(2):283–94.

13. Chang HC, Bhatt S, Dogra VS. Pearls and pitfalls in diagnosis of ovarian torsion. Radiographics 2008;28(5):1355–68.

14. Glanc P, Ghandehari H, Kahn D, et al. OP15.09: acute ovarian torsion: the impact of time delays to surgery. Ultrasound Obstet Gynecol 2015;46(S1):99.

15. Fleischer AC, Stein SM, Cullinan JA, et al. Color Doppler sonography of adnexal torsion. J Ultrasound Med 1995;14(7):523–8.

16. Vijayaraghavan SB. Sonographic whirlpool sign in ovarian torsion. J Ultrasound Med 2004;23(12):1643–9 [quiz: 50–1].

17. Jung SI, Park HS, Yim Y, et al. Added value of using a CT coronal reformation to diagnose adnexal torsion. Korean J Radiol 2015;16(4):835–45.

18. Sam JW, Jacobs JE, Birnbaum BA. Spectrum of CT findings in acute pyogenic pelvic inflammatory disease. Radiographics 2002;22(6):1327–34.

19. Barrett S, Taylor C. A review on pelvic inflammatory disease. Int J STD AIDS 2005;16(11):715–20 [quiz: 21].

20. Cicchiello LA, Hamper UM, Scoutt LM. Ultrasound evaluation of gynecologic causes of pelvic pain. Obstet Gynecol Clin North Am 2011;38(1):85–114, viii.

21. Gradison M. Pelvic inflammatory disease. Am Fam Physician 2012;85(8):791–6.

22. Vandermeer FQ, Wong-You-Cheong JJ. Imaging of acute pelvic pain. Clin Obstet Gynecol 2009;52(1):2–20.

23. Romosan G, Valentin L. The sensitivity and specificity of transvaginal ultrasound with regard to acute pelvic inflammatory disease: a review of the literature. Arch Gynecol Obstet 2014;289(4):705–14.

24. Kumar P, Sait SF, Sharma A, et al. Ovarian hyperstimulation syndrome. J Hum Reprod Sci 2011;4(2):70–5.

25. Kim IY, Lee BH. Ovarian hyperstimulation syndrome. US and CT appearances. Clin Imaging 1997;21(4):284–6.

26. Brown CE, Stettler RW, Twickler D, et al. Puerperal septic pelvic thrombophlebitis: incidence and response to heparin therapy. Am J Obstet Gynecol 1999;181(1):143–8.

27. Kamaya A, Shin L, Chen B, et al. Emergency gynecologic imaging. Semin Ultrasound CT MR 2008;29(5):353–68.

28. Kubik-Huch RA, Hebisch G, Huch R, et al. Role of duplex color Doppler ultrasound, computed tomography, and MR angiography in the diagnosis of septic puerperal ovarian vein thrombosis. Abdom Imaging 1999;24(1):85–91.

29. Sinha D, Yasmin H, Samra JS. Postpartum inferior vena cava and ovarian vein thrombosis–a case report and literature review. J Obstet Gynaecol 2005;25(3):312–3.

30. Sharma P, Abdi S. Ovarian vein thrombosis. Clin Radiol 2012;67(9):893–8.

31. Peri N, Graham D, Levine D. Imaging of intrauterine contraceptive devices. J Ultrasound Med 2007;26(10):1389–401.

32. Boortz HE, Margolis DJ, Ragavendra N, et al. Migration of intrauterine devices: radiologic findings and implications for patient care. Radiographics 2012;32(2):335–52.

33. Bennett GL, Slywotzky CM, Giovanniello G. Gynecologic causes of acute pelvic pain: spectrum of CT findings. Radiographics 2002;22(4):785–801.

34. Kim JW, Lee CH, Kim KA, et al. Spontaneous prolapse of pedunculated uterine submucosal leiomyoma: usefulness of broccoli sign on CT and MR imaging. Clin Imaging 2008;32(3):233–5.

35. Roy C, Bierry G, El Ghali S, et al. Acute torsion of uterine leiomyoma: CT features. Abdom Imaging 2005;30(1):120–3.

36. Jeffrey RB, Jain KA, Nghiem HV. Sonographic diagnosis of acute appendicitis: interpretive pitfalls. AJR Am J Roentgenol 1994;162(1):55–9.

37. Shaaban AM, Rezvani M, Olpin JD, et al. Nongynecologic findings seen at pelvic US. Radiographics 2017;37(7):2045–62.

38. Trinchieri A. Epidemiology of urolithiasis: an up-date. Clin Cases Miner Bone Metab 2008;5(2): 101–6.

39. Jandaghi AB, Falahatkar S, Alizadeh A, et al. Assessment of ureterovesical jet dynamics in obstructed ureter by urinary stone with color Doppler and duplex Doppler examinations. Urolithiasis 2013;41(2):159–63.

40. Cheng PM, Moin P, Dunn MD, et al. What the radiologist needs to know about urolithiasis: Part 1—Pathogenesis, types, assessment, and variant anatomy. AJR Am J Roentgenol 2012;198(6): W540–7.

41. Kranz J, Schmidt S, Lebert C, et al. The 2017 update of the German clinical guideline on epidemiology, diagnostics, therapy, prevention, and management of uncomplicated urinary tract infections in adult patients. Part II: therapy and prevention. Urol Int 2018;100(3):271–8.

42. Tyagi P, Moon CH, Janicki J, et al. Recent advances in imaging and understanding interstitial cystitis. F1000Res 2018;7 [pii:F1000].

Imaging of Acute Pelvic Pain
Pregnant (Ectopic and First-trimester Viability Updated)

Kyle K. Jensen, MD*, Mehtab Sal, BA, Roya Sohaey, MD

KEYWORDS

- Ultrasonography • Pregnancy • First trimester • Ectopic pregnancy • Early pregnancy loss
- Pregnancy failure • Viability • Intrauterine pregnancy

KEY POINTS

- In first-trimester pregnant patients, pelvic pain from pregnancy complications, pregnancy loss, or abnormal implantation is nonspecific, with symptoms ranging from mild to catastrophic, and ultrasonography should be performed early for better evaluation.
- On ultrasonography, first assess for the presence or absence of an intrauterine pregnancy (IUP). If there is an IUP, then assess for viability; if there is not an IUP, search for abnormal implantation.
- Abnormal implantation is seen in a small percentage of pregnancies; however, it accounts for a disproportionately high percentage of maternal morbidity and mortality.

 Video content accompanies this article at http://www.radiologic.theclinics.com.

INTRODUCTION

In the first trimester, patient symptoms associated with pregnancy complications, pregnancy loss, and abnormal implantation are nonspecific. Most often, patients present to their providers or the emergency room with some symptom combination of pain and bleeding. Symptom severity ranges from mild to catastrophic. Ultrasonography is almost always the first modality used to image symptomatic early pregnant patients. This article begins by addressing diagnoses encountered when an intrauterine pregnancy is present because that is the first important diagnosis to make when imaging a pregnant patient with pain. An update on viability parameters is presented. Next, this article discusses presentations, causes, findings, and management strategies for abnormally implanted pregnancies.

FIRST-TRIMESTER VIABILITY

Early first-trimester pregnancy failure occurs in approximately 10% of patients, accounting for 80% of all pregnancy losses.[1] Transvaginal ultrasonography (TVUS) and concentration of maternal serum beta unit of human chorionic gonadotropin (β-hCG) are key tests to assess for early pregnancy failure.

For a normal intrauterine pregnancy (IUP), developmental milestones include[2]:

- Gestational sac (GS) at 5 weeks
- Yolk sac at 5.5 weeks
- Visible embryo at 6 weeks

In 2013, new guidelines for evaluating early pregnancy loss were created by the Society of Radiologists in Ultrasound (SRU) Multispecialty Panel

Department of Diagnostic Radiology, Oregon Health & Science University, L340, 3181 Southwest Sam Jackson Park Road, Portland, OR 97239, USA
* Corresponding author.
E-mail address: jensenky@ohsu.edu

Radiol Clin N Am 58 (2020) 347–361
https://doi.org/10.1016/j.rcl.2019.11.003
0033-8389/20/© 2019 Elsevier Inc. All rights reserved.

(Table 1) because of updated research showing that the previously used cutoff values for crown rump length (CRL) and mean sac diameter (MSD) lead to false-positive interpretations of early pregnancy loss.[3] The goal of these guidelines is to eliminate false-positive interpretations, preventing inappropriate medical or surgical management of a potentially viable desired IUP.[1]

- SRU guidelines for definitive diagnosis of pregnancy failure[3]:
  o CRL at least 7 mm without cardiac activity
  o MSD at least 25 mm without embryo

More recent studies suggest limitations of the 2013 SRU guidelines, including the following from the 2018 American College of Obstetrics and Gynecology[1]:

- Strict measurement and observational cutoffs may limit clinical management because of patient preferences
  o For example, willingness to wait for 100% certainty of failure
- Few data points near cutoff values in studies used for SRU guidelines
- SRU guidelines are more conservative than data in literature and lead to patient stress and anxiety

o Literature: no embryo seen at 7-day follow-up of GS without embryo was 100% specific in a study of 359 patients
o SRU guidelines recommend 14-day follow-up of GS without embryo

Historically, a "discriminatory level" of β-hCG was used for evaluation of IUP development.[2] However, recent guidelines challenge the use of a discriminatory level:

- Absolute β-hCG level should not be used to determine when an IUP should be visualized[1,3]
  o Potential for false-positive interpretation of early pregnancy loss
    ▪ Instead, use accurate gestational age
- Historically: IUP seen on TVUS at β-hCG level of 1000 mIU/mL
  o However, follow-up IUP with cardiac activity has been seen when initial GS was empty and β-hCG level 2000 to 3000 mIU/mL
  o Multiple gestations have higher β-hCG levels than singleton at same gestational age
  o Updated use of β-hCG: more conservative value should be used (eg, >3500 mIU/mL) for potential ectopic[4]
    ▪ Goal: prevent termination of normal IUP (ie, false-positive)

Table 1
Ultrasonography assessment for early pregnancy loss

	Crown Rump Length Without Heartbeat (mm)	Mean Sac Diameter Without Embryo (mm)	GS Without YS; Length of Time for Follow-up US Not Showing Embryo with Heart Beat (d)	GS with YS; Length of Time for Follow-up US Not Showing Embryo with Heart Beat (d)	β-hCG	[a]Additional Findings
Diagnostic for Early Pregnancy Loss	>7	>25	14	>11	No single threshold value; correlated with trend of values on surveillance	
Suspicious for Early Pregnancy Loss	<7	16–24	7–13	7–10		

Abbreviations: US, ultrasonography; YS, yolk sac.
[a] Additional findings suspicious for, but not diagnostic of, early pregnancy loss: no embryo more than 6 weeks after LMP YS larger than 7 mm. Empty amnion: amnion adjacent to YS without embryo. Early oligohydramnios: less than 5 mm size difference between mean sac diameter and crown rump length.
Data from ACOG Practice Bulletin No. 200: Early Pregnancy Loss. Obstet Gynecol 2018;132(5):e197-e207; and Doubilet PM, Benson CB, Bourne T, Blaivas M, Society of Radiologists in Ultrasound Multispecialty Panel on Early First Trimester Diagnosis of M, Exclusion of a Viable Intrauterine; and P, Barnhart KT, Benacerraf BR, Brown DL, Filly RA, Fox JC, Goldstein SR, Kendall JL, Lyons EA, Porter MB, Pretorius DH, Timor-Tritsch IE. Diagnostic criteria for nonviable pregnancy early in the first trimester. N Engl J Med 2013;369(15):1443-1451. https://doi.org/10.1056/NEJMra1302417.

In hemodynamically stable patients, follow-up ultrasonography and/or serial β-hCG are most helpful

INTRAUTERINE PREGNANCY AND BLEEDING

Perigestational hemorrhage (PGH) occurs in asymptomatic and bleeding first-trimester patients. Various methods of analysis have been used, including subjective size determination, percentage surrounding the GS, and volumetric analysis, but these do not statistically correlate with chance of early pregnancy loss. Measuring the perigestational hemorrhage as a percentage fracture of the GS is most predictive of early pregnancy loss.[5]

As the size of PGH increases as a percentage fraction of GS, the rate of demise increases.[5]

- PGH size less than or equal to 10% of GS equals 5.8% demise
- PGH size greater than 50% of GS equals 23.3% demise (**Fig. 1**)
- Earlier diagnosis of PGH portends a worse outcome

- Less than or equal to 8 weeks: 17.3% demise
- Greater than 8 weeks: 3.6% demise
- PGH in patients greater than or equal to 35 years old equals higher loss than more than 35 years old

INTRAUTERINE PREGNANCY AND PAIN

Pelvic pain in the presence of an IUP adds several additional causes to the differential, including ovarian torsion (covered in a separate article in this issue), ruptured corpus luteum/hemorrhagic follicular cyst, and (rarely) red degeneration of a leiomyoma.

- Ruptured ovarian cyst (corpus luteum/hemorrhagic follicular cyst)[6]
  - Often imaging overlaps between the two: similar presentations
  - Ultrasonography findings (**Fig. 2**, Video 1):
    - Ovarian lesion with complex internal echogenicities and increased through transmission; partially collapsed with thick, irregular wall

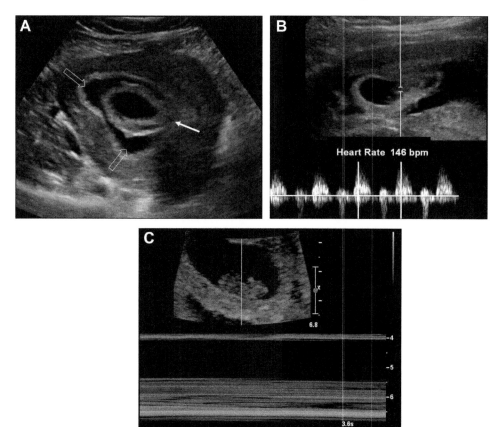

Fig. 1. Large perigestational hemorrhage and subsequent embryo demise. (*A*) The GS is barely attached to the uterus (*arrow*), surrounded by intrauterine blood (*open arrows*). (*B*) A living embryo was present. (*C*) On follow-up, there was embryo demise.

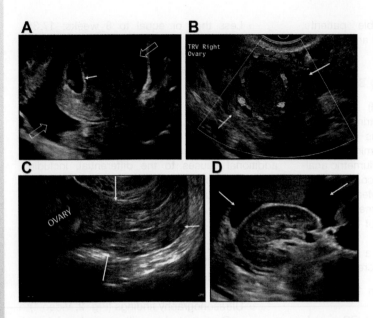

Fig. 2. Ruptured corpus luteum (CL) as cause of hemoperitoneum. (*A*) Transabdominal sagittal view of the uterus shows an IUP (*arrow*). However, the uterus is surrounded by fluid (*open arrows*). (*B*) Transvaginal ultrasonography of the right ovary (*arrows*) shows classic ring-of-fire color Doppler finding of a CL. (*C*) Adjacent to the ovary, there is a large heterogeneous masslike structure without flow, a blood clot in the adnexa. Subsequently, imaging of the upper abdomen was performed. (*D*) The hemorrhage extends to the right upper quadrant. Arrows point to blood anterior to the kidney.

- Early hemorrhage: blood can be anechoic
- First 24 hours: lacelike internal echogenicities
- Later: retracting clot with angular, curvilinear echogenic material
- While resolving: fluid-debris level during clot liquefaction
  - Computed tomography
    - Intermediate-density to high-density ovarian lesion (25–100 HU)
    - At rupture:
      - May have internal fluid/blood level
      - May be partially collapsed with irregular, thick wall
      - Hemoperitoneum, which can be extensive

TUBAL ECTOPIC PREGNANCY

Ectopic pregnancies account for 2% of all pregnancies, and approximately 90% are in the fallopian tube.[4,7] The prevalence of ectopic pregnancy in women presenting to the emergency department with pelvic pain, bleeding, or both is near 20%.[4,7,8] Severity of symptoms range from mild cramping and spotting to shock from internal hemorrhage. Ruptured ectopic pregnancy was the leading cause of hemorrhage-related mortality in pregnancy in 2011 to 2013.[9]

Risk Factors

Increased risk for tubal ectopic pregnancy (TEP) is associated with damage to the fallopian tube, although half of patients have no identifiable risk factors. The following risk factors are associated with TEP[4,8,10]:

- Prior pelvic inflammatory disease
- History of pelvic or tubal surgery
- Use of assisted reproductive technology (ART)
- History of prior TEP (10% chance for a second TEP, 25% chance of a third TEP)
- Indwelling intrauterine device (IUD) (53% incidence for TEP)

Imaging Technique

Transvaginal ultrasonography (TVUS) is the gold standard for imaging TEP.[4,11] However, all imaging should start with transabdominal ultrasonography (full bladder not required) in order to see whether there is a large mass or fluid extending into the abdomen, both of which can be missed with TVUS-only scanning.

Imaging protocols should include adequate documentation of the uterus and its contents, ovary, adnexa, and posterior cul-de-sac. Documentation of a dynamic examination using video clips/cine loops is recommended in order to show motion of structures in relation to each other. Probe pressure can aid in showing the relationship of adnexal masses to the ovary (ie, whether the mass moves with or separate from the ovary and uterus). External pressure with the nonscanning hand can be additive for this purpose as well.

Intrauterine Findings

The most reassuring sign that the patient does not have TEP is the presence of an IUP. However, uterine findings with TEP vary and include:

- Empty uterus with variable endometrial thickness
  - Thin empty endometrium
  - Diffusely echogenic endometrium from diffuse decidual reaction
  - Decidual cysts
    - Thin wall without peripheral flow (can mimic early IUP)
- Uterus with intracavitary blood
  - Diffusely distributed: endometrium distended by hypoechoic material
  - Focal collection: can mimic an IUP, so-called pseudosac
    - More centrally located than normal IUP
    - No yolk sac or embryo
    - Might move within endometrium with probe pressure
- Rarely, IUP can be seen along with TEP: heterotopic pregnancy[12,13]
  - Incidence of 1% in patients who have undergone in vitro fertilization
    - Otherwise, incidence is 1 in 4000 to 30,000
  - Look for TEP in symptomatic in vitro fertilization patients, even if IUP present

The adnexal findings with TEP can be divided into those that lead to a definitive diagnosis and those suggestive of the diagnosis[4,11,14,15]:

- Adnexal findings definitive of TEP
  - GS with yolk sac plus or minus embryo in adnexa
    - Separate from ovary
  - Document embryo cardiac activity if present
- Adnexal findings suspicious for TEP (more common) (**Fig. 3**, Video 2)
  - GS without yolk sac/embryo in adnexa, separate from ovary
    - Echogenic ringlike mass separate from ovary
    - Use probe pressure to show GS and ovary move separately
    - Find corpus luteum (CL) in ovary (often on same side as TEP)
    - GS echogenic wall is almost always brighter than CL
    - Color Doppler: ring-of-fire trophoblastic flow in TEP; however, CL may also have ring-of-fire peripheral flow appearance

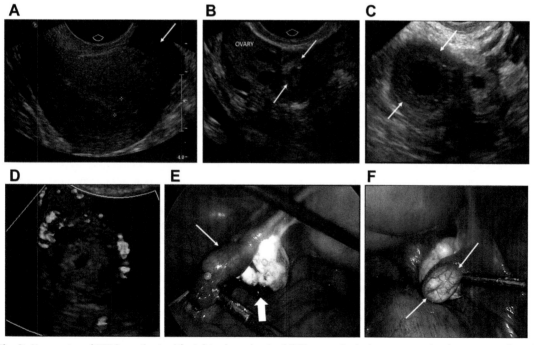

Fig. 3. Nonruptured TEP in patient with right adnexal pain. (*A*) Transvaginal ultrasonography shows a retroflexed uterus with thin endometrium (*calipers*) and surrounded by minimally complex pelvic fluid (*arrow*). (*B*) Adjacent to the right ovary there is an echogenic ring (*arrows*), the TEP (this shows the so-called sliding sign separate from the ovary). (*C*) Note that the tubal ectopic is more echogenic than the ovary and the CL (*arrows*). (*D*) Typical ring-of-fire peripheral flow is seen. This patient would have been a candidate for methotrexate (MTX) but opted for surgery. (*E*) Laparoscopic image shows a dilated intact fallopian tube (*arrow*) and a small amount of blood adherent to the right ovary (*thick arrow*). (*F*) The tube was incised and the intact GS (*arrows*) extracted.

- Pulse Doppler: high-velocity low-resistance flow in TEP, lower velocity and also low resistive flow in CL
- Nonspecific adnexal mass separate from ovary
  - Hematoma within dilated tube: small round, or tubular morphology
  - Ruptured tube with hematoma: large, any shape
  - Most often without vascular flow, although color Doppler may show otherwise hidden GS in blood clot
  - 80% positive predictive value as an isolated finding[15]
- Complex peritoneal fluid: pelvic fluid with echoes
  - Small amount of fluid is first seen in posterior cul-de-sac
    - Blood leaking from tube
    - Angle probe and look immediately posterior to cervix
  - Look in abdomen if large amount of fluid is seen in pelvis or large adnexal hematoma
    - Findings suggest ruptured TEP
- Differential diagnosis of adnexal findings: mimickers of TEP
  - CL: intact or ruptured
    - More hypoechoic than TEP
    - Hemorrhagic CL can contain echoes mimicking embryo
    - Moves with the ovary, not separate from ovary
    - When ruptured, can cause symptomatic hemoperitoneum
  - Paratubal cyst or hydrosalpinx
    - Thin-walled, anechoic, no peripheral blood flow
  - Endometrioma
    - Diffuse medium-level echoes, although decidualization with pregnancy causes heterogeneous appearance and internal flow

Management and Treatment

TEP is a nonviable pregnancy and management decisions depend on patient clinical status, history, and imaging findings. The options for treatment and management include medical, surgical, and surveillance.[4,16–18]

- Methotrexate (MTX) as medical treatment
  - MTX is a folate antagonist with cytotoxic effects on actively dividing cells (ie, trophoblasts)
  - Intramuscular injection is most common route

- Single-dose and multiple-dose protocols are described
  - Higher success rates with earlier TEP diagnosis
    - TEP less than 4 cm on ultrasonography
    - No embryo cardiac activity
    - hCG levels less than 5000 mIU/mL
  - Relative contraindications
    - Embryo cardiac activity
    - hCG level greater than 5000 mIU/mL
    - TEP greater than 4 cm
    - Patient does not accept blood transfusion
  - Absolute contraindications
    - Heterotopic pregnancy/IUP
    - Ruptured TEP
    - Hemodynamically unstable patient
    - Patient cannot participate in follow-up surveillance
    - Medical reason for MTX intolerance (ie, hepatic or renal disease)
  - Surveillance after MTX treatment
    - hCG followed until nonpregnant levels
      - hCG levels may initially increase but then progressively diminish
      - Should regress by at least 15% by 4 to 7 days after start of treatment
    - Ultrasonography surveillance is not routine
      - Imaging findings do not predict rupture or time to resolution
      - Initial findings may show a larger TEP even when treatment is successful
- Surgical treatment are salpingostomy (tube sparing) and salpingectomy (removal of tube)
  - No significant difference in rates of subsequent IUP with 2 different techniques
  - Salpingectomy preferred if severe tubal damage seen at time of surgery
  - hCG surveillance after salpingostomy recommended because residual trophoblastic tissue might be present
    - Prophylaxis with single-dose MTX after salpingostomy in some cases

NONTUBAL ABNORMALLY IMPLANTED PREGNANCY

Abnormally implanted pregnancies that are not in the fallopian tube account for less than 10% of all ectopic pregnancies. However, these pregnancies are associated with a disproportionately high incidence of maternal morbidity and mortality. The definition, causes, incidence, imaging characteristics, and treatment options for cesarean section scar pregnancy (CSSP), cervical ectopic pregnancy (CEP), interstitial pregnancy (IP) and angular pregnancy (AP), and ovarian ectopic pregnancy (OEP) are discussed here.

CESAREAN SECTION SCAR PREGNANCY
Definition

The GS implants on the area of dehiscence left behind after hysterotomy for cesarean delivery in a prior pregnancy. Implantation can be centrally located within the dehiscence/niche of the prior cesarean section scar or eccentrically, involving the area.[19–21] Note that a cesarean section scar pregnancy (CSSP) is potentially viable but highly associated with morbidly adherent placenta (MAP), also known as abnormally invasive placenta or placenta accreta spectrum (accreta, increta, percreta).

Two types of CSSP have been described[22] (Fig. 4):

- Type 1 is endogenic CSSP
  - GS progressing to the cervicoisthmic area (intrauterine)
  - Could result in a viable pregnancy
  - High risk for bleeding and MAP
- Type 2 is exogenic CSSP
  - GS progressing toward the maternal bladder and/or the abdominal cavity
  - High risk for uterine rupture and intraperitoneal hemorrhage

CSSP incidence[19–22]:

- Approximately 1 in 1700 pregnancies
- 1% to 3% of all ectopic pregnancies
- 6% of ectopic pregnancies in women with at least 1 prior cesarean section
- Mean gestational age at time of diagnosis is 7 ± 2.5 weeks

Presentation[22]:

- Low abdominal pain with or without bleeding in 25%

- One-third of cases are incidentally diagnosed and asymptomatic
- Uterine rupture is a rare presentation

Imaging Characteristics

In a nongravid uterus, the cesarean scar can be identified in 60% to 70% of cases and is a wedge-shaped or linear hypoechoic region in the lower uterine segment, seen best with TVUS or sonohysterography.[23] However, during pregnancy a CSSP is misdiagnosed in approximately 15% of cases.[22] Most often, the CSSP is thought to represent a normal IUP and its lower than expected location is not noticed by the sonographer because magnified images are obtained that focus only on the GS content (yolk sac, embryo, and so forth). Another cause for misdiagnosis is assuming that the low GS is an abortion in progress.[19]

Suggested ultrasonography criteria for the diagnosis or CSSP are[19–22]:

- Center of GS is lower than expected
  - Midpoint of GS is proximal to midpoint of uterus
    - GS is closer to cervical internal os than to fundus
  - Normal IUPs are located distal to midpoint of uterus
  - Criteria have shown sensitivity of 93% and specificity of 99%
- GS with triangular shape because it is implanted in triangular niche of cesarean scar
  - Early finding (<7 weeks)
- Difficult to differentiate type 1 from type 2 CSSP early in pregnancy
  - Asymmetric GS implantation with part of echogenic trophoblastic tissue in cesarean scar niche and otherwise growing toward fundus suggests type 1
  - Completely in the scar suggests type 2

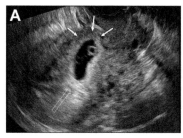 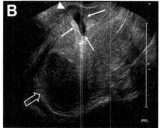

Fig. 4. Ectopic CSSP; endogenic (type 1) versus exogenic (type 2). (A) Sagittal transvaginal ultrasonography of an endogenic CSSP shows the GS partially implanted in the scar (arrows). The superior margin of the sac (open arrow) extends toward the fundus. (B) Sagittal transvaginal ultrasonography in another patient with exogenic CSSP shows the GS (arrows) fully implanted in the scar (arrows), bulging the outer contour of the uterus (arrowhead) as it extends toward the maternal bladder and not into the uterus (open arrow), which is filled with blood.

- Both with associated maternal morbidity but type 1 with chance for viable fetus
- Empty cervical canal
  - Differentiates CSSP from cervical ectopic or abortion in progress (both involve the cervical canal)
- Endometrium is otherwise empty of blood
  - Suspect diagnosis if most of intracavitary fluid is above a GS
- Doppler findings: typical peripheral trophoblastic flow seen on color Doppler
  - IUP in process of passing through lower uterine segment does not have flow
- Magnetic resonance (MR) imaging is helpful if ultrasonography is inconclusive; however, shown to be equally accurate

Prognosis

Untreated CSSP can lead to MAP (Fig. 5), uterine rupture, and hysterectomy. In a recent systemic review of patients with CSSP with embryo cardiac activity who continued the pregnancy, 15% required hysterectomy in the first or second trimester, 33% progressed to the third trimester, and 75% of those had MAP, usually percreta. In patients with CSSP without embryo cardiac activity, 69% had uncomplicated miscarriage.[19]

Treatment Options

The best treatment results for CSSP are with early and combined treatment with the goal of preserving fertility and preventing life-threatened complications.[22,24] In a recent systemic review of 751 cases of CSSP, 44% of patients had complications with treatment (most were severe) and the method with fewest complications was intragestational injection of MTX or KCl.[21]

Treatment options are as follows[19–25]:

- Systemic MTX (intramuscular route)
  - Single-dose or multiple-dose regimens necessary
  - Higher success rates associated with:
    - hCG level less than 12,000 mIU/mL, GA less than 8 weeks, no embryo cardiac activity
  - 25% to 30% fail treatment, 13% with complications
- Ultrasonography-guided injection of GS with MTX or KCl
  - Usually a single injection
    - 10% to 20% need 2 injections

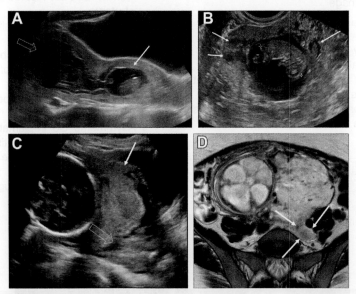

Fig. 5. Cesarean section scar ectopic in a patient with 2 prior cesarean sections. (A) The GS (arrow) containing a living embryo is located in the lower uterine segment. The uterus is otherwise distended with blood (open arrow points to fundus). (B) An otherwise normal early embryo (calipers) and prominent vessels (arrows) in the trophoblastic tissue of the GS seen on transvaginal images. The risk of uterine rupture and progression to MAP was discussed with the patient, who chose to continue the pregnancy. (C) Ultrasonography at 26 weeks shows placenta previa (open arrow points to placenta covering cervix) as well as focal loss of myometrium anteriorly, in expected area of cesarean section scar (arrow). (D) T2-weighted MR confirmed the finding in the anterior uterus (not shown) and in addition showed a focal posterior lateral percreta (arrows point to placenta extending beyond the margins of the uterus and into the parametrial fat).

○ 30% fail treatment

○ 17% need surgical intervention

- MTX (systemic or local) plus dilation and curettage (D&C)
  ○ Similar success rates to MTX alone
  ○ Look for myometrial thickness greater than 3.5 mm near bladder if this treatment is considered
- Hysteroscopy resection of CSSP
  ○ Considered primary treatment of type 1 CSSP
    ▪ Good visualization of GS and surrounding vessels, uterine wall
  ○ 3% complication rate
  ○ 17% need further intervention
- Laparoscopic resection of CSSP
  ○ For type 2 CSSP when GS growing toward bladder and abdominal cavity
  ○ Wedge resection of uterine wall usually necessary
- New minimally invasive treatment with cervical ripening balloon catheter[25]
  ○ Balloon at CSSP site compresses the GS
  ○ Ultrasonography surveillance performed
  ○ 37 cases reported and no complications[25]
- Uterine artery embolization (rarely used)
  ○ Adjuvant treatment to minimize bleeding and increase success rate of a primary treatment

Recommendation

All women with a prior cesarean delivery and a new pregnancy should undergo early TVUS assessment during the first trimester. CSSP should be specifically ruled out in these patients.

CERVICAL ECTOPIC PREGNANCY

Definition and presentation[26–28]:

- Implantation of fertilized ovum within the cervix, inferior to internal os
- CEP is not a viable pregnancy and must be treated

- Mean age of presentation: 7 to 8 weeks' gestation
- 85% present with vaginal bleeding

Incidence[26]:

- 1 in 20,000 pregnancies
- Less than 1% of all ectopic pregnancies

Risk Factors

Risk factors include any history that would lead to poor uterine implantation[27]:

- IUD in place
- Embryo transfer via ART
- Cervical or uterine anomalies
- Uterine myoma
- Uterine scarring (curettage history, cesarean section, Asherman syndrome)

Imaging Characteristics

TVUS is gold standard for diagnosis and MR is rarely needed. [28]

- Empty uterine cavity with enlarged cervix (**Fig. 6**)
  ○ Cervix is ballooned compared with uterine cavity
  ○ Hour-glass appearance of uterus
- Closed internal os
  ○ No sliding sign of detached IUP going through cervix
- Entire chorionic sac is below internal os
  ○ Typical echogenic ring of a GS
  ○ Shows blood flow on color Doppler

Prognosis[27]:

- With accurate and early diagnosis, treatments are often successful
- Failed treatment or late diagnosis leads to hysterectomy
  ○ Cervix has well-developed blood supply and muscles lack contracting properties

A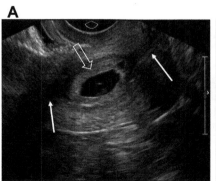

B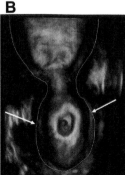

Fig. 6. CEP at 6 weeks. (*A*) Sagittal transvaginal ultrasonography of cervix shows the entire GS (*open arrow*) below the internal os and in the cervical canal (*arrows*). (*B*) Coronal three-dimensional (3D) ultrasonography shows a ballooned bulbous cervix (*arrows*) leading to a hour-glass appearance of the uterus (*outlined*).

○ Late diagnosis or misdiagnosis may result in massive hemorrhage
○ Hysterectomy rate less than 2%

Treatment strategies depend on sonographic findings and patient status[26,28]:

- Expectant management plus or minus systemic MTX for stable low-risk patients with low or decreasing hCG levels
- Sonographic findings associated with lower chance of success with systemic treatment alone:
  ○ GA greater than 9 weeks
  ○ Embryo CRL greater than 10 mm
  ○ Embryo with cardiac activity
- Ultrasonography-guided intra-GS injection considered for more advanced CEP:
  ○ Injection of MTX, prostaglandin, or KCl
  ○ Often in combination with systemic intramuscular MTX
- Treatment surveillance with ultrasonography and serial hCG levels is important after treatment
- Surgical treatment might be necessary:
  ○ Hemodynamic unstable patients
  ○ Failed minimally invasive treatment
  ○ Techniques include D&C and hysteroscopic resection of CEP

INTERSTITIAL/CORNUAL PREGNANCY AND ANGULAR PREGNANCY
Definition of Terms

Cornual pregnancy and IP terminology is mixed in the literature.[26,28,29] In addition, historically, the term cornual pregnancy was often used to describe a diagnosis only in women with müllerian duct anomalies, such as bicornuate or septate uterus. Therefore, the preferred term for the purpose of this article is IP, and several investigators have recommended avoiding the term cornual pregnancy altogether.

The definition of IP is one in which implantation occurs in the interstitial (intramural) segment of the fallopian tube, the 1-cm to 2-cm medial part of the fallopian tube that runs in the interstitial portion of the uterus.

An AP is an eccentric IUP located in the upper lateral uterus, near the ostia of the fallopian tube. The original classification for AP was surgical and defined as an eccentric pregnancy that displaced the round ligament upward and outward as seen at the time of surgery. However, the key difference with IP is that the GS is intrauterine.

Pathophysiology

Interstitial pregnancy occurs in the same high-risk patient population as tubal ectopic pregnancy.
Incidence[30]:

- 2% to 4% of all ectopic pregnancies are IPs
- However, mortality of 2% to 2.5% is 2 to 5 times higher than with TEP

Imaging Characteristics for Interstitial Pregnancy and Angular Pregnancy

Ultrasonography usually is the first and only modality necessary for diagnosis. Three-dimensional (3D) ultrasonography is helpful for showing the anatomic relationship of the GS with the endometrium and myometrium in multiple planes.
IP findings (**Figs. 7** and **8**, Video 3):

- Key finding: the pregnancy is extraendometrial
- Interstitial line sign[31]
  ○ Echogenic line in cornual region of uterus extends to midportion of GS
  ○ Represents the interstitial portion of the tube in small IPs and the endometrium in larger pregnancies

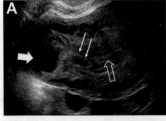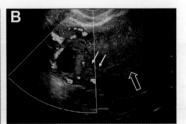

Fig. 7. Interstitial line seen in a 6-weeks IP implantation. (*A*) Axial transvaginal ultrasonography of the right uterus shows an eccentric lateral GS (*big arrow*), an empty endometrium (*open arrow*), and a subtle echogenic line (*arrows*) representing the interstitial line, between the two. (*B*) Color Doppler image at the same level shows typical peripheral trophoblastic vascularity of the interstitial implanted GS as well as the interstitial line (*arrows*) extending from the endometrium (*open arrows*) to the sac. This pregnancy was treated with ultrasonography-guided MTX injection.

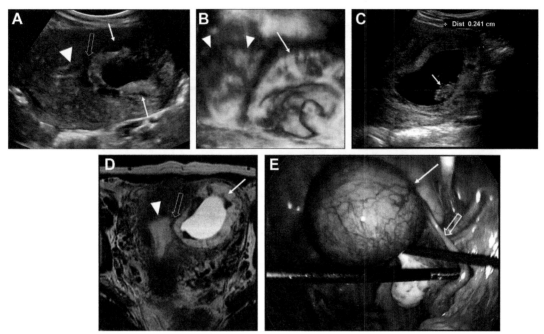

Fig. 8. IP at gestational age 8 weeks. (*A*) Axial transvaginal ultrasonography shows an eccentric left lateral GS (*arrows*) separate from the endometrium (*arrowhead*) by intervening hypoechoic myometrium (*open arrow*). (*B*) Coronal 3D ultrasonography confirms the suspicion that the GS (*arrow*) is separate from the endometrium (arrowheads point to fundus of normal triangular endometrium). No evidence for uterine duplication anomaly was seen. (*C*) Coronal ultrasonography of the GS shows an embryo (*arrow*) that had cardiac activity (not shown) as well as only 2.4 mm of left lateral myometrial coverage (*calipers*). The ultrasonography findings are diagnostic for IP; however, MR was obtained because this was a highly desirable pregnancy and the referring team wanted to rule out an AP. (*D*) T2-weighted coronal MR confirms the left IP (*arrow*) separate from the endometrium (*arrowhead*), with intervening medial myometrium (*open arrow*). (*E*) Laparoscopic image shows the cornual bulge of the pregnancy (*arrow*) separate from the fallopian tube (*open arrow*). This IP was treated with cornual wedge resection.

○ Interstitial line sign has a reported sensitivity of 80% and specificity of 98%
- Myometrium less than 5 mm and eccentric GS less than 1 cm from lateral wall of uterine cavity[32]
  ○ 88% to 93% specificity but only 40% sensitivity

AP findings (**Fig. 9**):

- Key: GS is within the endometrium, at the angle (an eccentric IUP)

Role of Magnetic Resonance

Helpful for difficult cases with primary goal to show relationship of GS to endometrium[29]

- MR findings with IP:
  ○ GS predominantly surrounded by myometrium (hypointense on T2)
  ○ Junctional zone intact (secondary finding)
- MR findings with AP:
  ○ GS predominantly surrounded by endometrium (hyperintense on T2)

Prognosis:

- IPs are not viable and if pregnancy is not treated there is high risk for uterine rupture[29]
- APs are potentially viable but are also considered high risk[33]
  ○ 38.5% rate of pregnancy failure
  ○ 13.6% rate of uterine rupture

Management:

AP management[34]:
- Careful surveillance in asymptomatic or minimally symptomatic patients
- Therapeutic abortion:
  ○ Intrauterine approach with ultrasonography guidance almost always successful because of the intrauterine location of the GS
IP management:
- Laparoscopic surgery is the most common approach[34]
  ○ Wedge resection of cornua for smaller IPs
  ○ Cornuostomy for larger IPs
- Successful medical treatment of smaller IPs has been reported[26,35]

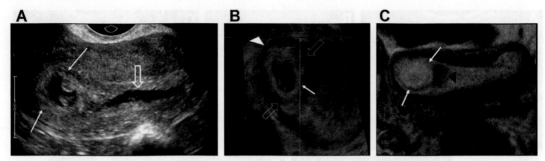

Fig. 9. AP at gestational age 7 weeks in patient presenting with bleeding. (*A*) Axial transvaginal ultrasonography shows an eccentric GS (*arrows*) and adjacent blood (*open arrow*) in the endometrial cavity. (*B*) Coronal 3D ultrasonography shows the sac (*arrow*) is located in the right cornual region but is surrounded by endometrium (*open arrows*) with thin lateral myometrial coverage (*arrowhead*). (*C*) T2-weighted MR confirms an intrauterine, albeit eccentric, GS (*arrows*) surrounded by the T2-hyperintense endometrium. A small blood clot (*arrowhead*) is seen attached to the sac. This desired pregnancy was monitored and failed at 9 weeks.

- o Single dose of intramuscular MTX
- o Not recommended if there is a living embryo
- Ultrasonography-guided injections of KCl or MTX[36]
- If hCG levels are decreasing spontaneously, watchful waiting might also be pursued[26,29,35]

OVARIAN ECTOPIC PREGNANCY
Definition

Implantation of GS within or on the surface of the ovary.[26]

Pathophysiology

Two mechanisms described[37]:

- Direct fertilization of ovum inside ovary
- Retrograde migration of fertilized ovum from fallopian tube to ovary

Epidemiology[26,38]:

- 3.6% of all ectopic pregnancies (1:7000 - 1:40000 pregnancies)

- Higher incidence in women using ART (6% of all ectopics if in vitro fertilization pregnancy)
- Use of IUDs and presence of endometriosis have also been implicated as risk factors
  - o In Ge and colleagues'[39] 2019 series of 12 OEPs, 33% had IUDs, 33% infertility, 25% endometriosis, and 16.6% with no known risk factors

Presentation[26,37–39]:

- Adnexal mass, adnexal pain
- Minimal vaginal bleeding
- Massive intraperitoneal bleeding and hypovolemic shock from rupture
  - o Early rupture common because tunica albuginea lacks muscle fibers and central ovary has loose connective tissue and rich vascularity

Imaging characteristics and challenges:

- Challenges:
  - o CL diagnosed as OEP (overdiagnosis)

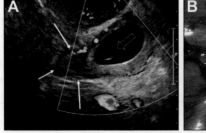
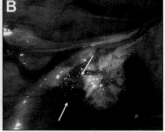

Fig. 10. OEP on surface of ovary in patient presenting with right adnexal pain. (*A*) On transvaginal ultrasonography of the right ovary (*arrows*), a GS with a yolk sac and living embryo is seen (*open arrow*). The ovarian tissue surrounds the sac and intraovarian ectopic pregnancy was suspected. (*B*) At laparoscopy, the GS was located between the fimbria of the fallopian tube and the ovary, and, after removal, residual trophoblastic tissue was present on the ovary surface (*arrows*).

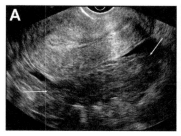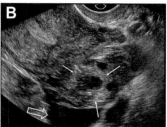

Fig. 11. OEP with rupture in patient presenting with severe abdominal pain and hypotension. (A) Transvaginal sagittal ultrasonography shows an empty uterus and large blood clot in the posterior cul-de-sac (arrows). (B) Transvaginal axial image of the left ovary shows an echogenic ring in the ovary (arrows) surrounded by follicles and free fluid (open arrow) adjacent to the ovary. This appearance is most often seen with a CL, and the scan was appropriately read as pregnancy of unknown location. The patient went for laparoscopy because of her unstable condition. The left ovary was removed and pathology confirmed an OEP.

- ■ CL internal debris may be misdiagnosed as yolk sac or embryo
  - ○ OEP diagnosed as CL (underdiagnosis)
  - ○ OEP diagnosed as distal tubal pregnancy (underdiagnosis)
- • Key sonographic features of OEP (Figs. 10 and 11)
  - ○ GS within or on the surface of the ovary
  - ○ Echogenic ring of GS is formed by trophoblastic tissue and is more echogenic than CL[39,40]
  - ○ OEP may contain yolk sac and embryo

Treatment[39]:

- • Nonruptured OEP typically treated with operative laparoscopy and ovarian wedge resection
- • Medical management with MTX rare; most cases go to laparoscopy for definitive diagnosis and treatment
- • Postoperative MTX indicated in cases of persistent trophoblastic tissue
- • Ruptured OEPs require laparoscopy, laparotomy, and often oophorectomy

SUMMARY

Ultrasonography is often the only modality needed to differentiate between the different causes of first-trimester pain and bleeding. When an IUP is definitively seen, then the question of viability can often be answered with high-quality imaging and an understanding of measurement criteria. When an IUP is not present, then the possibility of an abnormally implanted gestation should be seriously entertained. Although most ectopic pregnancies are in the fallopian tube, the nontubal implantations are associated with an unusually high incidence of maternal morbidity. Attention to the imaging findings described enables clinicians to make accurate diagnoses of these rarer abnormally implanted pregnancies as well.

DISCLOSURE

The authors have nothing to disclose.

SUPPLEMENTARY DATA

Supplementary data related to this article can be found online at https://doi.org/10.1016/j.rcl.2019.11.003.

REFERENCES

1. ACOG practice bulletin No. 200: early pregnancy loss. Obstet Gynecol 2018;132(5):e197–207.
2. Rodgers SK, Chang C, DeBardeleben JT, et al. Normal and abnormal US findings in early first-trimester pregnancy: review of the Society of Radiologists in Ultrasound 2012 Consensus Panel Recommendations. Radiographics 2015;35(7):2135–48.
3. Doubilet PM, Benson CB, Bourne T, et al, Society of Radiologists in Ultrasound Multispecialty Panel on Early First Trimester Diagnosis of Miscarriage and Exclusion of a Viable Intrauterine Pregnancy. Diagnostic criteria for nonviable pregnancy early in the first trimester. N Engl J Med 2013;369(15):1443–51.
4. ACOG practice bulletin No. 193 summary: tubal ectopic pregnancy. Obstet Gynecol 2018;131(3):613–5.
5. Heller HT, Asch EA, Durfee SM, et al. Subchorionic hematoma: correlation of grading techniques with first-trimester pregnancy outcome. J Ultrasound Med 2018;37(7):1725–32.
6. Potter AW, Chandrasekhar CA. US and CT evaluation of acute pelvic pain of gynecologic origin in nonpregnant premenopausal patients. Radiographics 2008;28(6):1645–59.
7. From the Centers for Disease Control and Prevention. Ectopic pregnancy–United States, 1990-1992. JAMA 1995;273(7):533. Available at: https://www.ncbi.nlm.nih.gov/pubmed/7837386.
8. Barnhart KT, Sammel MD, Gracia CR, et al. Risk factors for ectopic pregnancy in women with

symptomatic first-trimester pregnancies. Fertil Steril 2006;86(1):36–43.

9. Creanga AA, Syverson C, Seed K, et al. Pregnancy-related mortality in the United States, 2011-2013. Obstet Gynecol 2017;130(2):366–73.

10. Backman T, Rauramo I, Huhtala S, et al. Pregnancy during the use of levonorgestrel intrauterine system. Am J Obstet Gynecol 2004;190(1):50–4.

11. Wang PS, Rodgers SK, Horrow MM. Ultrasound of the first trimester. Radiol Clin North Am 2019;57(3):617–33.

12. Barrenetxea G, Barinaga-Rementeria L, Lopez de Larruzea A, et al. Heterotopic pregnancy: two cases and a comparative review. Fertil Steril 2007;87(2):417.e9-15.

13. Maymon R, Shulman A. Controversies and problems in the current management of tubal pregnancy. Hum Reprod Update 1996;2(6):541–51.

14. Barnhart K, van Mello NM, Bourne T, et al. Pregnancy of unknown location: a consensus statement of nomenclature, definitions, and outcome. Fertil Steril 2011;95(3):857–66.

15. Barnhart KT, Fay CA, Suescum M, et al. Clinical factors affecting the accuracy of ultrasonography in symptomatic first-trimester pregnancy. Obstet Gynecol 2011;117(2 Pt 1):299–306.

16. Cheng X, Tian X, Yan Z, et al. Comparison of the fertility outcome of salpingotomy and salpingectomy in women with tubal pregnancy: a systematic review and meta-analysis. PLoS One 2016;11(3):e0152343.

17. Practice Committee of American Society for Reproductive Medicine. Medical treatment of ectopic pregnancy: a committee opinion. Fertil Steril 2013;100(3):638–44.

18. Stovall TG, Ling FW. Single-dose methotrexate: an expanded clinical trial. Am J Obstet Gynecol 1993;168(6 Pt 1):1759–62 [discussion: 1762–55].

19. Cali G, Timor-Tritsch IE, Palacios-Jaraquemada J, et al. Outcome of cesarean scar pregnancy managed expectantly: systematic review and meta-analysis. Ultrasound Obstet Gynecol 2018;51(2):169–75.

20. Kaelin Agten A, Cali G, Monteagudo A, et al. The clinical outcome of cesarean scar pregnancies implanted "on the scar" versus "in the niche". Am J Obstet Gynecol 2017;216(5):510.e1-e6.

21. Timor-Tritsch IE, Monteagudo A, Bennett TA, et al. A new minimally invasive treatment for cesarean scar pregnancy and cervical pregnancy. Am J Obstet Gynecol 2016;215(3):351.e1-8.

22. Gonzalez N, Tulandi T. Cesarean scar pregnancy: a systematic review. J Minim Invasive Gynecol 2017;24(5):731–8.

23. Rasheedy R, Sammour H, Elkholy A, et al. Agreement between transvaginal ultrasound and saline contrast sonohysterography in evaluation of cesarean scar defect. J Gynecol Obstet Hum Reprod 2019. https://doi.org/10.1016/j.jogoh.2019.05.013.

24. Birch Petersen K, Hoffmann E, Rifbjerg Larsen C, et al. Cesarean scar pregnancy: a systematic review of treatment studies. Fertil Steril 2016;105(4):958–67.

25. Monteagudo A, Cali G, Rebarber A, et al. Minimally invasive treatment of cesarean scar and cervical pregnancies using a cervical ripening double balloon catheter: expanding the clinical series. J Ultrasound Med 2019;38(3):785–93.

26. Alalade AO, Smith FJE, Kendall CE, et al. Evidence-based management of non-tubal ectopic pregnancies. J Obstet Gynaecol 2017;37(8):982–91.

27. Cipullo L, Cassese S, Fasolino L, et al. Cervical pregnancy: a case series and a review of current clinical practice. Eur J Contracept Reprod Health Care 2008;13(3):313–9.

28. Dibble EH, Lourenco AP. Imaging unusual pregnancy implantations: rare ectopic pregnancies and more. AJR Am J Roentgenol 2016;207(6):1380–92.

29. Arleo EK, DeFilippis EM. Cornual, interstitial, and angular pregnancies: clarifying the terms and a review of the literature. Clin Imaging 2014;38(6):763–70.

30. Moawad NS, Mahajan ST, Moniz MH, et al. Current diagnosis and treatment of interstitial pregnancy. Am J Obstet Gynecol 2010;202(1):15–29.

31. Ackerman TE, Levi CS, Dashefsky SM, et al. Interstitial line: sonographic finding in interstitial (cornual) ectopic pregnancy. Radiology 1993;189(1):83–7.

32. Timor-Tritsch IE, Monteagudo A, Matera C, et al. Sonographic evolution of cornual pregnancies treated without surgery. Obstet Gynecol 1992;79(6):1044–9. Available at: https://www.ncbi.nlm.nih.gov/pubmed/1579304.

33. Jansen RP, Elliott PM. Angular intrauterine pregnancy. Obstet Gynecol 1981;58(2):167–75. Available at: https://www.ncbi.nlm.nih.gov/pubmed/7254728.

34. Cucinella G, Calagna G, Rotolo S, et al. Interstitial pregnancy: a 'road map' of surgical treatment based on a systematic review of the literature. Gynecol Obstet Invest 2014;78(3):141–9.

35. Jermy K, Thomas J, Doo A, et al. The conservative management of interstitial pregnancy. BJOG 2004;111(11):1283–8.

36. Monteagudo A, Minior VK, Stephenson C, et al. Non-surgical management of live ectopic pregnancy with ultrasound-guided local injection: a case series. Ultrasound Obstet Gynecol 2005;25(3):282–8.

37. Ishikawa H, Sanada M, Shozu M. Ovarian pregnancy associated with a fresh blastocyst transfer following in vitro fertilization. J Obstet Gynaecol Res 2015;41(11):1823–5.

38. Joseph RJ, Irvine LM. Ovarian ectopic pregnancy: aetiology, diagnosis, and challenges in surgical management. J Obstet Gynaecol 2012;32(5): 472–4.

39. Ge L, Sun W, Wang L, et al. Ultrasound classification and clinical analysis of ovarian pregnancy: a study of 12 cases. J Gynecol Obstet Hum Reprod 2019. https://doi.org/10.1016/j.jogoh.2019.04.003.

40. Comstock C, Huston K, Lee W. The ultrasonographic appearance of ovarian ectopic pregnancies. Obstet Gynecol 2005;105(1):42–5.

Nonfetal Imaging During Pregnancy
Acute Abdomen/Pelvis

Courtney C. Moreno, MD[a],*, Pardeep K. Mittal, MD[b], Frank H. Miller, MD[c]

KEYWORDS

- Magnetic resonance imaging • Pregnancy • Computed tomography • Abdominal pain
- Acute appendicitis

KEY POINTS

- Determining the cause of abdominal pain in pregnant women can be challenging because of anatomic changes that make physical examination findings less reliable.
- Noncontrast magnetic resonance imaging is increasingly performed to evaluate for causes of acute abdominal pain in pregnant women, either as the first-line test or as a second-line test following ultrasonography.
- Accurately determining the cause of abdominal pain in pregnant women is important so that timely treatment can be initiated to benefit the mother and the fetus.
- The imaging appearances of common causes of abdominal pain are reviewed with example images provided.

INTRODUCTION

Abdominal pain is a common occurrence in pregnant women, and potential causes range from those specific to pregnancy (eg, round ligament pain in the first trimester; contractions in later stages of pregnancy) to the wide range of disorders that are not specific to pregnancy but can also cause abdominal pain in men and women who are not pregnant (eg, acute appendicitis, cholecystitis, nephrolithiasis). However, physical examination findings may be less reliable, especially in later stages of pregnancy, because of changes in anatomy that occur as the fetus grows and the uterus enlarges. For example, the cecum and appendix may be pushed from the right lower quadrant to the right upper quadrant by the enlarging uterus, thus confounding the physical examination in a pregnant woman with clinically suspected acute appendicitis.[1]

In addition, physiologic changes result in symptoms that are considered normal during pregnancy, including nausea and vomiting in the first trimester and gastroesophageal reflux and constipation in later stages of pregnancy, but overlap with symptoms of more concerning causes of abdominal pain. Furthermore, normal physiologic changes of pregnancy, such as an increase in the pregnant woman's white blood cell count and mild anemia, may also confound the diagnosis of intra-abdominal disorder.[2]

Prompt and accurate diagnosis of the cause of abdominal pain in pregnancy is important so that appropriate management can be initiated for the health of the pregnant woman and the fetus. Recent years have seen a shift toward noncontrast

[a] Department of Radiology and Imaging Sciences, Emory University School of Medicine, 1364-A Clifton Road Northeast Suite AT-627, Atlanta, GA 30327, USA; [b] Department of Radiology, Medical College of Georgia, 1120 15th Street, BA-1411, Augusta, GA 30912, USA; [c] Body Imaging Section and Fellowship, MRI, Department of Radiology, Northwestern University Feinberg School of Medicine, 676 North Saint Clair, Suite 800, Chicago, IL 60611, USA
* Corresponding author.
E-mail address: courtney.moreno@emoryhealthcare.org

Radiol Clin N Am 58 (2020) 363–380
https://doi.org/10.1016/j.rcl.2019.10.005
0033-8389/20/© 2019 Elsevier Inc. All rights reserved.

magnetic resonance (MR) imaging for the evaluation of pregnant women with abdominal pain, either as a secondary test following an inconclusive ultrasonography scan or as the primary test for some indications, such as acute appendicitis.[3] This article presents a general approach to the imaging evaluation of pregnant women with abdominal pain and then reviews the imaging findings of a variety of causes of abdominal pain with an emphasis on MR imaging.

IMAGING APPROACH

If a pregnant woman presents with localizing abdominal pain and the differential diagnosis is narrow (eg, acute cholecystitis), ultrasonography could be performed as the first-line test because it is readily available, rapidly performed, inexpensive, and does not expose the fetus or mother to ionizing radiation.[4] Ultrasonography is reasonably accurate for diagnosing some causes of abdominal pain, such as hydronephrosis[5] or acute cholecystitis.[6] In centers with expertise, ultrasonography may the first-line test to assess for acute appendicitis in pregnant women.[7]

When ultrasonography is inconclusive or does not identify a cause of acute abdominal pain, or if the mother's symptoms are nonlocalizing and the differential diagnosis is broad, noncontrast MR imaging is the preferred modality because it also does not expose the fetus or mother to ionizing radiation and provides a comprehensive analysis of the abdomen and pelvis. In addition, noncontrast MR imaging may be the preferred test to evaluate for acute appendicitis in some institutions based on institutional expertise.[7] Noncontrast MR imaging is not associated with increased harm to the fetus or in early childhood.[8] On the contrary, gadolinium administered at any time during pregnancy was found to be associated with an increased risk of stillbirth, neonatal death, and rheumatological, inflammatory, and infiltrative skin conditions.[8] Given these recent data and theoretic concerns from prior animal studies, gadolinium use should be limited to rare situations in which benefits clearly outweigh the potential risks.[4]

A sample noncontrast MR protocol is provided in Box 1. T1-weighted sequences are helpful for general anatomic assessment and for the identification of blood products that, depending on age, may show high signal intensity on T1-weighted imaging. T2-weighted sequences, including MR cholangiopancreatography (MRCP), are helpful to assess for disorders related to fluid-containing structures (eg, choledocholithiasis, hydronephrosis). Thick-slab

---

> **Box 1**
> **Sample noncontrast magnetic resonance protocol for assessment of abdominal pain in pregnant women.**
>
> T2 (single shot; eg, half-Fourier acquisition single shot turbo spin echo [HASTE]/single shot fast spin echo [SSFSE]) axial and coronal, abdomen and pelvis
>
> T2 (single shot; eg, HASTE/SSFSE) sagittal pelvis
>
> T2 with fat saturation (single shot; eg, HASTE/SSFSE) axial and coronal, abdomen and pelvis
>
> MR cholangiopancreatography (thick slab and thin cuts)
>
> T1 with fat saturation gradient echo axial and coronal, abdomen and pelvis
>
> In-phase and opposed-phase axial abdomen and pelvis
>
> Diffusion-weighted abdomen and pelvis
>
> Steady-state free precession abdomen plus/minus pelvis

MRCP images provide an overview of the biliary system, whereas thin slices are helpful to assess for intraductal stones, which can be obscured by thick-slab volumetric techniques or maximum intensity projection images from three-dimensional MRCP. T2-weighted sequences with fat saturation are key to assess for inflammation because the fluid signal intensity of inflammation is more conspicuous against a background of low-signal-intensity fat. In-phase images are helpful to assess for susceptibility artifacts. For example, the identification of blooming air within the appendix can help when trying to find the appendix on MR. Opposed-phase images are helpful to assess for fat-water interfaces and fat-containing structures such as dermoids or renal angiomyolipomas. Diffusion-weighted images are helpful to highlight areas of inflammation, abscesses, and tumors.

In the setting of trauma, the risk/benefit profile of computed tomography (CT) may warrant performing a CT examination for pregnant women, with special attention to achieving a CT dose that is as low as is reasonably achievable. Because CT is typically more readily available and is performed with faster image acquisition times compared with MR, CT is often the preferred imaging modality for pregnant women who have experienced trauma. According to the America College of Obstetricians and Gynecologists, if CT is necessary in addition to ultrasonography or MR, or is more readily available for the diagnosis in question, it should not be withheld from pregnant women.[4] Although iodinated contrast material crosses the placenta and enters the fetal circulation or amniotic fluid, it has not been shown to have mutagenic or teratogenic effects or adverse effects on the fetal thyroid.[4]

ACUTE APPENDICITIS

Acute appendicitis is the most common indication for nonobstetric surgery in pregnant women.[9] Accurately diagnosing acute appendicitis in pregnant women is challenging because of anatomic changes rendering physical examination findings less reliable and physiologic changes in hematologic parameters such as the normal increase in serum white blood cell count that occurs in pregnant women. Accurate diagnosis is important because of the risk of fetal loss,[10] which is greater for complicated (6% fetal loss) versus simple (2%) appendicitis.[11] In addition, a negative appendectomy (defined as removal of a normal appendix in a patient suspected of having acute appendicitis) is also associated with an increased risk of fetal loss.[11]

In centers with expertise, ultrasonography may be the first-line test to diagnose acute appendicitis in pregnant women because CT (the current first-line test in patients who are not pregnant) would expose the fetus to ionizing radiation. Ultrasonography is performed with graded compression, and a noncompressible blind-ending tubular structure that measures 7 mm or more in diameter is diagnostic of acute appendicitis (Fig. 1).[12,13]

However, the appendix is not always identifiable with ultrasonography, and may not be identifiable in up to 97% of pregnant women during the second and third trimesters.[13] However, if the appendix is visible and diagnostic criteria for acute appendicitis are met, the positive predictive value of ultrasonography is high (94%).[14] However, the negative predictive value of ultrasonography is low (40%), and, if the appendix is not visualized with confidence, additional testing with noncontrast MR should be pursued.[14]

MR is increasingly performed to evaluate pregnant women with suspected acute appendicitis either as the second-line test following inconclusive ultrasonography or as the first-line test. In a 2014 survey sent to the membership of the Association of University Radiologists, the Association of Program Directors in Radiology, and the Society of Radiologists in Ultrasound, 73% of respondents reported using MR imaging to evaluate for suspected acute appendicitis after an inconclusive ultrasonography scan in the first trimester and 67% in the third trimester, compared with 46% and 29% in a survey conducted in 2007.[15]

T1-weighted and T2-weighted sequences are used to locate the appendix. Inflammatory changes are most conspicuous on T2-weighted images obtained with fat saturation (Figs. 2 and 3). The accuracy of MR imaging for the diagnosis of acute appendicitis in pregnant women is 88% to 99%[16–19] with 60% to 100% sensitivity, 92% to 100% specificity, 92% to 100% positive predictive value, and 94% to 100% negative predictive value.[16–20]

The appendix is visualized at MR in 60% to 76% of pregnant women with suspected acute appendicitis and may be more difficult to see in later stages of pregnancy.[21,22] In a series of 233 pregnant women with suspected appendicitis, a nonvisualized appendix or lack of inflammatory findings reliably excluded the diagnosis of acute appendicitis with high interradiologist agreement.[23] In an evaluation of 58 pregnant women with suspected appendicitis, no patients with a nonvisualized appendix were ultimately diagnosed with acute appendicitis.[21]

Alternative causes of abdominal pain are identifiable in 24% to 44% of MR examinations performed to assess for acute appendicitis,

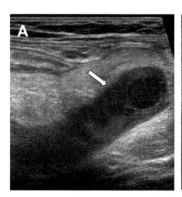
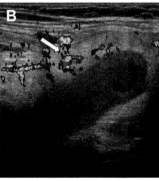

Fig. 1. Acute appendicitis. (A) Grayscale ultrasonography image shows a dilated, thick-walled, blind-ending, and noncompressible tubular structure in the right lower quadrant compatible with an inflamed appendix (arrow). Color Doppler ultrasonography image (B) shows associated hyperemia (arrow).

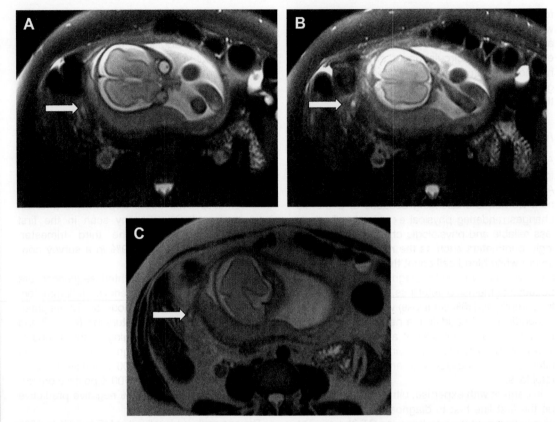

Fig. 2. Acute appendicitis. (*A*, *B*) Axial T2-weighted images obtained with fat saturation show inflammatory changes around the appendix (*arrows*). (*C*) Axial T2-weighted image without fat saturation shows the appendix (*arrow*), but inflammatory changes are much less conspicuous in this image without fat saturation.

including hydronephrosis, degenerating fibroid, cholelithiasis, and pyelonephritis.[18,21] In an evaluation of 79 pregnant women of whom 31 underwent MR imaging and 34 had pathology-confirmed appendicitis, patients who underwent MR had shorter length of stay (33.7 vs 64.8 hours, *P*<.001) but clinical outcomes and hospital charges were not affected.[24] MR was more cost-effective than CT imaging in a decision-

analytical model analyzing preoperative imaging strategies for pregnant women in the second or third trimester of pregnancy after an indeterminate ultrasonography scan.[25] The integration of MR imaging into the evaluation of pregnant women with suspected acute appendicitis resulted in a reduction of the negative laparotomy rate from 55% to 21% without a change in the perforation rate.[26]

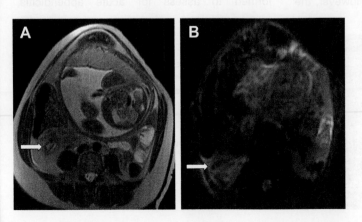

Fig. 3. Acute appendicitis. (*A*) Axial T2-weighted MR image shows a fluid-filled, dilated appendix (*arrow*) with periappendiceal fluid. (*B*) Axial T2-weighted image with fat saturation shows periappendiceal edema (*arrow*).

CHOLELITHIASIS

Acute cholecystitis is the second most common indication for nonobstetric surgery in pregnant women.[9] Gallstone formation is more common during pregnancy because of estrogen-related effects, including the formation of cholesterol-supersaturated bile and reduced gallbladder motility.[27]

Ultrasonography is the first-line imaging test to evaluate for acute cholecystitis.[28] Imaging findings of acute cholecystitis include gallbladder wall thickening (>3 mm), pericholecystic fluid, and a positive sonographic Murphy sign.[29] In a meta-analysis, the sensitivity and specificity of ultrasonography for the diagnosis of acute cholecystitis were 88% and 80%, respectively.[30] A pitfall is that gallbladder wall thickening can also be caused by chronic cholecystitis, liver disease, renal disease, and heart disease. Also, the sonographic Murphy sign may be unreliable if the patient has received pain medication before imaging.

As a general rule, the bile duct normally measures up to 5 mm in diameter up to age 50 years, with an additional 1 mm in diameter increase considered normal per decade beyond age 50 years.[31] A dilated bile duct may indicate a more distal gallstone within the duct or other obstructing lesion. MRCP is the preferred test to evaluate for choledocholithiasis, especially if not seen on ultrasonography. On MRCP, gallstones appear as rounded or angular geometric areas of low signal intensity (Fig. 4). The sensitivity and specificity of MRCP for choledocholithiasis are 93% and 96%, respectively.[32] Pitfalls include mistaking low signal intensity related to cholecystectomy clips in a slab MRCP image or flow-related artifact in thin-slice T2-weighted images for stricture or stones. Thin-cut MRCP images are helpful to localize stones, and steady-state images are helpful to confirm that an area of low signal intensity is a stone and not a flow void with low signal intensity.

Endoscopic ultrasonography and endoscopic retrograde cholangiopancreatography (ERCP) and cholecystectomy can be safely performed in pregnant women.[33] By comparison, conservative management of cholelithiasis and its complications is associated with frequent emergency department visits and recurrent biliary symptoms.[33]

SMALL BOWEL OBSTRUCTION

Although uncommon, the incidence of small bowel obstruction in pregnant women is increasing because of an increasing number of women of childbearing age undergoing bariatric surgical procedures and therefore being at increased risk for internal hernia or adhesive disease.[34,35] Adhesional disease (50%) is the most common cause of small bowel obstruction in pregnant women, followed by internal hernia (15%), intussusception (12%), and volvulus (9%).[34] MR is the preferred modality to evaluate for small bowel obstruction in pregnant women because of its lack of ionizing radiation, superior soft tissue resolution, and multiplanar capabilities. Dilated bowel should be traced to the point where it transitions to decompressed bowel, and this transition zone should be carefully interrogated to determine the cause of the obstruction (Fig. 5). In patients with adhesive disease, the culprit adhesion typically is not identifiable on imaging. However, once other causes of small bowel obstruction are ruled out in the transition zone (eg, hernia), adhesive disease may be assumed.

Internal hernias can be challenging to diagnose, and there is scant literature available on the appearance of internal hernias specifically in pregnant women. In the general population following Roux-en-Y gastric bypass, mesenteric swirling is the single best predictor of internal hernia (sensitivity, 61%–89%; specificity, 67%–94%).[36,37] However, some internal hernias are occult on imaging. Because internal hernia is the most common cause of small bowel obstruction following Roux-en-Y gastric bypass (42%), MR imaging showing a small bowel obstruction in a pregnant woman with prior gastric bypass should be interpreted with caution.[38] A potential pitfall is the misattribution of bowel wall thickening to infection in the setting of an imaging-occult internal hernia with ischemic bowel. In addition, the distinction between a partial and complete obstruction is not readily made with MR because currently no oral contrast agent exists that is distinguishable enough from physiologic fluid to allow assessment of whether an oral contrast agent passes beyond the transition point.

Internal hernia is managed operatively because of the high risk of bowel ischemia, whereas a small bowel obstruction caused by adhesive disease may initially be managed conservatively (eg, bowel rest and nasogastric tube placement). In a recent series reviewing pregnant women with small bowel obstructions, most patients (91%) eventually underwent surgical intervention, and the rate of fetal loss was 17% with a maternal mortality of 2%.[34]

INFLAMMATORY BOWEL DISEASE

Fertility rates of patients with inflammatory bowel disease in remission and who have never had prior

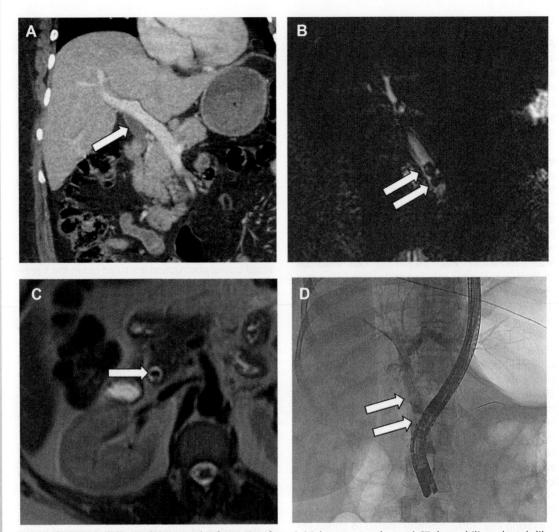

Fig. 4. Choledocholithiasis. (*A*) Coronal reformation from initial contrast-enhanced CT shows biliary ductal dilatation (*arrow*) but no obstructing lesion. Patient's pregnancy status was not known at time of initial CT imaging. (*B*) Thin-cut MRCP image in the coronal plane shows 2 stones in the bile duct (*arrows*). (*C*) Axial T2-weighted MR image confirms a stone in the bile duct (*arrow*). (*D*) Fluoroscopic image from endoscopic retrograde cholangiopancreatography shows several filling defects in the bile duct (*arrows*). The bile duct was swept with a 12-mm balloon, and 4 large stones were removed.

pelvic surgery are similar to the general population.[39] Patients with inflammatory bowel disease are advised to try to become pregnant while their disease is in remission because patients who become pregnant during a flare are more likely to experience poor fetal outcomes such as premature birth.[40] Most patients who become pregnant while in remission remain in remission, whereas most patients who become pregnant experiencing active disease continue to have active disease during pregnancy.[40,41]

Noncontrast MR is the preferred modality to assess for active inflammatory bowel disease and its complications in pregnant patients. Active inflammatory bowel disease appears as areas of bowel wall thickening and edema, with edema most conspicuous on T2 images obtained with fat saturation (**Figs. 6** and **7**). Diffusion-weighted imaging can be helpful. MR is also useful to assess for complications, including infected fluid collections, fistulae, and bowel obstruction. A pitfall of MR is that extraluminal air is less readily apparent compared with CT. Extraluminal air does not show signal in any pulse sequence. Assessment for extraluminal susceptibility artifacts that bloom on in-phase images may be helpful. In addition, direct demonstration of a bowel leak is typically not possible with MR imaging because there currently

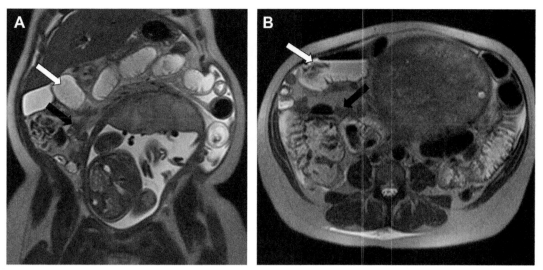

Fig. 5. Small bowel obstruction. (*A*) Coronal and (*B*) axial T2-weighted images show dilated small bowel (*white arrows*) with decompressed small bowel more distally (*black arrows*) compatible with a small bowel obstruction caused by adhesions.

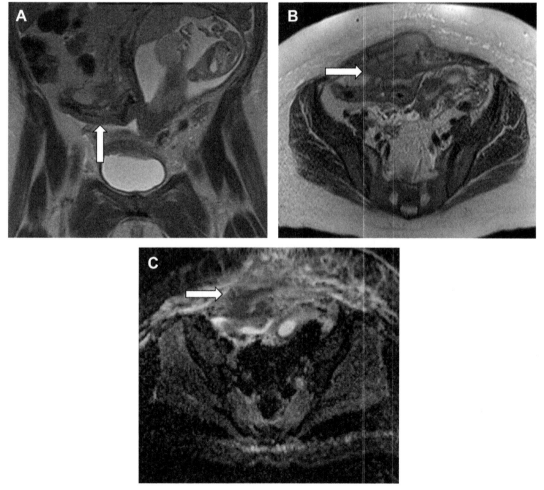

Fig. 6. Crohn disease. (*A*) Coronal T2-weighted image shows thick-walled distal ileum (*arrow*). (*B*) Axial T2-weighted image shows fistulization (*arrow*) to the anterior abdominal wall. (*C*) Axial apparent diffusion coefficient map diffusion-weighted image shows extensive restricted diffusion signal abnormality within the anterior abdominal wall and subcutaneous fat (*arrow*) indicating extensive inflammation.

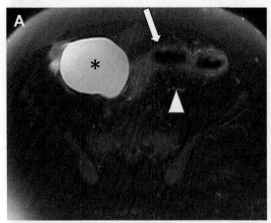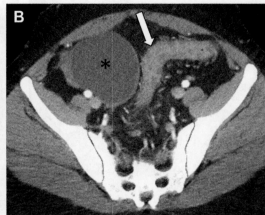

Fig. 7. Crohn disease. (*A*) Axial T2-weighted MR with fat saturation shows colonic inflammation (*arrow*) with prominent adjacent vasculature (comb-sign, *arrowhead*). Also 8-cm right ovarian cyst (*asterisk*). The patient miscarried and underwent a CT scan (*B*) approximately 3 weeks later, which showed persistent colonic wall thickening (*arrow*) and the right ovarian cyst (*asterisk*).

is not an oral contrast agent that is sufficiently distinguishable from intestinal contents to confirm a leak.

HELLP SYNDROME

HELLP (hemolysis, elevated liver function tests, and low platelets) syndrome occurs in approximately 0.9% of all pregnancies and in approximately 10% to 20% of patients with severe preeclampsia.[42,43] Approximately 70% of cases are diagnosed during the third trimester of pregnancy, most commonly between the 27th and 37th gestational weeks, whereas 30% of cases are diagnosed after delivery.[43,44] The association with preeclampsia is controversial because most, but not all, patients who develop HELLP syndrome also have preeclampsia.[45]

The cause of HELLP syndrome is uncertain, and a combination of genetic, maternal, and environmental factors triggered by an immunologic event has been proposed.[46] Patients most often present with upper abdominal pain, and many have nausea, vomiting, and headache.[43] These clinical symptoms may initially mimic a viral illness. The onset of HELLP syndrome is typically rapid, and may be preceded by hypertension, proteinuria, edema, and weight gain.[43]

The diagnosis of HELLP syndrome is established based on clinical presentation and laboratory abnormalities with imaging performed to assess for complications, including intraparenchymal hepatic hematoma or infarct and hepatic rupture (**Figs. 8–10**). In a study of 568 patients diagnosed with preeclampsia or HELLP syndrome, 3 patients (0.53%) had abdominal imaging findings.[47] On contrast-enhanced CT, areas of intraparenchymal hemorrhage are lower in attenuation than the adjacent liver.[47] On ultrasonography, intrahepatic hematoma may appear hypoechoic or as isoechoic heterogeneity.[47] Patients with HELLP syndrome may also show areas of liver infarction, which appear as areas of hypoenhancing liver parenchyma without the mass effect on liver parenchyma or vasculature that is seen with intraparenchymal hematoma.[48] Other nonspecific imaging findings have also been described in patients with HELLP syndrome and include hepatic steatosis, periportal edema, nonhemorrhagic free fluid, renal collecting system dilatation, and bowel dilatation and edema (see **Figs. 8–10**).[47,48] Other maternal complications include retinal detachment (0.9%), pulmonary edema (6%), acute renal failure (7.7%), placental abruption (16%), and disseminated intravascular coagulation (21%).[44]

Treatment of prenatal HELLP syndrome depends on gestational age with immediate delivery at 34 weeks' gestation or later, delivery within 48 hours after corticosteroid treatment at 27 to 34 weeks' gestation, or conservative management including corticosteroid treatment if less than27 weeks' gestation.[43] Reported maternal mortalities range from 1% to 25%, most commonly caused by cerebral stroke or hemorrhage or hepatic rupture.[43] Neonatal mortality ranges from 7% to 34%, primarily caused by prematurity, placental insufficiency, or placental abruption.[43]

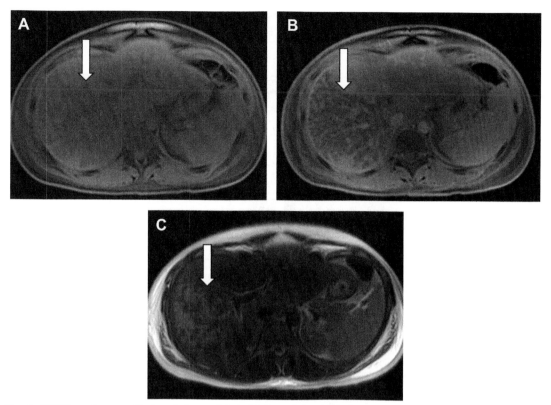

Fig. 8. HELLP syndrome with liver infarcts. (*A*) Axial T1-weighted MR image with fat saturation shows a large geographic area of abnormal low T1 signal intensity in the right hepatic lobe (*arrow*). (*B*) Axial T1-weighted image obtained after administration of intravenous contrast material shows large areas of hypoperfusion of the right hepatic lobe (*arrow*) compatible with liver infarct. (*C*) Axial T2-weighted image shows geographic areas of increased T2 signal intensity (*arrow*) in the right hepatic lobe.

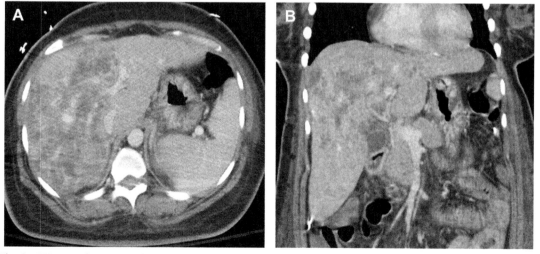

Fig. 9. HELLP syndrome with liver infarcts. A 38-year-old woman who underwent emergent delivery because of preeclampsia. (*A*) Axial and (*B*) coronal contrast-enhanced CT images show large areas of liver hypoenhancement compatible with liver infarcts.

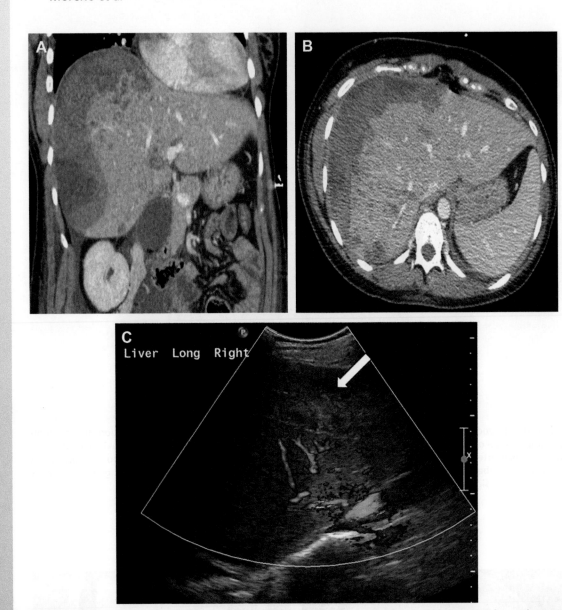

Fig. 10. HELLP syndrome with liver infarct and subcapsular hematoma. A 32-year-old woman who underwent emergent cesarean section (C-section) for preeclampsia. (*A*) Postpartum coronal and (*B*) axial contrast-enhanced CT images show geographic areas of hypoenhancement compatible with liver infarcts with associated subcapsular hematoma. (*C*) Longitudinal image obtained with power Doppler ultrasonography shows subcapsular hematoma (*arrow*).

ACUTE FATTY LIVER OF PREGNANCY

Acute fatty liver of pregnancy is a rare but potentially fatal condition occurring in approximately 1 in 10,000 to 1 in 20,000 pregnancies.[49,50] This condition occurs in late pregnancy with a median gestational age of 36 weeks, and most women (74% in one series) are diagnosed antenatally.[50] The cause of acute fatty liver of pregnancy is unknown, but an abnormality in fetal fatty acid metabolism has been proposed.[51]

The most common presenting signs and symptoms are nausea and vomiting, hypertension, and abdominal pain.[49] Imaging, specifically ultrasonography, plays a role in the diagnosis of acute fatty liver of pregnancy because a hyperechoic liver on ultrasonography is one of the diagnostic criteria according to the Swansea criteria.[52] To establish a diagnosis of acute fatty liver of pregnancy using the Swansea criteria, 6 or more of the following features must be identified in the absence of another explanation: encephalopathy, polydipsia/polyuria, abdominal pain, vomiting, hypoglycemia, increased bilirubin level, increased urate level, leukocytosis, increased ammonia level, increased transaminase levels, microvesicular steatosis on liver biopsy, coagulopathy, renal impairment, or ascites or hyperechoic liver on ultrasonography.[52]

In addition to hyperechogenicity on ultrasonography, other imaging features of hepatic steatosis include low attenuation on CT imaging and signal loss on opposed-phase MR imaging. CT criteria for hepatic steatosis include an absolute liver attenuation of less than 40 Hounsfield units (HU) (52.5% sensitivity; 100% specificity) or liver attenuation at least 10 HU less than that of the spleen (60.5% sensitivity, 100% specificity) on portal venous phase CT.[53] Liver attenuation of less than 40 HU on noncontrast CT is also considered to be diagnostic of hepatic steatosis.[54] Signal loss on opposed-phase images compared with in-phase images indicates hepatic steatosis with MR.

Complications of acute fatty liver of pregnancy include renal impairment, hemorrhage, pancreatitis, and hepatic encephalopathy requiring ventilator support for airway protection.[49,51] Supportive care and expeditious delivery are the treatment of acute fatty liver of pregnancy.[49,51] Because this condition occurs during late pregnancy, delivery is typically possible, occurring within 4 days of diagnosis in 98% of patients in one series.[50] Postnatal cases are typically diagnosed within 4 days of delivery.[50] In a study of 51 women with acute fatty liver of pregnancy, normalization of most laboratory values occurred within 7 to 10 days after delivery.[49] However, a 2% to 18% maternal fatality rate has been reported.[50,51] Sixty percent of women were admitted to the intensive care unit in one series with 1 patient requiring a liver transplant.[50] The neonatal mortality is approximately 10% to 23%.[50,51]

HYDRONEPHROSIS

Mild hydronephrosis occurs in up to 90% of pregnant women as a result of mass effect on the ureters caused by the gravid uterus, and smooth muscle relaxation caused by progesterone effects.[55] Pregnancy-related hydronephrosis is most commonly right sided or bilateral and is most commonly observed in the third trimester.[55] Ultrasonography is the first-line test to evaluate for collecting system dilatation. MR typically is not necessary to diagnose hydronephrosis, although it can be used to define the level of ureteral narrowing (Fig. 11). A pitfall in the evaluation of hydroureteronephrosis with MR is that small ureteral calculi are occult on MR.[56] Renal and ureteral calculi appear as areas of low signal intensity and typically are not directly visible unless large (eg, >1 cm).[56] However, MR can identify the secondary findings of ureteral colic (eg, hydroureteronephrosis) (see Fig. 11).[56]

Most cases of physiologic hydronephrosis of pregnancy are asymptomatic. However, pregnant

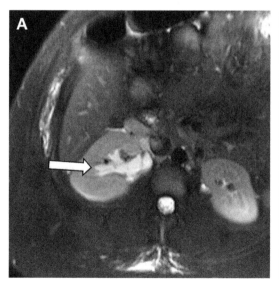
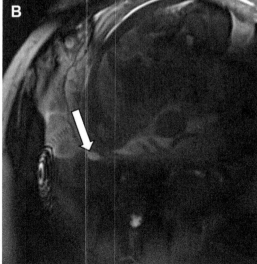

Fig. 11. Hydronephrosis, ureteral colic. (A, B) Axial T2-weighted images obtained with fat saturation show moderate right-sided hydronephrosis (A, arrow) and hydroureter (B, arrow). The patient subsequently passed a stone with relief of symptoms.

women with moderate or severe hydronephrosis may be symptomatic. The incidence of symptomatic hydronephrosis in pregnancy was 0.5% in one series.[57] Patients with symptomatic hydronephrosis of pregnancy may be initially managed conservatively, although nephroureteral stent placement may be necessary for patients whose symptoms do not improve with conservative management.[57]

PYELONEPHRITIS

Pyelonephritis is a complication in 1% to 2% of pregnancies.[58,59] The urinary tract infection typically begins in the urinary bladder and then reaches the kidneys via either ascending or hematogenous spread.[60] Although the incidence of bacteriuria is similar in pregnant and nonpregnant women, pregnant women are at increased risk for pyelonephritis caused by urinary stasis and changes in urine pH.[59] Pyelonephritis most commonly occurs during the second and third trimesters and may result in septicemia, renal dysfunction, anemia, or preeclampsia.[58,59] Patients may present with fever, flank pain, chills, nausea, and vomiting.[59] Dysuria is uncommon.[59]

Although ultrasonography may be ordered to assess for pyelonephritis, the interstitial edema of pyelonephritis is often occult on ultrasonography. The sensitivity of ultrasonography for pyelonephritis was 33% in one series.[61] In some patients, hypoechoic areas may be visible in areas of pyelonephritis and may be more readily apparent with harmonic imaging.[62] Color Doppler may show increased or decreased vascularity and power Doppler may show focal areas of decreased perfusion.

MR is the imaging test of choice for assessment of pyelonephritis in pregnant patients because of its superior soft tissue resolution. On MR, infection and inflammation appear as areas of increased T2-weighted signal (**Fig. 12**) with restricted diffusion.[63] Focal high-T2 signal intensity that is fluid signal intensity bright could indicate development of a focal abscess. Apparent diffusion coefficient values are lower in areas of acute pyelonephritis compared with normal renal parenchyma and are lower in areas of renal abscess compared with areas of pyelonephritis.[63–65]

Routine prenatal screening for asymptomatic bacteriuria is a standard part of prenatal care so that antibiotics that are safe for the fetus and mother can be administered before complications such as pyelonephritis develop.[58] Antibiotics are also used to treat pyelonephritis. Maternal pyelonephritis is a risk factor for adverse birth outcomes, including preterm delivery.[66]

ADRENAL HEMORRHAGE

Spontaneous adrenal hemorrhage is an uncommon cause of abdominal pain in pregnant women. The incidence of spontaneous adrenal hemorrhage is unknown, and this condition is largely the subject of case reports.[67,68] Patients typically present with acute onset of flank pain or upper abdominal pain that may be accompanied by nausea and a low-grade fever.[68] Causes include preeclampsia, eclampsia, sepsis, and trauma.[69]

Adrenal hemorrhage may be first detected on ultrasonography because ultrasonography is often the first-line imaging test in pregnant women with flank pain. On ultrasonography, adrenal hemorrhage appears as a nonspecific heterogeneous suprarenal mass. Noncontrast MR is typically next performed for better characterization. MR appearance varies based on acuity. Initially, blood

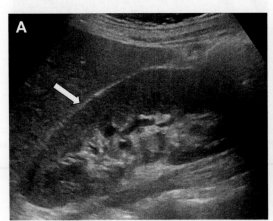
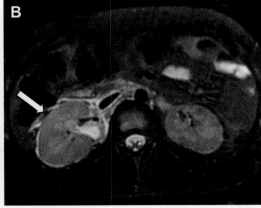

Fig. 12. Pyelonephritis. (*A*) Longitudinal gray-scale ultrasonography image shows a normal-appearing right kidney (*arrow*). (*B*) Axial T2-weighted MR image obtained with fat saturation 2 hours later shows perinephric edema and asymmetric enlargement of the right kidney (*arrow*).

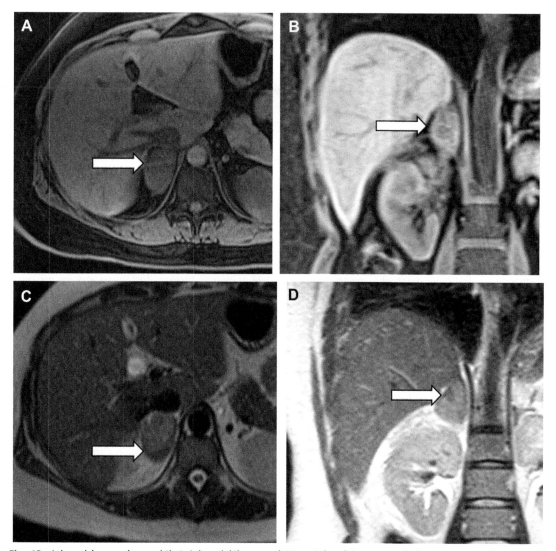

Fig. 13. Adrenal hemorrhage. (*A*) Axial and (*B*) coronal T1-weighted images with fat saturation of the upper abdomen show an enlarged right adrenal gland with intrinsic high T1 signal intensity (*arrows*). (*C*) Axial and (*D*) coronal T2-weighted images show heterogeneous T2 signal intensity (*arrows*).

products appear hypointense to isointense on T1-weighted images and hyperintense on T2-weighted images. In the subacute phase, blood products appear hyperintense on T1-weighted images (**Fig. 13**). Blooming susceptibility artifacts associated with subacute to chronic blood products are visible on in-phase imaging, and older blood products show low signal on T2-weighted images because of hemosiderin staining. Follow-up imaging should be obtained to evaluate for resolution of the adrenal hemorrhage and exclude an underlying mass.

Initial management of adrenal hemorrhage includes evaluation of laboratory values to assess adrenal function and serial serum hemoglobin levels to assess for continued bleeding.[67] Unilateral adrenal hemorrhage typically does not significantly impair adrenal function and can be managed conservatively, whereas bilateral adrenal hemorrhage can be fatal if untreated because of adrenal insufficiency.[67] Decreasing serum hemoglobin level and hematocrit indicating massive adrenal hemorrhage are an indication for emergent adrenalectomy or angioembolization to control bleeding.

OVARIAN TORSION

Ovarian torsion is an uncommon cause of abdominal pain in pregnant women. Women who have undergone assisted reproductive technologies,

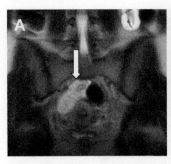
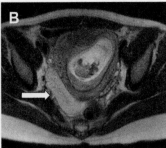

Fig. 14. Ovarian torsion. (*A*) Coronal T2-weighted image and (*B*) axial T2-weighted image show an enlarged right ovary (*arrows*).

especially those who have experienced ovarian hyperstimulation syndrome, are at increased risk.[70,71] Ovarian torsion most commonly occurs during the first trimester and is least common in the third trimester but can occur at any time during pregnancy.[70] Patients typically present with abdominal pain and most also report nausea and vomiting.[70]

If torsion is the leading diagnostic consideration, ultrasonography is the test of choice because ultrasonography can assess for abnormal ovarian enlargement; masses, including cysts that would predispose to torsion; blood flow within the ovary; and pain associated with the ovary.[72] The most common finding in ovarian torsion is an enlarged ovary measuring greater than 4 cm.[72] However, during pregnancy ovaries are hormonally suppressed and appear physiologically smaller, hence even subtle asymmetry in size in a symptomatic patient should be reported. Other ultrasonography findings of ovarian torsion include peripheral follicles, free fluid, and a twisted vascular pedicle.[72] The presence of ovarian blood flow does not rule out torsion. Doppler blood flow was falsely normal in 61% of pregnant women with ovarian torsion in one series.[71] Detection of blood flow within a torsed ovary indicates that the ovary may be viable.[72]

On MR, ovarian torsion typically also appears as an enlarged ovary (Fig. 14). In addition, the uterus may be deviated toward the side of the twisted ovary. A central afollicular stroma with peripheral follicles within an enlarged ovary is further suggestive of ovarian torsion, and these findings are best seen on T2-weighted images.[73] On T1-weighted images, a T1-hyperintense rim indicating subacute hematoma may also be visible.[73] A twisted vascular pedicle is diagnostic of ovarian torsion but is only visible in a minority of patients.[73] Treatment of ovarian torsion is typically laparoscopic detorsion if the ovary is still viable and oophorectomy if the ovary is nonviable.[66,67]

TRAUMA

In pregnant women who have experienced significant trauma, low-dose contrast-enhanced CT is typically the first-line test because of its wide availability and short image acquisition time. The solid abdominal organs should be evaluated similarly to a nonpregnant patient for evidence of trauma such as splenic or liver laceration (Fig. 15). In addition, the placenta should be evaluated because women who have experienced trauma such as a motor vehicle collision are at increased risk for placental abruption. Placental abruption is defined as premature separation of the placenta.[74]

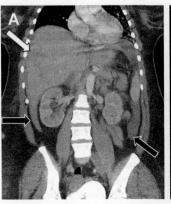
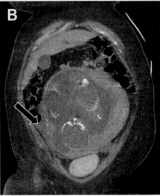

Fig. 15. Liver lacerations after motor vehicle collision. (*A*, *B*) Coronal reformations from contrast-enhanced CT show linear areas of low attenuation in the liver compatible with lacerations (*white arrow*) and blood products tracking along the right and left paracolic gutters and adjacent to the uterus (*black arrows*).

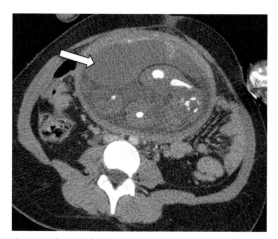

Fig. 16. Placental abruption. Axial contrast-enhanced CT image obtained following a motor vehicle collision shows large areas of full-thickness placental hypoenhancement (*arrow*). Placental abruption was confirmed intraoperatively during emergent C-section.

Placental enhancement is normally homogeneous in the first trimester and then becomes mildly heterogeneous in later stages of pregnancy.[75,76] However, large geographic areas of full-thickness placental hypoenhancement at contrast-enhanced CT are abnormal and are concerning for placental abruption (**Fig. 16**).[75,76] A potential pitfall is a uterine contraction, which can appear as a rounded myometrial bulge that forms an obtuse angle with the placenta and may be mistaken for placental injury.[75] By comparison, areas of placental injury typically do not form an obtuse angle with the remainder of the placenta.[75] An additional pitfall is retroplacental hematoma, which may have similar attenuation to myometrium and be mistaken for myometrium.[75]

Management of placental abruption depends on severity of the abruption, fetal evaluation, and gestational age. For example, a nearly full-term fetus with a large abruption may undergo urgent delivery. By comparison, a fetus that is in an earlier stage of pregnancy with reassuring heart rate and a small area of abruption may be managed conservatively.

SUMMARY

Determining the cause of abdominal pain in pregnant women is challenging because of anatomic and physiologic changes that occur with pregnancy. Imaging, including noncontrast MR, plays an important role in the evaluation of pregnant women with concerning abdominal pain. Accurate MR diagnosis is important so that appropriate treatment can be initiated for the health of the fetus and the mother.

DISCLOSURE

The authors have nothing to disclose.

REFERENCES

1. Lee KS, Rofsky NM, Pedrosa I. Localization of the appendix at MR imaging during pregnancy: utility of the cecal tilt angle. Radiology 2008;249:134–41.
2. Lurie S, Rahamim E, Piper I, et al. Total and differential leukocyte count percentiles in normal pregnancy. Eur J Obstet Gynecol Reprod Biol 2008;136:16–9.
3. Shur J, Bottomly C, Patel JH. Imaging of acute abdominal pain in the third trimester of pregnancy. BMJ 2018;361:k2511.
4. Committee on Obstetric Practice. Committee opinion no. 723: guidelines for diagnostic imaging during pregnancy and lactation. Obstet Gynecol 2017;130:e210–6.
5. Smith-Bindman R, Aubin C, Bailitz J, et al. Ultrasonography versus computed tomography for suspected appendicitis. N Engl J Med 2014;371:1100–10.
6. Wertz JR, Lopez JM, Olson D, et al. Comparing the diagnostic accuracy of ultrasound and CT in evaluating acute cholecystitis. AJR Am J Roentgenol 2018;211:W92–7.
7. Expert Panel on Gastrointestinal Imaging, Garcia EM, Camacho MA, Karolyi DR, et al. ACR Appropriateness Criteria right lower quadrant pain-suspected appendicitis. J Am Coll Radiol 2018;15:S373–87.
8. Ray JG, Vermeulen MJ, Bharatha A, et al. Association between MRI exposure during pregnancy and fetal and childhood outcomes. JAMA 2016;316:952–61.
9. Juhasz-Boss I, Solomayer E, Strik M, et al. Abdominal surgery in pregnancy-an interdisciplinary challenge. Dtsch Arztebl Int 2014;111:465–72.
10. Prodromidou A, Machairas N, Kostakis ID, et al. Outcomes after open and laparoscopic appendectomy during pregnancy: a meta-analysis. Eur J Obstet Gynecol Reprod Biol 2018;225:40–50.
11. McGory ML, Zingmond DS, Tillou A, et al. Negative appendectomy in pregnant women is associated with a substantial risk of fetal loss. J Am Coll Surg 2007;205:534–40.
12. Puylaert JB. Acute appendicitis: US evaluation using graded compression. Radiology 1986;158:355–60.
13. Lehnert BE, Gross JA, Linnau KF, et al. Utility of ultrasound for evaluating the appendix during the second and third trimester of pregnancy. Emerg Radiol 2012;19:293–9.
14. Segev L, Segev Y, Rayman S, et al. The diagnostic performance of ultrasound for acute appendicitis

in pregnant and young nonpregnant women: a case-control study. Int J Surg 2016;34:81–5.

15. Hansen W, Moshiri M, Paladin A, et al. Evolving practice patterns in imaging pregnant patients with acute abdominal and pelvic conditions. Curr Probl Diagn Radiol 2017;46:10–6.

16. Patel D, Fingard J, Winters S, et al. Clinical use of MRI for the evaluation of acute appendicitis during pregnancy. Abdom Radiol (NY) 2017;42:1857–63.

17. Wi SA, Kim DJ, Cho ES, et al. Diagnostic performance of MRI for pregnant patients with clinically suspected appendicitis. Abdom Radiol (NY) 2018;43:3456–61.

18. Kereshi B, Lee KS, Siewert B, et al. Clinical utility of magnetic resonance imaging in the evaluation of pregnant females with suspected acute appendicitis. Abdom Radiol (NY) 2018;43:1446–55.

19. Burke LM, Bashir MR, Miller FH, et al. Magnetic resonance imaging of acute appendicitis in pregnancy: a 5-year multiinstitutional study. Am J Obstet Gynecol 2015;213:693.e1-6.

20. Duke E, Kalb B, Arif-Tiwari H, et al. A systematic review and meta-analysis of diagnostic performance of MRI for evaluation of acute appendicitis. AJR Am J Roentgenol 2016;206:508–17.

21. Al-Katib S, Sokhandon F, Farah M. MRI for appendicitis in pregnancy: is seeing believing? Clinical outcomes in cases of appendix nonvisualization. Abdom Radiol (NY) 2016;41:2455–9.

22. Theilen LH, Mellnick VM, Longman RE, et al. Utility of magnetic resonance imaging for suspected appendicitis in pregnant women. Am J Obstet Gynecol 2015;212:345.e1-6.

23. Tsai R, Raptis C, Fowler KJ, et al. MRI of suspected appendicitis during pregnancy: interradiologist agreement, indeterminate interpretation and the meaning of non-visualization of the appendix. Br J Radiol 2017;90:20170383.

24. Fonseca AL, Schuster KM, Kaplan LJ, et al. The use of magnetic resonance imaging in the diagnosis of suspected appendicitis in pregnancy: shortened length of stay without increase in hospital charges. JAMA Surg 2014;149:687–93.

25. Kastenberg ZJ, Hurley MP, Luan A, et al. Cost-effectiveness of preoperative imaging for appendicitis after indeterminate ultrasonography in the second or third trimester of pregnancy. Obstet Gynecol 2013;122:821–9.

26. Rapp EJ, Naim F, Kadivar K, et al. Integrating MR imaging into the clinical workup of pregnant patients suspected of having appendicitis is associated with a lower negative laparotomy rate: single-institution study. Radiology 2013;267:137–44.

27. de Bari O, Wang TY, Liu M, et al. Cholesterol cholelithiasis in pregnant women: pathogenesis,

prevention, and treatment. Ann Hepatol 2014;13:728–45.

28. Revzin MV, Scoutt LM, Garner JG, et al. Right upper quadrant pain: ultrasound first! J Ultrasound Med 2017;36:1975–85.

29. Smith EA, Dillman JR, Elsayes KM, et al. Cross-sectional imaging of acute and chronic gallbladder inflammatory disease. AJR Am J Roentgenol 2009;192:188–96.

30. Shea JA, Berlin JA, Escarce JJ, et al. Revised estimates of diagnostic test sensitivity and specificity in suspected biliary tract disease. Arch Intern Med 1994;154:2573–81.

31. Wu CC, Ho YH, Chen CY. Effect of aging on common bile duct diameter: a real-time ultrasonographic study. J Clin Ultrasound 1984;12:473–8.

32. Giljaca V, Gurusamy KS, Takwoingi Y, et al. Endoscopic ultrasound versus magnetic resonance cholangiopancreatography for common bile duct stones. Cochrane Database Syst Rev 2015;2:CD011549.

33. Othman M, Stone E, Hashimi M, et al. Conservative management of cholelithiasis and its complications in pregnancy is associated with recurrent symptoms and more emergency department visits. Gastrointest Endosc 2012;76:564–9.

34. Webster PJ, Bailey MA, Wilson J, et al. Small bowel obstruction in pregnancy is a complex surgical problem with a high risk of fetal loss. Ann R Coll Surg Engl 2015;97:339–44.

35. Kakarla N, Dailey C, Marino T, et al. Pregnancy after gastric bypass surgery and internal hernia formation. Obstet Gynecol 2005;105:1195.

36. Lockhart ME, Tessler FN, Canon CL, et al. Internal hernia after gastric bypass: sensitivity and specificity of seven CT signs with surgical correlation and controls. AJR Am J Roentgenol 2007;188:745–50.

37. Dilauro M, McInnes MDF, Schieda N, et al. Internal hernia after laparoscopic Roux-en-Y gastric bypass: optimal CT signs for diagnosis and clinical decision making. Radiology 2017;282:752–60.

38. Koppman JS, Li C, Gandsas A. Small bowel obstruction after laparoscopic Roux-en-Y gastric bypass: a review of 9,527 patients. J Am Coll Surg 2008;206:571–84.

39. Mahadevan U. Fertility and pregnancy in the patient with inflammatory bowel disease. Gut 2006;55:1198–206.

40. Hashash JG, Kane S. Pregnancy and inflammatory bowel disease. Gastroenterol Hepatol 2015;11:96–102.

41. Abhyankar A, Ham M, Moss AC. Meta-analysis: the impact of disease activity at conception on disease activity during pregnancy in patients with inflammatory bowel disease. Aliment Pharmacol Ther 2013;38:460–6.

42. Aloizos S, Seretis C, Liakos N, et al. HELLP syndrome: understanding and management of a pregnancy-specific disease. J Obstet Gynaecol 2013;33:331–7.

43. Haram K, Svendsen E, Abildgaard U. The HELLP syndrome: clinical issues and management. A review. BMC Pregnancy Childbirth 2009;9:8.

44. Sibai BM, Ramadan MK, Usta I, et al. Maternal morbidity and mortality in 442 pregnancies with hemolysis, elevated liver enzymes, and low platelets (HELLP syndrome). Am J Obstet Gynecol 1993; 169:1000–6.

45. Gomes CF, Sousa M, Lourenco I, et al. Gastrointestinal diseases during pregnancy: what does the gastroenterologist need to know? Ann Gastroenterol 2018;31:385–94.

46. Abildgaard U, Heimdal K. Pathogenesis of the syndrome of hemolysis, elevated liver enzymes, and low platelet count (HELLP): a review. Eur J Obstet Gynecol Reprod Biol 2013;166:117–23.

47. Nunes JO, Turner MA, Fulcher AS. Abdominal imaging features of HELLP syndrome: a 10-year retrospective review. AJR Am J Roentgenol 2005;185:1205–10.

48. Perronne L, Dohan A, Bazeries P, et al. Hepatic involvement in HELLP syndrome: an update with emphasis on imaging features. Abdom Imaging 2015;40:2839–49.

49. Nelson DB, Yost NP, Cunningham FG. Acute fatty liver of pregnancy: clinical outcomes and expected duration of recovery. Am J Obstet Gynecol 2013; 209:456.e1-7.

50. Knight M, Nelson-Piercy C, Kurinczuk JJ, et al. A prospective national study of acute fatty liver of pregnancy in the UK. Gut 2008;57:951–6.

51. Ko HH, Yoshida E. Acute fatty liver of pregnancy. Can J Gastroenterol 2006;20:25–30.

52. Ch'ng CL, Morgan M, Hainsworth I, et al. Prospective study of liver dysfunction in pregnancy in Southwest Wales. Gut 2002;51:876–80.

53. Lawrence DA, Oliva IB, Israel GM. Detection of hepatic steatosis on contrast-enhanced CT images: diagnostic accuracy of identification of areas of presumed focal fatty sparing. AJR Am J Roentgenol 2012;199:44–7.

54. Boyce CJ, Pickhardt PJ, Kim DH, et al. Hepatic steatosis (fatty liver disease) in asymptomatic adults identified by unenhanced low-dose CT. AJR Am J Roentgenol 2010;194:623–8.

55. Fainaru O, Almog B, Gamzu R, et al. The management of symptomatic hydronephrosis in pregnancy. BJOG 2002;109:1385–7.

56. Kalb B, Sharma P, Salman K, et al. Acute abdominal pain: is there a potential role for MRI in the setting of the emergency department in a patient with renal calculi? J Magn Reson Imaging 2010; 32:1012–23.

57. Tsai Y-L, Tsai Y-L, Seow K-M, et al. Comparative study of conservative and surgical management for

58. Hill JB, Sheffield JS, McIntire DD, et al. Acute pyelonephritis in pregnancy. Obstet Gynecol 2005;105: 18–23.

59. Matuskiewicz-Rowinska J, Malyszko J, Wieliczko M. Urinary tract infections in pregnancy: old and new unresolved diagnostic and therapeutic problems. Arch Med Sci 2015;11:67–77.

60. Craig WD, Wagner BJ, Travis MD. Pyelonephritis: radiologic-pathologic review. Radiographics 2008; 28:255–77.

61. Yoo JM, Koh JS, Han CH, et al. Diagnosing acute pyelonephritis with CT, Tc-DMSA SPECT, and Doppler ultrasound: a comparative study. Korean J Urol 2010;51:260–5.

62. Kim B, Lim HK, Choi MH, et al. Detection of parenchymal abnormalities in acute pyelonephritis by pulse inversion harmonic imaging with or without microbubble ultrasonographic contrast agent: correlation with computed tomography. J Ultrasound Med 2001;20:5–14.

63. Rathod SB, Kumbhar SS, Nanivadekar A, et al. Role of diffusion-weighted MRI in acute pyelonephritis: a prospective study. Acta Radiol 2015;56:244–9.

64. Faletti R, Cassinis MC, Gatti M, et al. Acute pyelonephritis in transplanted kidneys: can diffusion-weighted magnetic resonance imaging be useful for diagnosis and follow-up? Abdom Radiol (NY) 2016;41:531–7.

65. Faletti R, Gatti M, Bassano S, et al. Follow-up of acute pyelonephritis: what causes the diffusion-weighted magnetic resonance imaging recovery to lag clinical recovery? Abdom Radiol (NY) 2018;43: 639–46.

66. Farkash E, Weintraub AY, Sergienko R, et al. Acute antepartum pyelonephritis in pregnancy: a critical analysis of risk factors and outcomes. Eur J Obstet Gynecol Reprod Biol 2012;162:24–7.

67. Gupta A, Minhas R, Quant HS. Spontaneous adrenal hemorrhage in pregnancy: a case series. Case Rep Obstet Gynecol 2017;2017:3167273.

68. Gavrilova-Jordan L, Edmister W, Farrell MA, et al. Spontaneous adrenal hemorrhage during pregnancy: a review of the literature and a case report of successful conservative management. Obstet Gynecol Surv 2005;60:191–5.

69. Bockorny B, Posteraro A, Bilgrami S. Bilateral spontaneous adrenal hemorrhage during pregnancy. Obstet Gynecol 2012;120:377–81.

70. Smorgick N, Pansky M, Feingold M, et al. The clinical characteristics and sonographic findings of maternal ovarian torsion in pregnancy. Fertil Steril 2009;92:1983–7.

71. Hasson J, Tsafrir Z, Azem F, et al. Comparison of adnexal torsion between pregnant and

nonpregnant women. Am J Obstet Gynecol 2010; 202:536.e1-6.

72. Chang HC, Bhatt S, Dogra VS. Pearls and pitfalls in diagnosis of ovarian torsion. Radiographics 2008; 28:1355–68.

73. Duigenan S, Oliva E, Lee SI. Ovarian torsion: diagnostic features on CT and MRI with pathologic correlation. AJR Am J Roentgenol 2012;198: W122–31.

74. Oyelese Y, Ananth CV. Placental abruption. Obstet Gynecol 2006;108:1005–16.

75. Wei SH, Helmy M, Cohen AJ. CT evaluation of placental abruption in pregnant trauma patients. Emerg Radiol 2009;16:365–73.

76. Raptis CA, Mellnick VM, Raptis DA, et al. Imaging of trauma in the pregnant patient. Radiographics 2014; 34:748–63.

Nonfetal Imaging During Pregnancy: Placental Disease

Priyanka Jha, MBBS[a],*, Gabriele Masselli, MD[b], Michael A. Ohliger, MD, PhD[a], Liina Põder, MD[a]

KEYWORDS

- Hemorrhage • MR imaging • Placenta • Ultrasound • Placenta accreta spectrum disorder
- Placental masses • Placenta previa • Abruption

KEY POINTS

- Placenta is a vital organ connecting the maternal and fetal circulations.
- Placenta accreta spectrum disorders and placental masses are the most common indications for dedicated placental imaging with ultrasound or MR imaging.
- Placental accreta spectrum disorders present with characteristic imaging findings of irregular lakes, myometrial thinning, abnormal intraplacental vascularity, and placental bulge on ultrasound and MR imaging. Imaging is helpful in assessing the extent of involvement and presurgical planning.
- Antepartum hemorrhage is an important cause of maternal and fetal morbidity and mortality, and most of the cases are due to placenta abnormalities including placenta previa and placental abruption. MR imaging can help distinguish hematomas from other causes of antepartum bleeding, such as vasa previa, degenerated uterine fibroid, cervical pathology, and placental tumors.
- Placental masses are most commonly identified during the routine fetal ultrasound examinations. Imaging evaluation should focus on the effect of the mass on fetal well-being in this scenario.

INTRODUCTION

Placenta is a vital organ that allows exchange of nutrients and gases between the mother and the developing fetus.[1] The placenta develops by 10 to 14 weeks of pregnancy and is fully functional by the end of the first trimester to support the hormonal needs of continuing the pregnancy and the metabolic needs of the developing fetus. As such, disease states that affect the placenta can have important consequences for both the mother and the fetus.[1,2]

Ultrasound (US) is the first line of imaging for most placental diseases. Per guidelines, all pregnancies should have an "anatomy scan," also called as a level one scan, at 18 to 20 weeks of gestation.[3] Although most of this scan focuses on assessing the anatomic development of the fetus, evaluating the placenta is a crucial component of this examination.[3] MR imaging has an increasingly important role as an adjunct modality for imaging for placental disease processes as well and can be particularly helpful for troubleshooting and advanced evaluation.[4,5]

The most common placental pathologies for which imaging is necessary include placenta accreta spectrum disorders (PASD) and placental masses. Both processes are relatively uncommon; however, the adverse consequences to both the fetus and the mother are substantial and hence should be specifically sought after and never overlooked. This review addresses the normal anatomy of the placenta, imaging technique and protocols, imaging findings and summarizes the key information that needs to be conveyed to the clinical providers.

[a] Department of Radiology and Biomedical Imaging, University of California San Francisco, 505 Parnassus Avenue, Box 0628, San Francisco, CA, USA; [b] Department of Radiology, Umberto I Hospital, Sapienza University, Via Silvestro Gherardi 38, 00146 Rome, Italy
* Corresponding author.
E-mail address: priyanka.jha@ucsf.edu

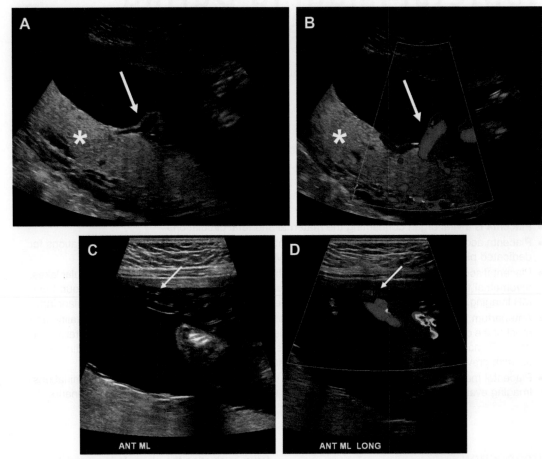

Fig. 1. Different types of cord insertion. (*A*) Grayscale and (*B*) color Doppler images demonstrate central cord insertion (*arrow*) to posterior placenta (*asterisk*). (*C*) Transabdominal grayscale and (*D*) color Doppler images demonstrate cord insertion into the chorioamniotic membranes and uterus away from the placenta (*arrow*). The cord travels within the membranes toward the placenta diagnostic of a velamentous cord insertion. (*E, F*) When fetal MR imaging is performed for other reasons, cord insertion may be easily detectable as on these coronal T2-weighted images demonstrating velamentous cord insertion (*arrow*) into the uterus and the cord traveling in the fetal membranes (*short arrows*) toward the placenta. (*G, H*) Transabdominal grayscale and color Doppler images demonstrate marginal cord insertion at the edge (*arrow*) of the posterior placenta (*asterisk*).

NORMAL ANATOMY AND IMAGING TECHNIQUE

The normal placenta is a discoid structure with tapering edges, which attaches to the myometrium in a uniformly layering fashion. It measures up to 4 cm in maximum thickness. The umbilical cord mostly inserts centrally into the placenta but can be marginal or velamentous as well (**Fig. 1**). Normally, the lower placental edge should be at least 2 cm from the margin of the internal cervical os.[6] If less than 2 cm from the internal os, this counts as placenta previa. When the placenta covers the internal os, this constitutes complete previa (**Fig. 2**). Sometimes, variant anatomy such as succenturiate lobe (portion of the placenta separate from the main

placental mass) and vasa previa (**Fig. 3**) are present, which are extremely important to detect and relay to the clinicians because of the risk of retention of this lobe during delivery and both conditions being at high risk for significant hemorrhage.[7]

The normal placenta is homogeneous, slightly hyperechoic relative to the myometrium on grayscale US (**Fig. 4**).[1] On high-frequency and high-resolution images, the placenta may seem slightly less hyperechoic and overall the myometrium seems more closer in echogenicity to the placenta. Hence, this relative difference in echogenicity is based on sonographic technical parameters (see **Fig. 4**). Very few lakes may be present, especially adjacent to the placental cord insertion.[8] On color Doppler imaging, few

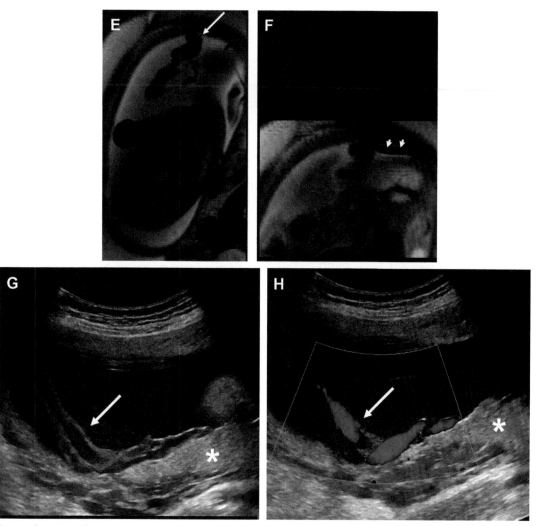

Fig. 1. (continued)

small caliber intraplacental vessels and subplacental vascularity can be seen.[8] On MR imaging, placenta is mostly isointense to the myometrium on T1-weighted images and hyperintense to the myometrium on T2-weighted (T2W) images (Fig. 5). Sometimes, the pregnant uterus can develop vascular congestion, in which case the myometrium demonstrates T2-hyperintense appearance. In such cases, the placenta relatively seems iso- to hypointense to the myometrium (see Fig. 5). With increasing gestational age, structure of the cotyledons becomes more apparent and results in decreased signal intensity to intermediate signal intensity compared with the surrounding myometrium (Fig. 6).[9,10] First and second trimester placentas are very homogeneous in their appearance but with development of this lobular pattern, the placenta becomes less homogeneous in appearance, as thin hypointense septa become apparent between the lobules on T2W images (see Fig. 6). Placental septa and cotyledons are more often visible when MR imaging is performed with a 3 T system.[7]

The placental-myometrial interface is demonstrated as a retroplacental clear space on US and as T2-hypointense interface on MR imaging. Given the isointensity of the placenta to the myometrium on T1-weighted images, the interface is not well seen and is best evaluated on T2W sequences. The normal subplacental vascularity can be seen as multiple flow voids in this subplacental space. A few flow voids can be present within the placenta adjacent to the umbilical cord insertion. The myometrium has a variable thickness and thins as the pregnancy progresses. The underlying myometrial wall thins as the pregnancy advances, and

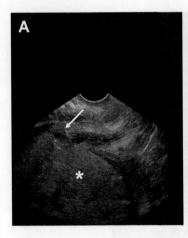
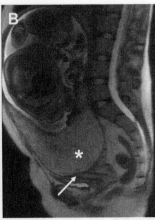

Fig. 2. Complete placenta previa. (*A*) Endovaginal image of placenta (*asterisk*) completely covering internal os (*arrow*). (*B*) Sagittal T2-weighted MR image demonstrates placenta (*asterisk*) completely covering the internal os (*arrow*).

this finding alone does not imply PASD.[11] The myometrium naturally thins at sites of compression, such as adjacent to the maternal spine and aorta, appearing as a single thin layer of uniform signal on T2W images. In addition, the myometrium is expected to thin as the gestation progresses, especially at the site of previous scars.[12]

IMAGING PROTOCOLS
Ultrasound

US images should evaluate the entire placenta, and images should be acquired documenting that the entire placenta has been evaluated. Grayscale as well as Doppler imaging should be used. Based on body habitus and depth of the placenta, evaluation with a curvilinear 2 to 6 Megahertz (mHz) and 9 mHz linear transducers can be performed.[13,14] In all pregnancies, placenta should be evaluated for the location of implantation, proximity to the cesarean section scar (if applicable), placenta previa or vasa previa, succenturiate lobe, and shape and thickness of the placenta. After this general evaluation, particularly in patients with history of uterine intervention such as cesarean section, myomectomy, embolization, or Asherman syndrome, attention should be drawn to specific findings of PASD such as placental heterogeneity, irregular lacunes or placental lakes, loss of retroplacental clear space/subplacental lucency, myometrial thinning, abnormal subplacental and intraplacental vascularity, placental bulge, and extrauterine invasion (such as that into the bladder or the parametrium). Studies have shown improved patient outcomes when targeted evaluation of the placenta is performed in patients with suspected PASD.[15] Details of these findings are discussed later in this article. In addition, with placental evaluation, it is imperative to evaluate the area of the internal os with color Doppler imaging to evaluate for any aberrant vessels at this location. If any vessels are present, they can be further evaluated with spectral Doppler to look for their maternal versus fetal origin, based on heart rate observations. Vessels demonstrating arterial waveforms at fetal heart rate are highly suspicious for vasa previa.

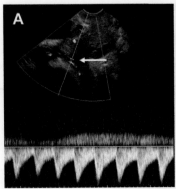
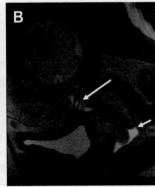

Fig. 3. Vasa previa. (*A*) Endovaginal image demonstrates a crossing vessel over internal os (*arrow*) with fetal heart rate diagnostic of vasa previa. (*B*) MR imaging sagittal ssFSE performed on the same day correlated with this finding (*arrow*). Patient had ruptured membranes, and fluid around the vessels outlined the finding. Fluid is seen in the upper vagina from ruptured membranes (*short arrow*). ssFSE, single-shot fast spin echo.

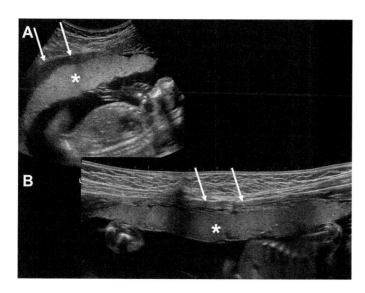

Fig. 4. Normal sonographic appearance of the placenta. (*A*) Transabdominal US demonstrated homogeneously hyperechoic second trimester placenta (*asterisk*) in relationship to hypoechoic myometrium (*arrows*). (*B*) High-resolution image performed with a linear transducer shows the normal placenta (*asterisk*) to be slightly less hyperechoic, and the myometrium (*arrows*) does not seem as hypoechoic in comparison to the placenta. The overall relative signal of these structures depends on imaging parameters.

MR Imaging

The authors' institutional MR imaging protocol for placental imaging is summarized in **Table 1**. In brief, a combination of T2 (not fat suppressed) and T1 images are necessary. Most of the findings for PASD and placental masses are evident on nonfat-suppressed T2W images. T1 images are essential to evaluate for intrinsic hyperintensity secondary to hemorrhage in PASD and to detect the presence of fat in placental masses. Occasionally, fat-suppressed T1 images may be needed, when evaluating for the presence of fat in placental masses. The role of diffusion-weighted imaging in placental imaging is still evolving. In the author's experience, DWI is particularly helpful in cases with severe myometrial vascular congestion, to help delineate the placental-myometrial interface. In this scenario, the placenta demonstrates hyperintensity, whereas the myometrium does not and hence making their interface better visualized.

Technical details of MR imaging for the placenta are summarized in Michael A. Ohliger and Hailey H. Choi's article, "Imaging Safety and Technical Considerations in the Reproductive Age Female," in this issue.

IMAGING FINDINGS/PATHOLOGY
Placenta Accreta Spectrum

PASD is a spectrum of disorders where the placenta adheres to the underlying myometrium and hence does not separate at the time of delivery, leading to massive hemorrhage, which can be life threatening to the mother. The spectrum includes accreta (where the placenta is attached directly to the myometrium, without intervening decidua), increta (with myometrial invasion), and percreta, where the placenta extends outside the uterine serosa and possibly into adjacent organs such as the bladder and the parametrium. International Federation of

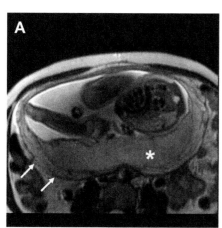
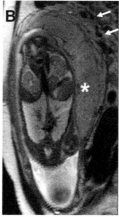

Fig. 5. Normal MR imaging appearance of the placenta. (*A*) Sagittal and (*B*) axial T2W MR images in second trimester demonstrate a homogeneous placenta (*asterisk*), slightly hyper to isointense to myometrium (*arrows*). The signal of myometrium varies on T2W images that depend on the degree of physiologic vascular engorgement. As seen in (*B*), numerous flow voids may be present in the physiologically engorged myometrium (*arrows*).

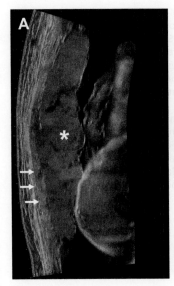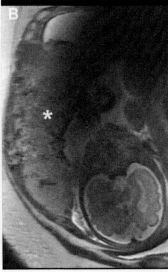

Fig. 6. Normal appearance of a "mature" placenta in late gestation. (A) Transabdominal image performed with high-resolution linear transducer of a patient in the third trimester demonstrates the placenta (*asterisk*) to be hyperechoic relative to the myometrium (*arrows*) and overall more heterogeneous in appearance. (B) Sagittal T2W MR image in a patient in her third trimester demonstrates the placenta (*asterisk*) to be more heterogeneous in signal as well.

Gynecology and Obstetrics has proposed a combined clinical-pathologic classification, which includes both intraoperative observations as well as findings on gross pathology.[16] Often relying on pathology alone can lead to erroneous estimation of the severity of the findings, leading to this combined system.[16] No single imaging feature has been shown to be diagnostic for PASD, and usually a combination of multiple findings exists, alerting the reviewers to the correct diagnosis.

Ultrasound

On US some of the commonly reported signs are the presence of multiple placental lakes with irregular margins (**Fig. 7**), the loss of retroplacental clear space, between the placenta and the myometrium (see **Fig. 7**), and presence of placenta previa (see **Fig. 7**). Other features include heterogeneous placenta, asymmetry of placental thickness, myometrial thinning, bladder wall interruption, myometrial, and bladder wall hypervascularity (see **Fig. 7**).

Prominent placental lacunes This is the most commonly reported US finding of abnormal placentation, which is present irrespective of the depth of invasion (see **Fig. 7**).[14,17] Placental lacunes are vascular anechoic or hypoechoic structures located within the center of the cotyledons. Although a few of these are often present in normal placentae, imaging findings of PASD represent a spectrum of worsening appearance, as they become larger, irregular, and concentrated in the area of invasion and can demonstrate slow internal flow on real-time imaging.[14,17] These are

also often referred as "placental lakes" and give the placenta the classic "moth-eaten" appearance.[14,17]

Loss of retroplacental clear space The normal placental-myometrial interface seems hypoechoic on gray-scale US, which represents the normal decidua basalis. With PASD, this clear space is obliterated (see **Fig. 7**),[13,17–19] and approximately 70% of cases will show this finding.[17] In some cases, this area can have prominent subplacental vascularity.

Myometrial thinning In cases of PAS, myometrium may be thinned to submillimeter levels and actually becomes undetectable in more severe cases (see **Fig. 7**).[14,17] It is reported to occur in about 50% of cases, which may be reflective of US changes that happen at the more invasive end of the spectrum.[14,17]

Placental bulge sign With deeper depths of invasion, the placenta may bulge outward, creating an hourglass or snowman configuration of the uterine contour. Along with myometrial thinning, this finding highly suggests myometrial invasion (**Figs. 8 and 9**).

Bladder wall interruption Bladder wall interruption is defined as the interruption of the hyperechoic fat plane between the uterus and the bladder, which can involve the bladder wall and extend into the bladder lumen in the most severe cases.[14,20,21] Prominent vessels may be identified at the bladder wall, but these are not specific for invasion (see **Fig. 7**).[14] Spectral interrogation of these vessels can be performed, and if fetal heart

Table 1
MR imaging protocol for placental imaging at 3 T

	Coverage	TR	TE	Flip	NEX	Slice	Matrix	FOV	Phase	Oversample
Patient should drink water before commencing study										
Coronal, axial, and sagittal single-shot fast spin echo (ssFSE)	Uterus to below cervix	2000	100	X	X	4/0	384x256	36	R > L	PE FOV 1.0
Axial LAVA FLEX or mDIXON DUAL ECHO	Center over the placenta	4.2	1.2	15	1	3/0	260x256	34	A > P	PE FOV 1.1
Coronal ssFSE (nonpropeller)	High-resolution imaging (reduced field of view), center over the placenta	2000	100	X	X	4/0	384x256	26–28	R > L	PE FOV 1.0
Axial T2 FSE (nonpropeller)	No fat saturation, high-resolution imaging (reduced field of view), center over the placenta	4000	120	120	2	4/0	320x256	24	R > L	NPW
Sagittal T2 FSE propeller	No fat saturation, high-resolution imaging (reduced field of view), center over the placenta	11,000	74		2	4/0	256x256	24		
Axial and sagittal diffusion-weighted imaging (DWI)	Multiple b-values of 0, 50, 500, 1000: ADC maps Routine field of view	5000	30.5		2	6/0	80x80	34		PE FOV 1

Abbreviations: ADC, apparent diffusion coefficient; FOV, field of view; NEX, number of excitations; TE, the echo time; TR, the repetition time.

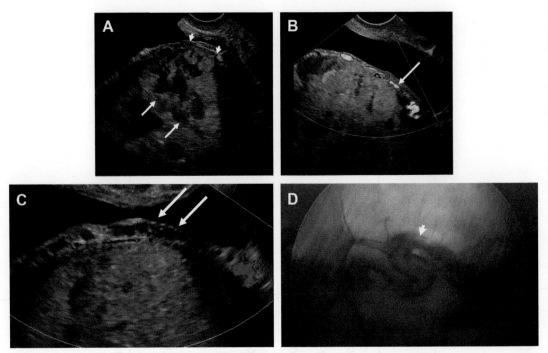

Fig. 7. US features of placenta accreta spectrum (PAS). (*A*) Endovaginal grayscale image demonstrates complete placenta previa with multiple placental lakes with irregular margins (*arrows*) and loss of retroplacental clear space (*short arrows*). (*B*) Endovaginal image with color Doppler demonstrates loss of retroplacental clear space and increased retroplacental vascularity (*arrow*). (*C*) Endovaginal image demonstrates extensive bladder wall hypervascularity (*arrows*). (*D*) Intraoperative cystoscopy image obtained during delivery demonstrates prominent submucosal vascularity (*arrowhead*).

rate can be demonstrated, it highly suggests bladder invasive PASD.

Asymmetric thickness Invasive placentas often appear thickened in the portion implanted on the cervix, and overall the placental thickness is increased in the areas involved by PASD.[22]

MR imaging

MR imaging is now recognized for its strengths in assessment of invasive placentation.[4] MR imaging provides supplemental knowledge in addition to US, particularly in cases of posterior and lateral invasion, areas that may be technically challenging for US imaging[23,24] (see **Fig. 8**). At the authors' institution, any patient with suspicion for

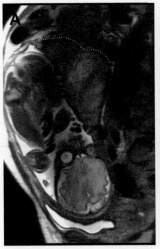 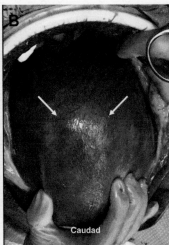

Fig. 8. MR imaging appearance of placenta accreta spectrum. (*A*) Sagittal T2W image demonstrates posterior placenta with bulge (*dotted line*) into the myometrium. (*B*) During the surgery a subtle blue bulge was noted on the posterior uterus (*arrows*). Cesarean hysterectomy specimen confirmed placenta increta on pathology.

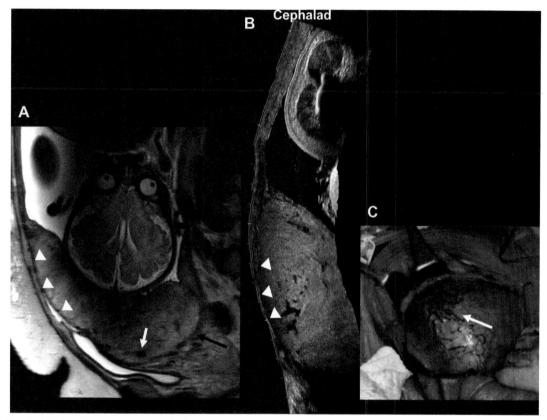

Fig. 9. MR imaging appearance of placenta accreta spectrum with intraoperative correlation. (*A*) Sagittal T2W MR image demonstrates complete placenta previa (*black arrow*) with bulging of lower uterine segment and barely visible retroplacental myometrium (*arrowheads*). T2-dark bands are present in the placenta (*white arrow*). (*B*) Intraoperative US confirms the bulge and retroplacental thinning of myometrium (*arrowheads*). (*C*) Intraoperative picture demonstrates a uterine bulge with blue tinge (*arrow*) corresponding to imaging findings. Gross pathology confirmed placenta increta.

invasive placenta based on US findings undergoes MR imaging of the placenta and uterus.[23,24] If normal placentation is confidently diagnosed with US, patients may not be referred for additional imaging. Although MR imaging has similar overall sensitivity and specificity to US, it has been shown to have a high predictive accuracy in assessing both the depth and topography of placental invasion.[4] It has also been beneficial in cases with clinical suspicion for accreta and discordant US findings and in cases in which percreta is suspected.[23] MR imging is also helpful for surgical planning. Knowing the location of the placenta and its relationship to cervix, bladder, and pelvic sidewall allows for preoperative planning for stents, embolization, and extent of dissection anticipated. Recent work by Bourgioti and colleagues[25,26] has demonstrated MR imaging to be capable of assessing extrauterine spread as well as predict adverse maternal and neonatal outcomes. Similar to US, myometrial

thinning, asymmetric placental thickening, and bladder wall interruption are also present on MR imaging. Most commonly reported MR imaging findings for PASD, in addition to findings recognized on US, are described below.

T2-dark bands Dark intraplacental bands are linear or polygonal areas of very low signal intensity on T2W images (see **Fig. 9**).[12,27] They can be of variable thickness with a maximum diameter ranging from 6 mm to 20 mm or more and are thought to represent areas of fibrin deposition due to repetitive intraplacental hemorrhage or infarcts.[4,12,27–29] Small intraplacental dark bands may occasionally be noted in mature noninvasive placentas (>30 weeks of gestation), typically on the fetal surface of the placenta, whereas the abnormal T2-dark bands usually contact the maternal surface of the placenta.[30] This feature is considered one of the most consistent abnormal MR imaging findings in patients with PASD.[6,25,28–31]

Placental bulge sign One of the most commonly reported MR imaging signs of PASD is abnormal uterine bulging. When an abnormal placenta implants in the lower uterine segment, the uterus develops an hourglass or snowman configuration, rather than the typical inverted pear shape (see **Figs. 8** and **9**). This finding is best seen in coronal and sagittal images but can be seen on axial images too when the bulging is lateral in location.[11,30,32] The presence of uterine bulging has been shown to be associated with deeper depths of invasion.[6,27,32–34] The investigators have noted the presence of the bulge in patients with increta[5] as well as placenta percreta[35] on MR imaging.

Loss of retroplacental T2-hypointense line The hypointense interface between placenta and myometrium on T2W images corresponds to the retroplacental hypoechoic zone described in obstetric US and is best seen on T2W sequences.[12] This interface is lost in cases of PASD. This finding is usually present along with focal myometrial defects and thinning.[31] In cases of placenta percreta, placental tissue can be seen extending through the myometrium with disruption of this T2-hypointense line.[36]

Myometrial thinning Myometrium can be thinned at the placental attachment to less than 1 mm in thickness and even essentially becomes imperceptible with PASD.[37] This is also best assessed on T2W sequences.[11,38,39] However, because there is some expected thinning of the myometrium as pregnancy progresses, myometrial visualization becomes difficult as the pregnancy progresses.[11,12] When the myometrium is well demonstrated, focal interruptions of the wall are seen at sites of invasion with placental tissue extending through the breach in case of percreta (**Fig. 10**).[4,33,40]

Abnormal intraplacental vascularity and subplacental vascularity Abnormal vessels are located in the placental parenchyma along with a prominent network of vessels in the placental bed with disruption of the uteroplacental interface in cases of PASD. These vessels may extent to the underlying myometrium, can reach up to the uterine serosa, and may be accompanied by extensive neovascularization around the bladder, uterus, and vagina. A novel "stripped fetal vessel" sign has been proposed, which refers to a large caliber intraplacental vessel that travels between the fetal and maternal placental surfaces without change in caliber.[41]

The term "placental bed" refers to that part of the decidua and adjacent myometrium that

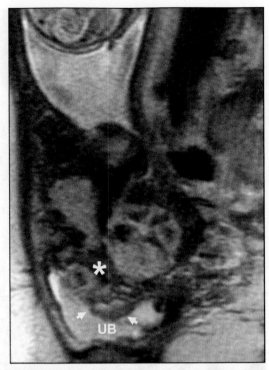

Fig. 10. MR imaging appearance of placenta accreta spectrum with placenta percreta. T2W sagittal image demonstrates extremely heterogeneous placenta (*asterisk*) invading (*short arrows*) into the lumen of urinary bladder (UB).

underlies the placenta and whose primary function is the maintenance of an adequate blood supply to the intervillous space of the placenta.[42] Although it is common to see flow voids here even in normal pregnancies, in PASD these vessels are seen to directly enter the placenta and can even course up to the umbilical cord insertion.

PLACENTAL ABRUPTION

Placental abruption represents premature separation of the placenta from the uterine wall. Although rare (affecting <1% of pregnancies), third-trimester abruption is associated with an increased risk of preterm delivery and fetal death. Imaging appearance of placental abruption can be classified based on the location of the hematoma as retroplacental, marginal subchorionic, preplacental, and intraplacental (**Fig. 11**).

US is frequently performed to confirm the presence of abruption and assess the extent of subchorionic or retroplacental hematoma.[43] However, in up to 50% of cases of abruption US is negative for different reasons: (1) acute hemorrhage echo texture is very similar to that of the adjacent placenta and is therefore very

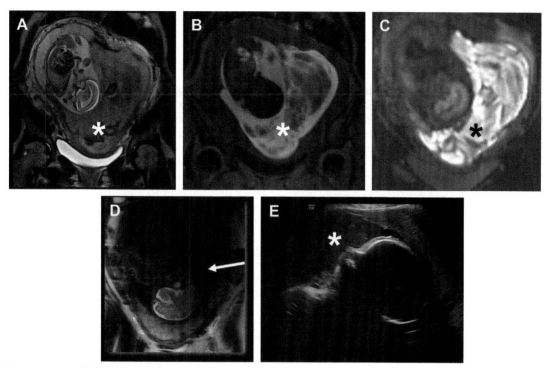

Fig. 11. Coronal MR (*A*) T2-weighted, (*B*) T1-weighted, and (*C*) DWI demonstrate hyperacute placental abruption (*asterisk*) with intermediate signal intensity on T2-weighted images, high signal intensity on T1-weighted images, and reduced diffusion on high B-value images. (*D*) In a different patient, hemorrhage can be of very low signal intensity on T2-weighted images as seen on this case of intraamniotic hemorrhage of subacute chronicity (*arrow*). (*E*) Corresponding transabdominal US demonstrates diffuse echoes throughout the amniotic sac, correlating to large amount of intraamniotic hemorrhage (*asterisk*).

difficult to detect; (2) the imaging appearance of an abnormally thick and heterogeneous placenta is rare, being present only in large acute clots; and (3) many subacute clots result in falsely negative because blood dissects out from beneath the placenta and drains through the cervix.[44,45] MR images have intrinsic high soft tissue contrast and can accurately depict placental-related hemorrhage with a reported high sensitivity of 95% to 100% and high specificity of 100%.[45] By considering the signal intensity changes on T1-weighted, T2W, and diffusion-weighted images, with special reference to the paramagnetic effects of methemoglobin, it is possible to estimate the age of the bleeding (see **Fig. 11**).[46] Hyperacute hemorrhage is usually hyperintense on T2W and diffusion-weighted images, being iso- to hypointense on T1-weighted images (see **Fig. 11**).[46] Acute hemorrhage remains iso- to hypointense on T1-weighted images but now becomes hypointense on T2W and diffusion-weighed images.[46] Subacute hemorrhage is T1-hyperintense due to presence of methemoglobin. Chronic hemorrhage is hypointense on all T1-weighted, T2W, and diffusion-weighted images.[46]

PLACENTAL MASSES

Uncommonly, the placenta can develop masses, the most common of which is a chorioangioma. Broadly, placental masses can be classified as nontrophoblastic or trophoblastic in origin.[47] Trophoblastic masses include molar pregnancy, intraplacental choriocarcinoma, and complete hydatidiform mole with twin fetus. Nontrophoblastic masses include chorioangioma, placental teratoma, and placental mesenchymal defect.[47] Placenta can get metastases from maternal primaries such as lung and breast cancer but also fetal malignancy such as neuroblastoma.[47]

Nontrophoblastic Placental Masses

Chorioangioma
The most common nontrophoblastic mass to develop in the placenta is a chorioangioma.[47] As the name suggests, this is a benign proliferation of the vascular channels supported by chorionic stroma.[48] Interestingly, these masses occur at an unusual frequency in higher altitudes, and hypoxic origin of these masses has been postulated.[48] Most of these masses are small and

asymptomatic, being incidentally identified on US performed for fetal well-being. The masses are contiguous with fetal circulation, and resultant arteriovenous shunting within the placenta can be linked to several pregnancy complications, including fetal anemia, thrombocytopenia, nonimmune fetal hydrops, polyhydramnios, antepartum hemorrhage with premature placental detachment, preterm labor, intrauterine fetal growth restriction (IUGR), and increased perinatal mortality.[48]

On US, chorioangiomas appear as echogenic masses, which are characteristically located adjacent to the placental cord insertion and protrude into the amniotic cavity (Fig. 12). On Doppler interrogation, internal vascularity pulsating at fetal heart rate can be demonstrated, which is a hallmark for this diagnosis.[48] Larger masses start developing cystic areas and can even cause chorioamniotic separation, secondary to profuse mucin secretion (see Fig. 12).[47] Once diagnosed, careful assessment for polyhydramnios and fetal anemia using middle cerebral arterial Doppler assessment should be performed. On MR imaging, these masses are isointense to the placenta on T1-weighted images and are heterogeneous being mostly hyperintense to the placenta on T2W images (see Fig. 12).[47] Intrinsic T1 hyperintensity can develop at the periphery of the tumor related to hemorrhage.

Placental teratoma

Teratomas are extremely rare benign tumors of the placenta with a very favorable outcome. These masses include components from all 3 germ cell lines and always lie between the amnion and the chorion, usually on the fetal surface of the placenta.[49] The sonographic and MR imaging findings include demonstration of tissues of variable echogenicities or signal intensities demonstrating intratumoral fat, calcifications, and fluid.[50] On US, fat in a teratoma is hyperechoic to the normal placenta, whereas intratumoral calcifications are echogenic and demonstrate shadowing.[50] Gestational trophoblastic disorders can too present as hyperechoic masses but are unlikely to demonstrate calcification.[50] One of the major differentials for a teratoma includes a fetus acardiac amorphous (fetus in fetu). This entity demonstrates well-formed elements such as partial or complete formation of a vertebral column, ribs, pelvis, and skull base and sometimes a short umbilical cord may be present connecting this to the placenta.[50]

Placental mesenchymal defect

Placental mesenchymal defect (PMD) is a rare vascular anomaly of the placenta presenting as placentomegaly, multicystic mass, and villous hyperplasia.[51] Although this finding may be completely incidental, preterm delivery, IUGR, fetal anomalies (such as fetal liver cysts or vascular malformations), fetal overgrowth with Beckwith-Wiedemann syndrome, and even fetal demise have been associated with this abnormality.[51,52] Sonographic features include a multicystic mass, which can closely mimic a partial mole appearing given the presence of an enlarged placenta with multiple cystic masses (Fig. 13).[53] Differentiation from a molar pregnancy is important for appropriate management so that the pregnancy is not erroneously terminated. On color Doppler imaging, some of these cystic spaces demonstrate slow color flow, also called as a "stained-glass" appearance to the placenta (see Fig. 13).[54] In early pregnancy, lack of flow or slow flow can help differentiate PMD from chorioangioma and molar pregnancies, but this distinction can be difficult in later trimester due to overall increased flow to the placenta. MR imaging also shows corresponding findings of thickened placenta with multiple cystic spaces (see Fig. 13). Ultimately, chromosomal abnormality helps differentiate these entities, with PMD usually having a 46 XX karyotype, where partial moles are triploid.[47]

Trophoblastic placental masses

Trophoblastic masses include hyaditiform mole and intraplacental choriocarcinoma. Unusual cases such as complete hyaditiform mole with coexisting twin live fetus can also mimic a placental mass. All the masses on the trophoblastic spectrum are associated with disproportionally elevated beta-human chorionic gonadotropin (β-hCG) levels.

Intraplacental choriocarcinoma This is a rare variant of the choriocarcinoma spectrum, which is known to be associated with massive fetomaternal hemorrhage, likely due to villous erosion by the growing tumor, leading to fetal anemia and eventual fetal demise.[55] It should be considered in the differential for massive fetomaternal hemorrhage of unknown cause in the setting of an elevated β-hCG. On US, small intraplacental choriocarcinomas can be occult and isoechoic to the placenta.[55] They can also present as hyperechoic masses, whereas some may have cystic changes.[55] Retroplacental hemorrhage with placental abruption can develop, which is responsible for the associated fetomaternal hemorrhage.[56] Metastases to both mother and fetus can be present.[56]

Complete hydatidiform mole with twin live fetus This is a rare entity in which a normal

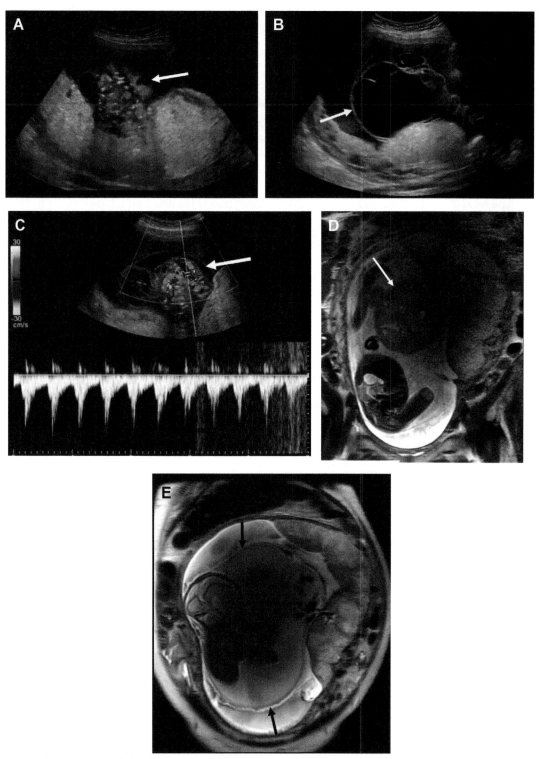

Fig. 12. Chorioangioma. (*A*) Large mixed, solid, and cystic mass (*arrows*) is seen arising from the placenta and protruding into the amniotic cavity. Echogenic foci throughout the mass represent scattered calcifications. (*B*) The mass is characteristically located adjacent to the placental cord insertion. (*C*) On spectral Doppler interrogation, the mass demonstrates internal vascularity pulsating at the fetal heart rate, also characteristic of a chorioangioma. (*D*, *E*) Coronal T2W images demonstrate a heterogenous, exophytic mass (*arrow*) arising from the placenta. (*E*) Separated amnion (*black arrows*) is seen consistent with chorioamniotic separation resulting from excessive mucin secretion by chorioangiomas.

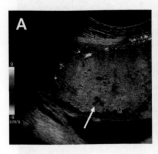
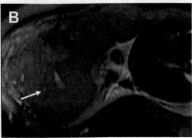

Fig. 13. Placental mesenchymal dysplasia. (*A*) On color Doppler US, the placenta is noted to be thickened with multiple tiny cystic spaces (*arrow*), which suggests PMD. (*B*) T2W MR imaging redemonstrates the thickened placenta with diffuse scattered T2-hypointense cystic spaces (*arrow*).

karyotype fetus develops along with an abnormal molar pregnancy.[57] This entity poses a significant clinical challenge, leading to both maternal and fetal morbidity. Maternal risks include preeclampsia, hyperthyroidism, and possibly malignancy; fetal complications include elevated risk of spontaneous abortion and neonatal thyrotoxicosis.[47,57] Although the normal fetus can have a favorable outcome, nearly 33% of the mothers develop persistent gestational trophoblastic disease after delivery.[58]

US findings include a multilocular cystic mass on grayscale images. On Doppler US, overall hypervascularity is seen without demonstrable flow in the cystic components (**Fig. 14**), a finding that helps differentiate from PMD.[11,23] Identifying this mass as separate from the placenta of the normal twin is very important and helps establish the diagnosis. This distinction is best established in the early gestational period and gets progressively more difficult with advancing gestation. PMD on the other hand is integrally intraplacental in location. MR imaging also demonstrates the cystic nature of the mass and can show the membrane separating the molar pregnancy from the normal pregnancy (see **Fig. 14**).[47] T1-weighted images best depict the hyperintensity associated with hemorrhage, which is common with molar pregnancies, and

often poorly identified on US (see **Fig. 14**). Typically, there is significant increase in size of this cystic mass of CHMTF from second to third trimester, in contrast to PMD, which most commonly decreases in size as the pregnancy evolves.[47]

PEARLS, PITFALLS, VARIANTS

Imagers should be aware of common pitfalls that can happen in imaging for PASD. Loss of retroplacental clear space from excess probe pressure is a well-known scenario, which can lead to overcalling accreta. Hence, when this finding is present in isolation without other features of PASD, probe pressure should be reduced and reimaging performed. Myometrial contractions can mimic masses (**Fig. 15**). In addition, the presence of contractions can lead to obscuration of this clear space (see **Fig. 15**).

MR imaging pitfalls include the presence of bulging of the uterus in patients without PASD. Similar to other scenarios, this should be interpreted in combination with other findings.[5] A relatively homogeneous placenta without T2-dark bands or abnormal vascularity may be placenta implanted in the region of scar that is ballooning with the pressure of gestation, without the presence of PASD. Occasionally,

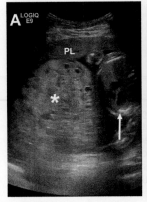
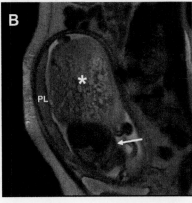

Fig. 14. Complete hyaditiform mole with twin fetus. (*A*) Transabdominal US at 24 weeks and (*B*) corresponding sagittal T2W MR image demonstrates a large cystic mass (*asterisk*), separate from placenta and a normally developed cotwin (*arrow*).

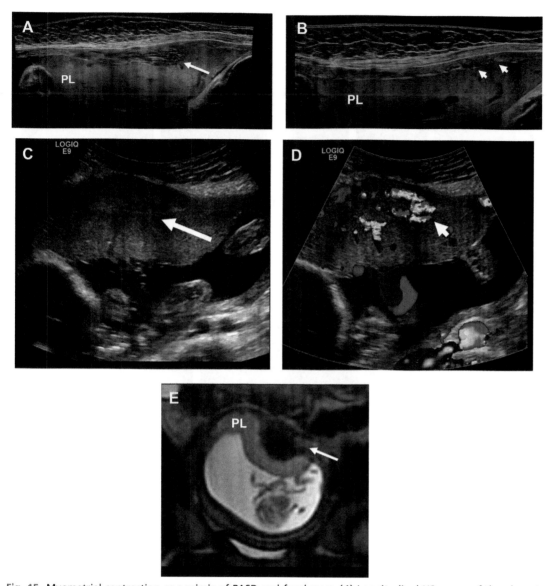

Fig. 15. Myometrial contraction as a mimic of PASD and focal mass. (*A*) Longitudinal US sweep of the placenta (PL) demonstrates retroplacental ill-defined focal masslike area (*arrow*), mimicking a retroplacental mass and obscuring the retroplacental interface. (*B*) This finding resolved later in the study (*arrowheads*) compatible with a contraction. (*C, D*) Transabdominal US grayscale image demonstrates focal retroplacental irregular mass-like area (*arrow*), which demonstrated focal area of hypervascularity (*short arrow*) on color Doppler image. This finding suggests focal contraction and can be misinterpreted as a mass. (*E*) Coronal T2W MR image demonstrates a retroplacental low-signal irregular mass (*arrow*) in keeping with a typical MR imaging appearance of focal myometrial contraction, which is a physiologic finding throughout the pregnancy.

nongravid uterus may also have this appearance. Cervical varices are another common pitfall that can be misinterpreted as placental pathology. These patients present with vaginal bleeding, which can be profuse. Often the indication for imaging is suspicion for vasa previa and placenta previa. On US, varices are seen as tubular, anechoic to hypoechoic structures, which should connect to maternal vasculature (**Fig. 16**). Most

commonly, these can be traced to connect to maternal myometrial vessels. Given the physiologic venous engorgement during pregnancy, some of these vessels become variceal and can even prolapse into the cervix and upper vagina. Spectral interrogation demonstrates venous waveforms. MR imaging features are those of a vessel, seen as a flow void in the region of the cervix and connecting to myometrial

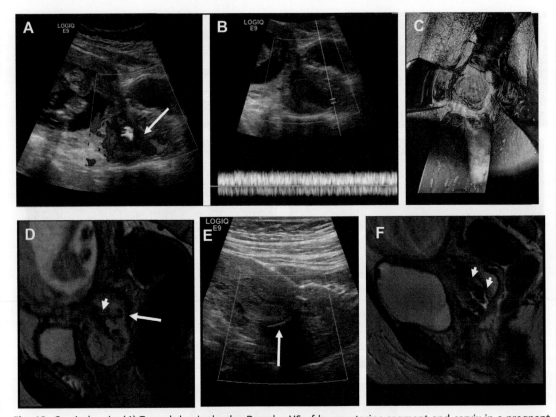

Fig. 16. Cervical varix. (*A*) Transabdominal color Doppler US of lower uterine segment and cervix in a pregnant woman presenting with multiple episodes of vaginal bleeding demonstrates prolapsed vascular structure in the cervical canal (*arrow*). (*B*) Spectral Doppler confirms venous flow that suggests a cervical varix. (*C*) On speculum examination a "blue bag of worms" appearance of the cervix was noted. (*D*) Sagittal T2W MR image shows edematous cervical stroma (*arrow*) with central flow voids (*short arrow*). (*E*) After transvaginal cerclage placement (*arrow*), color Doppler US shows no demonstrable color Doppler flow in the cervical canal. (*F*) Corresponding MR images shows decreased stromal T2 signal and collapsed vascular structures, which supports a thrombosed varix post cerclage placement.

vessels (see **Fig. 15**). Differential includes the marginal vein of the placenta, which is located at the edge of the placental disc and does not connect to myometrial vasculature. Varices can develop throughout the pelvis during pregnancy and can develop in unusual locations such as along the round ligaments, where they can present as palpable abnormalities and mimic an inguinal hernia (**Fig. 17**).

Thrombohematomas, also known as Breus mole, can mimic a placental mass.[47] Presence of myometrial contractions can also lead to globular appearance of subjacent placenta, which can mimic a placental mass; however, the "masslike" area will be very similar to the placenta in echogenicity.[47] Doppler imaging can be useful in this circumstance where the underlying area has similar vascularity. This should be addressed by the reimaging after the contraction has resolved.

WHAT THE REFERRING PHYSICIAN NEEDS TO KNOW

Imaging of PASD is focused on diagnosing the presence and extent of involvement, depth of placental invasion, if possible, extrauterine extension, and presurgical planning. Once the presence of PASD has been established, the radiologist should focus on assessing the location of the placenta and depth of invasion. Presence of placental bulge sign has been shown to be a marker for at least myometrial invasive disease. When combined with serosal hypervascularity, findings are highly suspicious for placenta percreta with extrauterine extension. Assessment of the extent of abnormal serosal vascularity can help predict the needs for additional hemostatic measures such as interventional radiology embolization. Proximity of the placenta with the bladder, specially posteriorly,

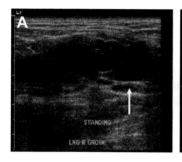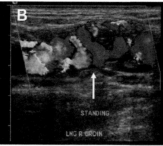

Fig. 17. Round ligament varices in a patient presenting with right groin lump, which developed and progressed during pregnancy. Clinical concern was for inguinal hernia. (*A*) Transabdominal US showed tubular structures (*arrow*), which demonstrated flow on (*B*) color Doppler images (*arrow*). Findings in keeping with pregnancy-related round ligament varices.

prompts cystoscopy at the time of delivery, possible placement of ureteral stents, creation of bladder patch at surgery, and urology involvement with worse involvement.

MR imaging allows to distinguish hematomas from other causes of antepartum bleeding and pain, such as vasa previa, degenerated uterine fibroid, cervical pathology, and placental tumors. Moreover, MR imaging helps to determine the age of the blood products based on MR signal characteristics of hemoglobin. Consequently, placental bleeding can be categorized into hyperacute, acute, early subacute, late subacute, and chronic hematomas. Hyperacute and acute placental hematomas are considered unstable hematomas with higher risk of rapid progression or rebleeding, which may require change in management.

In cases with placental masses, the goal of imaging is to characterize the mass and evaluate fetal well-being. Chorioangiomas can cause fetal anemia, polyhydramnios, chorioamniotic separation, and even hydrops. The larger the size of the mass, the higher the risk of complications. If a fetal intervention is anticipated, as in the setting of fetal anemia, knowing the location of the placenta and cord insertion is helpful to assess the feasibility and access for in utero transfusion.

SUMMARY

In summary, the placenta should be evaluated at the time of fetal evaluation with US. Potential risk factors for PASD should be elicited and if present, features of PASD should be evaluated for their presence. Prenatal diagnosis of PASD is essential for appropriate management and activation of multidisciplinary teams. Placental masses are uncommon and can be divided into trophoblastic and nontrophoblastic masses. Molar pregnancies and choriocarcinomas are trophoblastic masses. Although most nontrophoblastic placental masses are benign, the management focuses on the fetal well-being.

REFERENCES

1. Norton M. Callen's ultrasonography in obstetrics and gynecology. 6th edition. Philadelphia: Elsevier; 2017.
2. Myatt L, Thornburg KL. Effects of prenatal nutrition and the role of the placenta in health and disease. Methods Mol Biol 2018;1735:19–46.
3. AIUM-ACR-ACOG-SMFM-SRU practice parameter for the performance of standard diagnostic obstetric ultrasound examinations. J Ultrasound Med 2018; 37(11):E13–24.
4. D'Antonio F, Iacovella C, Palacios-Jaraquemada J, et al. Prenatal identification of invasive placentation using magnetic resonance imaging: systematic review and meta-analysis. Ultrasound Obstet Gynecol 2014;44(1):8–16.
5. Jha P, Rabban J, Chen L-M, et al. Placenta accreta spectrum: value of placental bulge as a sign of myometrial invasion on MR imaging. Abdom Radiol (NY) 2019;44(7):2572–81.
6. Masselli G, Gualdi G. MR imaging of the placenta: what a radiologist should know. Abdom Imaging 2013;38(3):573–87.
7. Elsayes KM, Trout AT, Friedkin AM, et al. Imaging of the placenta: a multimodality pictorial review. Radiographics 2009;29(5):1371–91.
8. Philips J, Gurganus M, DeShields S, et al. Prevalence of sonographic markers of placenta accreta spectrum in low-risk pregnancies. Am J Perinatol 2019;36(8):733–80.
9. Blaicher W, Brugger PC, Mittermayer C, et al. Magnetic resonance imaging of the normal placenta. Eur J Radiol 2006;57(2):256–60.
10. Gowland PA, Freeman A, Issa B, et al. In vivo relaxation time measurements in the human placenta using echo planar imaging at 0.5 T. Magn Reson Imaging 1998;16(3):241–7.
11. Leyendecker JR, DuBose M, Hosseinzadeh K, et al. MRI of pregnancy-related issues: abnormal placentation. AJR Am J Roentgenol 2012;198(2): 311–20.
12. Derman AY, Nikac V, Haberman S, et al. MRI of placenta accreta: a new imaging perspective. AJR Am J Roentgenol 2011;197(6):1514–21.

13. Jauniaux E, Bhide A, Kennedy A, et al. FIGO consensus guidelines on placenta accreta spectrum disorders: Prenatal diagnosis and screening. Int J Gynaecol Obstet 2018;140(3):274–80.

14. Jauniaux E, Collins S, Burton GJ. Placenta accreta spectrum: pathophysiology and evidence-based anatomy for prenatal ultrasound imaging. Am J Obstet Gynecol 2018;218(1):75–87.

15. Melcer Y, Jauniaux E, Maymon S, et al. Impact of targeted scanning protocols on perinatal outcomes in pregnancies at risk of placenta accreta spectrum or vasa previa. Am J Obstet Gynecol 2018;218(4): 443.e1–8.

16. Jauniaux E, Chantraine F, Silver RM, et al. FIGO consensus guidelines on placenta accreta spectrum disorders: Epidemiology. Int J Gynaecol Obstet 2018;140(3):265–73.

17. Jauniaux E, Collins SL, Jurkovic D, et al. Accreta placentation: a systematic review of prenatal ultrasound imaging and grading of villous invasiveness. Am J Obstet Gynecol 2016;215(6):712–21.

18. Alfirevic Z, Tang A-W, Collins SL, et al. Pro forma for ultrasound reporting in suspected abnormally invasive placenta (AIP): an international consensus. Ultrasound Obstet Gynecol 2016; 47(3):276–8.

19. Collins SL, Ashcroft A, Braun T, et al. Proposal for standardized ultrasound descriptors of abnormally invasive placenta (AIP). Ultrasound Obstet Gynecol 2016;47(3):271–5.

20. Finberg HJ, Williams JW. Placenta accreta: prospective sonographic diagnosis in patients with placenta previa and prior cesarean section. J Ultrasound Med 1992;11(7):333–43.

21. Shih JC, Jaraquemada JMP, Su YN, et al. Role of three-dimensional power Doppler in the antenatal diagnosis of placenta accreta: comparison with gray-scale and color Doppler techniques. Ultrasound Obstet Gynecol 2009;33(2):193–203.

22. Bhide A, Laoreti A, Kaelin Agten A, et al. Lower uterine segment placental thickness in women with abnormally invasive placenta. Acta Obstet Gynecol Scand 2019;98(1):95–100.

23. Budorick NE, Figueroa R, Vizcarra M, et al. Another look at ultrasound and magnetic resonance imaging for diagnosis of placenta accreta. J Matern Fetal Neonatal Med 2017;30(20):2422–7.

24. Aitken K, Allen L, Pantazi S, et al. MRI significantly improves disease staging to direct surgical planning for abnormal invasive placentation: a single centre experience. J Obstet Gynaecol Can 2016;38(3): 246–251 e1.

25. Bourgioti C, Zafeiropoulou K, Fotopoulos S, et al. MRI features predictive of invasive placenta with extrauterine spread in high-risk gravid patients: a prospective evaluation. AJR Am J Roentgenol 2018;211(3):701–11.

26. Bourgioti C, Zafeiropoulou K, Fotopoulos S, et al. MRI prognosticators for adverse maternal and neonatal clinical outcome in patients at high risk for placenta accreta spectrum (PAS) disorders. J Magn Reson Imaging 2018;50(2):602–18.

27. Lax A, Prince MR, Mennitt KW, et al. The value of specific MRI features in the evaluation of suspected placental invasion. Magn Reson Imaging 2007; 25(1):87–93.

28. Ueno Y, Kitajima K, Kawakami F, et al. Novel MRI finding for diagnosis of invasive placenta praevia: evaluation of findings for 65 patients using clinical and histopathological correlations. Eur Radiol 2014;24(4):881–8.

29. Goergen SK, Posma E, Wrede D, et al. Interobserver agreement and diagnostic performance of individual MRI criteria for diagnosis of placental adhesion disorders. Clin Radiol 2018;73(10):908.e1-9.

30. Azour L, Besa C, Lewis S, et al. The gravid uterus: MR imaging and reporting of abnormal placentation. Abdom Radiol (NY) 2016;41(12):2411–23.

31. Bour L, Placé V, Bendavid S, et al. Suspected invasive placenta: evaluation with magnetic resonance imaging. Eur Radiol 2014;24(12):3150–60.

32. Familiari A, Liberati M, Lim P, et al. Diagnostic accuracy of magnetic resonance imaging in detecting the severity of abnormal invasive placenta: a systematic review and meta-analysis. Acta Obstet Gynecol Scand 2018;97(5):507–20.

33. Alamo L, Anaye A, Rey J, et al. Detection of suspected placental invasion by MRI: do the results depend on observer' experience? Eur J Radiol 2013;82(2):e51–7.

34. Baughman WC, Corteville JE, Shah RR. Placenta accreta: spectrum of US and MR imaging findings. Radiographics 2008;28(7):1905–16.

35. Chen X, Shan R, Zhao L, et al. Invasive placenta previa: Placental bulge with distorted uterine outline and uterine serosal hypervascularity at 1.5T MRI - useful features for differentiating placenta percreta from placenta accreta. Eur Radiol 2018;28(2): 708–17.

36. Rahaim NSA, Whitby EH. The MRI features of placental adhesion disorder and their diagnostic significance: systematic review. Clin Radiol 2015; 70(9):917–25.

37. Twickler DM, Lucas MJ, Balis AB, et al. Color flow mapping for myometrial invasion in women with a prior cesarean delivery. J Matern Fetal Med 2000; 9(6):330–5.

38. Lim PS, Greenberg M, Edelson MI, et al. Utility of ultrasound and MRI in prenatal diagnosis of placenta accreta: a pilot study. AJR Am J Roentgenol 2011; 197(6):1506–13.

39. Maldjian C, Adam R, Pelosi M, et al. MRI appearance of placenta percreta and placenta accreta. Magn Reson Imaging 1999;17(7):965–71.

40. Kim JA, Narra VR. Magnetic resonance imaging with true fast imaging with steady-state precession and half-Fourier acquisition single-shot turbo spin-echo sequences in cases of suspected placenta accreta. Acta Radiol 2004;45(6):692–8.

41. Konstantinidou AE, Bourgioti C, Fotopoulos S, et al. Stripped fetal vessel sign: a novel pathological feature of abnormal fetal vasculature in placenta accreta spectrum disorders with MRI correlates. Placenta 2019;85:74–7.

42. Robert Pijnenborg IB. Roberto Romero placental bed disorders: basic science and its translation to obstetrics. Oxford (UK): Cambridge University Press; 2010.

43. Fadl SA, Linnau KF, Dighe MK. Placental abruption and hemorrhage-review of imaging appearance. Emerg Radiol 2019;26(1):87–97.

44. Jha P, Melendres G, Bijan B, et al. Trauma in pregnant women: assessing detection of post-traumatic placental abruption on contrast-enhanced CT versus ultrasound. Abdom Radiol (NY) 2017;42(4):1062–7.

45. Masselli G, Brunelli R, Parasassi T, et al. Magnetic resonance imaging of clinically stable late pregnancy bleeding: beyond ultrasound. Eur Radiol 2011;21(9):1841–9.

46. Masselli G, Brunelli R, Di Tola M, et al. MR imaging in the evaluation of placental abruption: correlation with sonographic findings. Radiology 2011;259(1):222–30.

47. Jha P, Paroder V, Mar W, et al. Multimodality imaging of placental masses: a pictorial review. Abdom Radiol (NY) 2016;41(12):2435–44.

48. Sirotkina M, Douroudis K, Westgren M, et al. Association of chorangiomas to hypoxia-related placental changes in singleton and multiple pregnancy placentas. Placenta 2016;39:154–9.

49. Shimojo H, Itoh N, Shigematsu H, et al. Mature teratoma of the placenta. Pathol Int 1996;46(5):372–5.

50. Ahmed N, Kale V, Thakkar H, et al. Sonographic diagnosis of placental teratoma. J Clin Ultrasound 2004;32(2):98–101.

51. Moscoso G, Jauniaux E, Hustin J. Placental vascular anomaly with diffuse mesenchymal stem villous hyperplasia. A new clinico-pathological entity? Pathol Res Pract 1991;187(2–3):324–8.

52. Tortoledo M, Galindo A, Ibarrola C. Placental mesenchymal dysplasia associated with hepatic and pulmonary hamartoma. Fetal Pediatr Pathol 2010;29(4):261–70.

53. Starikov R, Goldman R, Dizon DS, et al. Placental mesenchymal dysplasia presenting as a twin gestation with complete molar pregnancy. Obstet Gynecol 2011;118(2 Pt 2):445–9.

54. Kuwata T, Takahashi H, Matsubara S. 'Stained-glass' sign for placental mesenchymal dysplasia. Ultrasound Obstet Gynecol 2014;43(3):355.

55. Aso K, Tsukimori K, Yumoto Y, et al. Prenatal findings in a case of massive fetomaternal hemorrhage associated with intraplacental choriocarcinoma. Fetal Diagn Ther 2009;25(1):158–62.

56. Liu J, Guo L. Intraplacental choriocarcinoma in a term placenta with both maternal and infantile metastases: a case report and review of the literature. Gynecol Oncol 2006;103(3):1147–51.

57. Unsal MA, Guven S. Complete hydatidiform mole coexisting with a live fetus. Clin Exp Obstet Gynecol 2012;39(2):262–4.

58. Piura B, Rabinovich A, Hershkovitz R, et al. Twin pregnancy with a complete hydatidiform mole and surviving co-existent fetus. Arch Gynecol Obstet 2008;278(4):377–82.

Fertility-Sparing Approaches in Gynecologic Oncology
Role of Imaging in Treatment Planning

Erica B. Stein, MD[a],*, Jean M. Hansen, DO, MS[b],
Katherine E. Maturen, MD, MS[a,b]

KEYWORDS

- Cervical cancer • Endometrial cancer • Ovarian cancer • Trachelectomy • Parametrial invasion
- Stromal invasion

KEY POINTS

- Some early stage gynecologic cancers may be successfully treated while preserving the patient's fertility.
- Multiparametric pelvic MR imaging plays a key role in determining eligibility for fertility preservation.
- Understanding eligibility criteria and how to optimize MR imaging protocols enables radiologists to deliver clinically relevant information and add value with imaging.

INTRODUCTION

Many women of reproductive age who are diagnosed with cancer are interested in maintaining their future fertility. For women diagnosed with cervical, endometrial, or ovarian neoplasm, there are various fertility-sparing options for carefully selected patients with early stage cancer. The emerging specialty of oncofertility bridges oncology with reproductive research so that patients have all the necessary information available when making important decisions about future fertility.[1–3] Approaches may include cryopreservation of eggs or embryos, surrogacy, or organ-sparing surgical techniques. This review focuses on the latter.

If patients are deemed eligible, fertility-sparing options may include conization or trachelectomy for cervical cancer, medical hormonal treatment of endometrial cancer (EC), and cystectomy or unilateral salpingo-oophorectomy for ovarian neoplasm. If pelvic radiation is necessary, ovarian transposition is another option, to relocate the ovaries outside of the radiation field.

Determining which patients are eligible for fertility-sparing treatments relies heavily on accurate cancer staging. When multiparametric MR imaging is performed, the radiologist can answer specific questions about local extent of cervical cancer and EC and can assist in better characterizing sonographically indeterminate adnexal masses. Optimized MR imaging protocols are critical to image the tumors in the appropriate plane and answer the clinically relevant questions for our gynecology/oncology colleagues.

MR IMAGING PROTOCOLS

Patients are asked to fast 4 to 6 hours before their MR imaging examination to help reduce bowel

[a] Department of Radiology, Michigan Medicine, 1500 East Medical Center Drive, Ann Arbor, MI 48109, USA;
[b] Department of Obstetrics/Gynecology, Michigan Medicine, L4000 UH South, 1500 East Medical Center Drive, Ann Arbor, MI 48109, USA
* Corresponding author. Michigan Medicine, 1500 East Medical Center Drive, UH B1 D502, Ann Arbor, MI 48109.
E-mail address: erst@med.umich.edu

Radiol Clin N Am 58 (2020) 401–412
https://doi.org/10.1016/j.rcl.2019.10.006
0033-8389/20/© 2019 Elsevier Inc. All rights reserved.

peristalsis. Administration of an antiperistaltic agent, such as glucagon, is recommended for all female gynecologic MR imaging. The preferred method of administration is via the intramuscular route, because the medication has rapid absorption and a longer duration (30–60 minutes compared with 10 minutes when using the intravenous route). Additionally, patients should empty their bladder before the scan, because a full bladder can result in motion-related artifact.

A multichannel phased-array receiver coil is used at a field strength of greater than or equal to 1.5 T and patients are imaged in the supine position. Vaginal gel is optional for patients with cervical cancer.

MR imaging sequences may vary across institutions, but there are several key sequences that are integral to improving detection and characterization of masses, such as high-resolution small field-of-view T2-weighted imaging (T2WI). Sagittal high-resolution small field-of-view T2WI is particularly helpful for local tumor staging of cervical cancer and EC. In the setting of cervical cancer, additional high-resolution short-axis oblique T2WI perpendicular to the endocervical canal is performed and high-resolution long-axis oblique T2WI parallel to the endocervical canal is optional. When the clinical indication is for EC staging, the high-resolution short-axis oblique T2WI is performed perpendicular to the endometrial cavity, with optional long-axis oblique T2WI parallel to the endometrial cavity. If the clinical indication is for characterization of an adnexal mass, high-resolution small field-of-view true axial T2WI is performed. Alternatively, some institutions perform an oblique plane T2WI parallel to the endometrial cavity, referred to as the "ovarian axis", which can assist in visualizing the gonadal vessels and confirming ovarian origin of a mass.[4,5]

Dynamic contrast-enhanced (DCE) MR imaging is a technique where sequential image sets are rapidly acquired through the volume of interest following the intravenous administration of gadolinium contrast. In cases of cervical cancer and EC, DCE MR imaging is acquired in the sagittal plane, with delayed postcontrast T1-weighted imaging (T1WI) in the axial plane. With cervical cancer, DCE MR imaging has been shown to improve tumor-to-cervical stromal contrast in patients with small tumors less than 2 cm in size.[6,7] Similarly, DCE is helpful in delineating extent of myoinvasion for staging EC. For adnexal mass characterization, DCE MR imaging is acquired in the axial plane, imaged for a minimum of 3 minutes following contrast administration, and with a temporal resolution less than 15 seconds.[8–11]

DCE MR imaging is particularly helpful in characterizing sonographically indeterminate adnexal masses. Regions of interest are placed on the most rapidly enhancing component of the ovarian mass and the outer myometrium. The time-intensity curve of the ovarian mass is compared with the myometrial reference, which generally has a steep initial slope and a shoulder. Three unique time-intensity curves have been described in adnexal lesions.[12] A type I curve is defined as slow progressive enhancement without plateau and is suggestive of benignity. A type II curve demonstrates an initial slope less than that of myometrium but with a distinct shoulder, and has been associated with intermediate-risk lesions, such as borderline ovarian tumor. A type III curve demonstrates a rapid initial wash-in with a slope that is greater than adjacent myometrium, suggestive of probable malignancy.

When high temporal resolution DCE is not available, a multiphasic acquisition obtained at intervals of 30 seconds or more may still provide useful information about enhancement kinetics. When a mass enhances less than the myometrium (or much less than pelvic arteries) in the arterial phase, an aggressive ovarian malignancy is unlikely.[13]

CERVICAL CANCER AND FERTILITY-SPARING OPTIONS

Cervical cancer is commonly diagnosed in women of reproductive age, typically attributed to sexual activity and transmission of the human papilloma virus infection, a strongly associated risk factor. In a select patient population, fertility-sparing techniques may be applied, to allow for future fertility in these women.

Cone biopsy, or conization, refers to the en bloc removal of the squamocolumnar junction, which includes the ectocervix and endocervical canal. This technique may constitute definitive treatment of patients with stage IA1 tumors with negative margins and absence of lymphovascular space invasion. Patients with stage IA1 tumors with lymphovascular space invasion or stage IA2 tumors require lymph node assessment in the form of either pelvic lymphadenectomy or pelvic sentinel lymph node biopsies in conjunction with conization, radical trachelectomy, or hysterectomy. Stage IA tumors are not visible at MR imaging and are diagnosed by microscopy.

Radical trachelectomy is performed vaginally or abdominally, via an open or minimally invasive approach. The operation involves surgical removal of the cervix, the parametria, and the upper vagina. The upper vagina is then sutured to the lower uterine body. A cerclage or "purse string" stitch is placed by the surgeon in the lower uterine body to prevent pregnancy loss.

There are specific eligibility criteria (Table 1) required for consideration of radical trachelectomy for fertility-sparing treatment of cervical cancer, but individual practice patterns vary. Patients must desire fertility preservation and the preoperative evaluation must suggest that the patient is at low risk for needing postoperative radiation therapy.[14] The tumor must be confined to the cervix, should be less than or equal to 2 cm in size, and the superior aspect must be greater than or equal to 1 cm from the internal os (Fig. 1), although tumors 2 to 4 cm are not an absolute contraindication. Histology should be squamous cell carcinoma, adenocarcinoma, or adenosquamous carcinoma. Broadly, exclusion criteria include tumor size greater than 2 cm, parametrial spread, lymphovascular space invasion, and nodal or distant metastatic disease.

Tumor size, location relative to the internal cervical os, parametrial extension, and nodal metastases can all be assessed with pelvic MR imaging. On T2WI, cervical cancer typically appears as an intermediate signal intensity lesion that may or may not disrupt the low-signal intensity cervical stroma. Most tumors are either isointense or hypointense relative to adjacent stroma on the delayed postcontrast imaging. Small tumors may enhance earlier than adjacent cervical stroma, which is better delineated with DCE MR imaging. Cervical tumors typically demonstrate high signal intensity on high-b-value diffusion weighted imaging (DWI) with corresponding low signal on the apparent diffusion coefficient maps, relative to cervical stroma (Fig 2).

Tumor size should be reported in all three dimensions, with craniocaudal axis relative to the endocervical canal and distance from the internal os. At least 1 cm length between the superior margin of the cervical tumor and the internal os is desired, to allow for a negative margin and safe surgical anastomosis.[15] Some institutions have decreased this minimum length to 0.5 cm.[16] At MR imaging, the internal os anatomic landmark is defined as the waist of the uterus, the point at which the low signal intensity cervical stroma becomes intermediate signal intensity myometrium. The internal os is also the entrance site of the uterine vessels (Fig. 3). A cervical tumor that extends to or involves the internal os is ineligible for fertility-sparing techniques (Fig. 4).

Many patients may have a history of prior cone biopsy or other excisional procedure, which may affect the cervical length. The total length of the

Table 1
Eligibility and exclusion criteria

Gynecologic Cancer	Inclusion/Eligibility Criteria	Exclusion Criteria
Cervical	Tumor confined to cervix Tumor ≤2 cm in size Distance ≥1 cm between tumor and internal os Cervical stromal invasion <50% Favorable histology (squamous cell carcinoma, adenocarcinoma, adenosquamous)	Parametrial spread Tumor >2 cm in size Distance <1 cm between tumor and internal os Cervical stromal invasion >50% Lymphovascular space invasion (pathology diagnosis) Nodal or distant metastatic disease Aggressive histologic subtypes (eg, neuroendocrine tumor, adenoma malignum)
Endometrial	Absence of myometrial and cervical invasion No genetic predisposition for ovarian cancer Favorable histology (grade I endometrioid adenocarcinoma or premalignant condition)	Synchronous primary ovarian cancer or ovarian metastatic disease Nodal or distant metastatic disease Aggressive histologic subtypes (grade 2 and 3 endometrioid adenocarcinoma, serous, clear cell)
Ovarian	Any stage malignant germ cell tumor, sex-cord stromal tumor, or borderline tumor Stage I epithelial cell tumor Absence of extraovarian disease	Nodal or distant metastatic disease

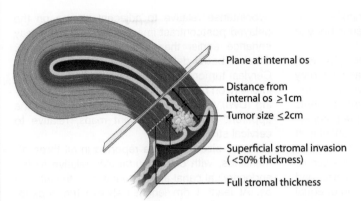

Fig. 1. Sagittal illustration of the cervix and uterine body highlighting important eligibility criteria for trachelectomy: tumor size ≤2 cm, distance from internal os ≥1 cm, and superficial stromal invasion (<50% stromal thickness).

Labels on figure:
— Plane at internal os
— Distance from internal os ≥1cm
— Tumor size ≤2cm
— Superficial stromal invasion (<50% thickness)
— Full stromal thickness

cervix should ideally be greater than 2.5 cm. Additional cone biopsy may be deferred in patients with a short cervix, given potential future complications of cervical incompetence and preterm delivery.[6,17,18]

At T2WI, cervical stromal invasion is present when the intermediate signal intensity tumor disrupts the low-signal intensity cervical stroma. Deep stromal invasion is defined as a cervical tumor that invades the outer third of the cervical stroma (Fig. 5). Given association between deep stromal invasion and higher recurrence rate and shorter survival, ideal tumors for a fertility-preserving approach involve less than half of the stromal thickness (see Fig. 1).[14,19] Because this parameter is difficult to assess clinically and by MR imaging, preoperative suspicion of deep stromal invasion is a relative rather than absolute contraindication and is balanced against other factors in surgical decision-making.[20,21]

By contrast, parametrial invasion is a definite contraindication to radical trachelectomy and denotes at least stage IIB disease. At MR imaging, parametrial invasion is present if the tumor disrupts the low signal intensity cervical stromal ring (Fig. 6). Lymph node or distant metastases are also a contraindication to fertility-preserving surgery. Pelvic or para-aortic lymph nodes larger than 1 cm in short axis are suspicious. Additional

morphologic features concerning for nodal metastatic disease include irregular borders, loss of fatty hilum, presence of necrosis, and signal intensity that is similar to the primary tumor.[22] Both computed tomography and MR imaging are limited in detecting metastatic disease in normal-sized lymph nodes, but fluorodeoxyglucose PET is often used clinically to assess for extracervical disease.

ENDOMETRIAL CANCER AND FERTILITY-SPARING OPTIONS

EC is most commonly diagnosed in postmenopausal women. EC is less commonly diagnosed in premenopausal women, but incidence has increased in recent years.[23] One of the main risk factors for the development of EC is prolonged unopposed estrogen exposure, which is seen in the setting of obesity, nulliparity, and polycystic ovarian syndrome.[24–26]

EC often presents with abnormal uterine bleeding and as a result is often diagnosed at early stages when the tumor is confined to the uterine body. Most women have low-grade, early stage endometrioid carcinoma and the long-term prognosis is excellent. The standard surgical management for early disease is total hysterectomy and bilateral salpingo-oophorectomy. Nodal

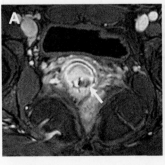
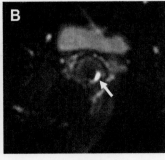

Fig. 2. Endocervical adenocarcinoma status postconization, eligible for trachelectomy. (A) Axial postcontrast T1WI with fat saturation shows a small hypoenhancing tumor at the ectocervix (arrow). (B) Axial DWI shows corresponding hyperintense signal (arrow). This patient is eligible for trachelectomy because tumor is ≤2 cm in size, distance from tumor to internal os is ≥1 cm, and there is no deep stromal invasion.

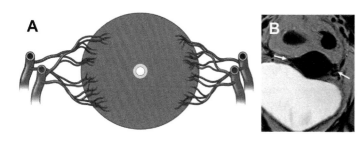

Fig. 3. Internal cervical os. (A) Axial illustration of the internal cervical os, demonstrating entrance of uterine vessels. (B) Oblique short-axis T2WI without fat saturation shows level of internal os with uterine vessels on either side (arrows).

assessment is also performed in many centers, with various approaches including sentinel lymph node mapping or pelvic and para-aortic lymphadenectomy.

Fertility-sparing options exist as an alternate to the standard surgical management in young women who desire future fertility. Conservative medical treatment includes oral progestins or levonorgestrel-coated intrauterine device.[27,28] Treatment response is evaluated every 3 to 6 months with endometrial biopsy or dilation and curettage and MR imaging if desired.[29–31] If there is no genetic predisposition for ovarian cancer and the patient is premenopausal, the ovaries may be preserved.[29] Total hysterectomy is recommended for patients following child-bearing given high risk of recurrence.[29,31]

There are specific eligibility criteria (see **Table 1**) for consideration of fertility-sparing options in premenopausal women with newly diagnosed EC. The pathology of the tumor must be a well-differentiated (FIGO grade 1) endometrioid adenocarcinoma or a premalignant condition (eg, atypical hyperplasia).[29,31] Histologic specimen must be obtained with dilation and curettage, providing a more accurate diagnosis than routine endometrial pipelle biopsy.[32]

Absence of myometrial and cervical invasion, well-assessed by MR imaging, is a prerequisite for consideration of fertility preservation (**Fig. 7**). Endometrial tumors typically demonstrate signal characteristics that are similar to or lower than adjacent normal myometrium on T2WI and stand out relative to adjacent low-signal junctional zone (inner myometrium). Most tumors enhance more slowly and less intensely compared with the adjacent myometrium. Maximal tumor-to-myometrial contrast occurs at approximately 90 to 120 seconds following intravenous administration of gadolinium with DCE.[33,34] Endometrial tumors impede diffusion, characterized by high signal intensity on the high-b-value DWI and low signal on apparent diffusion coefficient maps.[35–38] The normal endometrium also exhibits moderately high signal on DWI because of its cellularity, but ECs restrict diffusion even more strongly.

An uninterrupted low signal intensity junctional zone on T2WI is helpful to exclude myometrial involvement by tumor and to confirm that tumor is limited to the endometrial canal (**Fig. 8**). An analogous clue on DCE is a continuous rim of subendometrial enhancement of the inner junctional zone, best delineated within the first minute following contrast administration.[34,39,40]

To be considered for fertility-preservation, there can be no evidence of synchronous primary ovarian cancer or ovarian metastatic disease (**Fig. 9**). Ovarian involvement from either

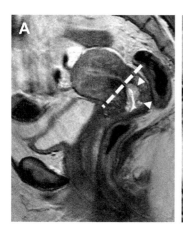
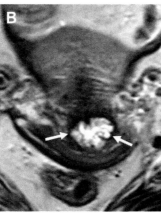

Fig. 4. Mucinous endocervical cancer, ineligible for trachelectomy. (A) Sagittal T2WI without fat saturation shows an endophytic mass (arrowheads) that extends within 1 cm of the internal os (dotted line). (B) Oblique short-axis T2WI without fat saturation shows evidence of deep stromal invasion (arrows). This patient is ineligible for trachelectomy given involvement of the internal os and deep stromal invasion.

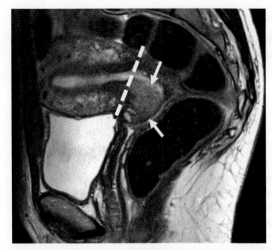

Fig. 5. Squamous cell carcinoma of the cervix, ineligible for trachelectomy. Sagittal T2WI without fat saturation shows a large infiltrative mass (*arrows*) with deep stromal invasion and involvement of the internal os (*dotted line*). This patient is ineligible for trachelectomy given tumor size greater than 2 cm, deep stromal invasion, and involvement of the internal os.

metastasis or primary neoplasm excludes the patient from conservative management.[3] Absence of nodal metastatic disease is the last criterion needed for consideration of fertility-preservation in the setting of EC. Nodal metastases are rare in early stage disease.[24,29,41,42]

OVARIAN CANCER AND FERTILITY-SPARING OPTIONS

The most common ovarian cancer type is high-grade serous carcinoma, which typically presents at an advanced stage with disseminated peritoneal disease. However, other histologies, such as borderline epithelial neoplasms and germ cell

tumors, are more common in younger women, and may sometimes be treated with a fertility-sparing surgical approach (see **Table 1**).[29,43–46] Standard surgical management includes resection of the ovarian tumor, surgical staging if early disease, or cytoreductive surgery when more advanced.[47] The more conservative fertility-sparing approach involves unilateral salpingo-oophorectomy with preservation of the contralateral ovary and uterus. Intraoperative frozen section evaluation by the pathologist is critical when fertility-sparing technique is desired.

Clinical evaluation for women with pelvic masses includes physical examination, pelvic ultrasound, and serum tumor marker assessment. Transvaginal ultrasound remains the modality of choice to evaluate for benign versus malignant features.[48] However, approximately 25% of masses remain sonographically indeterminate, and this is where MR imaging has a role in added characterization.[49–52]

Benign Ovarian Lesions

Imaging characteristics that favor a benign ovarian mass are: purely cystic, purely endometriotic, or purely fatty masses. Thin, smooth walls and septa are generally benign findings. Solid elements that exhibit homogenously low signal (less than skeletal muscle) on T2WI and DWI are a benign feature of fibrous tissue as may be seen in sex-cord stromal tumors.[8,53–56] On DCE (discussed previously in MR imaging protocols section) a type I time-intensity curve, characterized by slow progressive enhancement is predictive of benignity.[8,57] DWI should always be interpreted together with T1WI and T2WI, because benign and malignant masses can impede diffusion. However, if technically adequate DWI demonstrates no focal restricted diffusion within a mass, this is a reassuring sign of benignity.

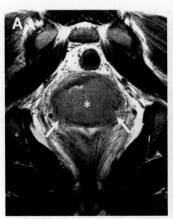
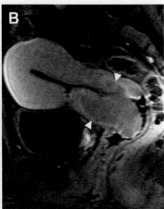

Fig. 6. Squamous cell carcinoma of the cervix, ineligible for trachelectomy. (*A*) Oblique short-axis T2WI without fat saturation shows a large infiltrative intermediate signal mass (*asterisk*) with deep stromal invasion and disruption of the hypointense cervical stromal ring (*arrows*) denoting parametrial extension (at least stage IIB). (*B*) Sagittal postcontrast T1WI with fat saturation shows the large cervical mass (*arrowheads*) that spans from external to internal os with deep stromal invasion. This patient is ineligible for many reasons including large tumor size greater than 2 cm, involvement of the internal os, deep stromal invasion, and parametrial extension.

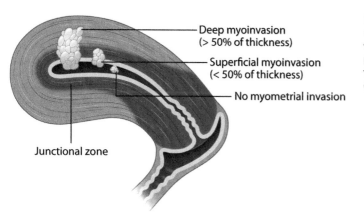

Fig. 7. Sagittal illustration of the uterus showing endometrial cancer with no myometrial invasion, with superficial myoinvasion (<50% stromal thickness), and deep myoinvasion (>50% stromal thickness).

Malignant Ovarian Lesions

Malignant ovarian masses at MR imaging typically demonstrate mixed cystic and solid composition, with brisk enhancement of the solid components. At DCE, malignant masses typically demonstrate a type III curve (rapid and more intense enhancement relative to adjacent myometrium).

Borderline Ovarian Tumors

Histologically, these tumors have features of malignancy but there is no evidence of ovarian stromal invasion. Serous histology is more common than mucinous. The solid components in serous borderline ovarian tumors tend to have a frond-like or papillary morphology with type II enhancement curves relative to myometrium (Fig. 10).[8,58] Borderline ovarian tumors may present with peritoneal deposits that are visible at MR imaging, classified as either invasive or noninvasive depending on the depth of invasion at pathologic inspection.

Stage I Epithelial Tumors

Most patients with epithelial ovarian tumors are postmenopausal and present at an advanced stage. A small percentage of cases occur in premenopausal women at an earlier stage and fertility-sparing options may be offered. Women with unilateral ovarian tumor involvement (stage IA or IC) and favorable histology (eg, serous, mucinous, grade 1 endometrioid) may be candidates for fertility preservation. Women with a more aggressive histology (eg, clear cell or serous carcinoma) that present at an earlier stage also may be candidates.[3] A patient may be excluded from fertility preservation in the setting of bilateral ovarian involvement (stage IB) or extraovarian spread of disease.[46,59]

Malignant Germ Cell Tumors

Most germ cell tumors are benign mature cystic teratomas. Only 5% of germ cell tumors are malignant, with dysgerminomas and immature teratomas being the most common, followed by yolk

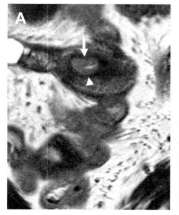
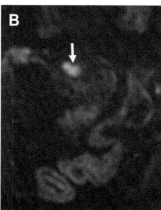

Fig. 8. Endometrial cancer, eligible for conservative medical management. (A) Oblique short-axis T2WI without fat saturation shows a small intermediate signal tumor (arrow) without myoinvasion; the low signal junctional zone (arrowhead) is not interrupted. (B) Oblique short-axis DWI shows hyperintense signal (arrow). This patient is eligible for conservative medical management given absence of myoinvasion.

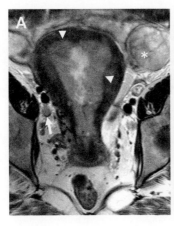
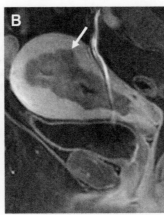

Fig. 9. Grade I endometrioid endometrial cancer with left ovarian and nodal metastases, ineligible for conservative medical management. (*A*) Oblique long-axis T2WI without fat saturation shows a large intermediate signal mass distending the endometrial canal (*arrowheads*), left ovarian metastasis (*asterisk*), and right pelvic lymph node metastasis (*arrow*). (*B*) Sagittal postcontrast delayed T1WI with fat saturation shows relative hypo-enhancement of the tumor relative to adjacent myometrium with greater than 50% myoinvasion (*arrow*). This patient is ineligible for conservative medical management despite low-grade neoplasm because of presence of myoinvasion and left ovarian and nodal metastases.

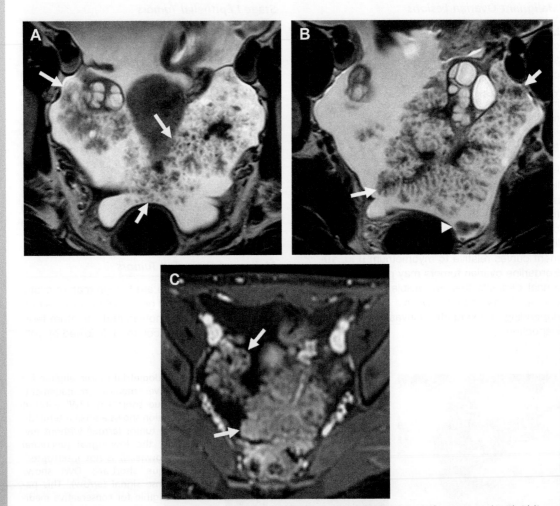

Fig. 10. Bilateral serous borderline ovarian tumors, eligible for unilateral salpingo-oophorectomy. (*A, B*) Oblique T2WI without fat saturation shows bilateral adnexal masses exhibiting frond-like morphology (*arrows*) intimately associated with the ovaries, small peritoneal deposit (*arrowhead*), and moderate ascites. (*C*) Axial postcontrast T1WI with fat saturation shows enhancement of the frond-like soft tissue components (*arrows*). The patient underwent left salpingo-oophorectomy, omentectomy, peritoneal stripping, and a right ovarian wedge resection with debulking. The remnant right ovary, right fallopian tube, and uterus were preserved.

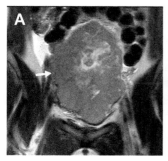
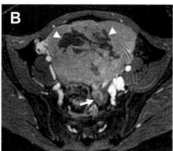

Fig. 11. Dysgerminoma of the right ovary, eligible for unilateral salpin go-oophorectomy. (*A*) Coronal T2WI without fat saturation shows a large predominantly solid pelvic mass (*arrow*). (*B*) Axial postcontrast T1WI with fat saturation shows central necrosis of the solid mass (*arrowheads*) and normal left ovary (*arrow*). This patient underwent right salpingo-oophorectomy, omentectomy, and lymphadenectomy with preservation of the left ovary, left fallopian tube, and uterus.

sac and mixed tumors.[3,60] Most patients present with early stage ovary-confined disease that is eligible for fertility preservation. Those patients with more advanced-stage disease still have a favorable prognosis given chemosensitivity of the primary tumor, which may still allow for fertility preservation surgery.[61] Malignant germ cell tumors are variable in appearance. Dysgerminomas typically present as a solid mass (**Fig. 11**), whereas immature teratomas often contain fat and/or calcifications, and yolk sac tumors may present as a mixed cystic and solid mass.[60]

Sex-Cord Stromal Tumors

Granulosa cell tumors are the most common sex-cord stromal tumor, with a bimodal distribution (juvenile and adult forms). The juvenile form is more aggressive, but fertility-sparing surgery remains the standard treatment.[56] Juvenile granulosa cell tumors may be solid or spongiform and are usually unilateral (**Fig. 12**). There is an association with endometrial hyperplasia, endometrial polyps, and endometrial carcinoma because of the production of estrogen by the primary ovarian mass.

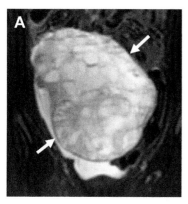
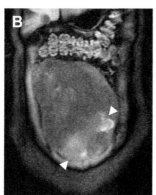
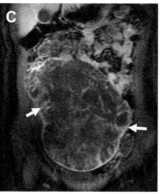

Fig. 12. Juvenile granulosa cell tumor of the right ovary, eligible for unilateral salpingo-oophorectomy. (*A*) Coronal T2WI with fat saturation shows a large multiseptated mass (*arrows*) and ascites. (*B, C*) Precontrast and postcontrast T1WI with fat saturation shows intratumoral hemorrhage (*arrowheads*) and irregular enhancing septations (*arrows*). This patient underwent right salpingo-oophorectomy with preservation of the left ovary, left fallopian tube, and uterus.

SUMMARY

Advances in imaging technology and research have improved the ability to make important distinctions in gynecologic imaging. Armed with understanding of the oncologic context and eligibility criteria for fertility-sparing approaches, radiologists have the opportunity to contribute rich information to interdisciplinary treatment planning in gynecologic oncology and to impact the outcomes of young women with cancer.

DISCLOSURE

Dr K.E. Maturen receives educational royalties from Elsevier and Wolters Kluwer. The authors would like to acknowledge and thank Ms. Danielle Dobbs of the University of Michigan Media Division for her original medical illustrations.

REFERENCES

1. Woodruff TK. The Oncofertility Consortium: addressing fertility in young people with cancer. Nat Rev Clin Oncol 2010;7(8):466–75.

2. Carter J, Rowland K, Chi D, et al. Gynecologic cancer treatment and the impact of cancer-related infertility. Gynecol Oncol 2005;97(1):90–5.

3. McEvoy SH, Nougaret S, Abu-Rustum NR, et al. Fertility-sparing for young patients with gynecologic cancer: how MRI can guide patient selection prior to conservative management. Abdom Radiol (NY) 2017;42(10):2488–512.

4. Forstner R, Thomassin-Naggara I, Cunha TM, et al. ESUR recommendations for MR imaging of the sonographically indeterminate adnexal mass: an update. Eur Radiol 2017;27(6):2248–57.

5. Spencer JA, Ghattamaneni S. MR imaging of the sonographically indeterminate adnexal mass. Radiology 2010;256(3):677–94.

6. Akita A, Shinmoto H, Hayashi S, et al. Comparison of T2-weighted and contrast-enhanced T1-weighted MR imaging at 1.5 T for assessing the local extent of cervical carcinoma. Eur Radiol 2011;21(9):1850–7.

7. Balleyguier C, Sala E, Da Cunha T, et al. Staging of uterine cervical cancer with MRI: guidelines of the European Society of Urogenital Radiology. Eur Radiol 2011;21(5):1102–10.

8. Thomassin-Naggara I, Aubert E, Rockall A, et al. Adnexal masses: development and preliminary validation of an MR imaging scoring system. Radiology 2013;267(2):432–43.

9. Thomassin-Naggara I, Balvay D, Aubert E, et al. Quantitative dynamic contrast-enhanced MR imaging analysis of complex adnexal masses: a preliminary study. Eur Radiol 2012;22(4):738–45.

10. Thomassin-Naggara I, Balvay D, Rockall A, et al. Added value of assessing adnexal masses with advanced MRI techniques. Biomed Res Int 2015; 2015:785206.

11. Thomassin-Naggara I, Toussaint I, Perrot N, et al. Characterization of complex adnexal masses: value of adding perfusion- and diffusion-weighted MR imaging to conventional MR imaging. Radiology 2011; 258(3):793–803.

12. Sadowski EA, Robbins JB, Rockall AG, et al. A systematic approach to adnexal masses discovered on ultrasound: the ADNEx MR scoring system. Abdom Radiol (NY) 2018;43(3):679–95.

13. Pereira PN, Sarian LO, Yoshida A, et al. Accuracy of the ADNEX MR scoring system based on a simplified MRI protocol for the assessment of adnexal masses. Diagn Interv Radiol 2018;24(2):63–71.

14. Sedlis A, Bundy BN, Rotman MZ, et al. A randomized trial of pelvic radiation therapy versus no further therapy in selected patients with stage IB carcinoma of the cervix after radical hysterectomy and pelvic lymphadenectomy: a Gynecologic Oncology Group Study. Gynecol Oncol 1999;73(2): 177–83.

15. Rob L, Skapa P, Robova H. Fertility-sparing surgery in patients with cervical cancer. Lancet Oncol 2011; 12(2):192–200.

16. Rob L, Charvat M, Robova H, et al. Less radical fertility-sparing surgery than radical trachelectomy in early cervical cancer. Int J Gynecol Cancer 2007;17(1):304–10.

17. Charles-Edwards EM, Messiou C, Morgan VA, et al. Diffusion-weighted imaging in cervical cancer with an endovaginal technique: potential value for improving tumor detection in stage Ia and Ib1 disease. Radiology 2008;249(2):541–50.

18. Downey K, Shepherd JH, Attygalle AD, et al. Preoperative imaging in patients undergoing trachelectomy for cervical cancer: validation of a combined T2- and diffusion-weighted endovaginal MRI technique at 3.0 T. Gynecol Oncol 2014; 133(2):326–32.

19. Delgado G, Bundy B, Zaino R, et al. Prospective surgical-pathological study of disease-free interval in patients with stage IB squamous cell carcinoma of the cervix: a Gynecologic Oncology Group study. Gynecol Oncol 1990;38(3):352–7.

20. Lakhman Y, Akin O, Park KJ, et al. Stage IB1 cervical cancer: role of preoperative MR imaging in selection of patients for fertility-sparing radical trachelectomy. Radiology 2013;269(1):149–58.

21. Mitchell DG, Snyder B, Coakley F, et al. Early invasive cervical cancer: tumor delineation by magnetic resonance imaging, computed tomography, and clinical examination, verified by pathologic results, in the ACRIN 6651/GOG 183 Intergroup Study. J Clin Oncol 2006;24(36):5687–94.

22. McMahon CJ, Rofsky NM, Pedrosa I. Lymphatic metastases from pelvic tumors: anatomic classification, characterization, and staging. Radiology 2010; 254(1):31–46.

23. Pellerin GP, Finan MA. Endometrial cancer in women 45 years of age or younger: a clinicopathological analysis. Am J Obstet Gynecol 2005;193(5):1640–4.

24. Morice P, Leary A, Creutzberg C, et al. Endometrial cancer. Lancet 2016;387(10023):1094–108.

25. Haoula Z, Salman M, Atiomo W. Evaluating the association between endometrial cancer and polycystic ovary syndrome. Hum Reprod 2012;27(5):1327–31.

26. Navaratnarajah R, Pillay OC, Hardiman P. Polycystic ovary syndrome and endometrial cancer. Semin Reprod Med 2008;26(1):62–71.

27. Minig L, Franchi D, Boveri S, et al. Progestin intrauterine device and GnRH analogue for uterus-sparing treatment of endometrial precancers and well-differentiated early endometrial carcinoma in young women. Ann Oncol 2011;22(3):643–9.

28. Rodolakis A, Biliatis I, Morice P, et al. European Society of Gynecological Oncology Task Force for Fertility Preservation: clinical recommendations for fertility-sparing management in young endometrial cancer patients. Int J Gynecol Cancer 2015;25(7): 1258–65.

29. Colombo N, Creutzberg C, Amant F, et al. ESMO-ESGO-ESTRO consensus conference on endometrial cancer: diagnosis, treatment and follow-up. Int J Gynecol Cancer 2016;26(1):2–30.

30. Kim MK, Seong SJ, Song T, et al. Comparison of dilatation & curettage and endometrial aspiration biopsy accuracy in patients treated with high-dose oral progestin plus levonorgestrel intrauterine system for early-stage endometrial cancer. Gynecol Oncol 2013;130(3):470–3.

31. Koh WJ, Abu-Rustum NR, Bean S, et al. Uterine neoplasms, Version 1.2018, national comprehensive cancer network clinical practice guidelines in oncology. J Natl Compr Canc Netw 2018;16(2):170–99.

32. Leitao MM Jr, Kehoe S, Barakat RR, et al. Comparison of D&C and office endometrial biopsy accuracy in patients with FIGO grade 1 endometrial adenocarcinoma. Gynecol Oncol 2009;113(1):105–8.

33. Park SB, Moon MH, Sung CK, et al. Dynamic contrast-enhanced MR imaging of endometrial cancer: optimizing the imaging delay for tumour-myometrium contrast. Eur Radiol 2014;24(11):2795–9.

34. Yamashita Y, Harada M, Sawada T, et al. Normal uterus and FIGO stage I endometrial carcinoma: dynamic gadolinium-enhanced MR imaging. Radiology 1993;186(2):495–501.

35. Fujii S, Matsusue E, Kigawa J, et al. Diagnostic accuracy of the apparent diffusion coefficient in differentiating benign from malignant uterine endometrial cavity lesions: initial results. Eur Radiol 2008;18(2): 384–9.

36. Lin G, Ng KK, Chang CJ, et al. Myometrial invasion in endometrial cancer: diagnostic accuracy of diffusion-weighted 3.0-T MR imaging–initial experience. Radiology 2009;250(3):784–92.

37. Shen SH, Chiou YY, Wang JH, et al. Diffusion-weighted single-shot echo-planar imaging with parallel technique in assessment of endometrial cancer. AJR Am J Roentgenol 2008;190(2):481–8.

38. Tamai K, Koyama T, Saga T, et al. Diffusion-weighted MR imaging of uterine endometrial cancer. J Magn Reson Imaging 2007;26(3):682–7.

39. Manfredi R, Mirk P, Maresca G, et al. Local-regional staging of endometrial carcinoma: role of MR imaging in surgical planning. Radiology 2004;231(2): 372–8.

40. Fujii S, Kido A, Baba T, et al. Subendometrial enhancement and peritumoral enhancement for assessing endometrial cancer on dynamic contrast enhanced MR imaging. Eur J Radiol 2015;84(4): 581–9.

41. Panici PB, Maggioni A, Hacker N, et al. Systematic aortic and pelvic lymphadenectomy versus resection of bulky nodes only in optimally debulked advanced ovarian cancer: a randomized clinical trial. J Natl Cancer Inst 2005;97(8):560–6.

42. ASTEC Study Group, Kitchener H, Swart AM, et al. Efficacy of systematic pelvic lymphadenectomy in endometrial cancer (MRC ASTEC trial): a randomised study. Lancet 2009;373(9658):125–36.

43. Colombo N, Parma G, Zanagnolo V, et al. Management of ovarian stromal cell tumors. J Clin Oncol 2007;25(20):2944–51.

44. Colombo N, Peiretti M, Garbi A, et al. Non-epithelial ovarian cancer: ESMO clinical practice guidelines for diagnosis, treatment and follow-up. Ann Oncol 2012;23(Suppl 7):vii20–6.

45. Ledermann JA, Raja FA, Fotopoulou C, et al. Newly diagnosed and relapsed epithelial ovarian carcinoma: ESMO Clinical Practice Guidelines for diagnosis, treatment and follow-up. Ann Oncol 2018; 29(Supplement_4):iv259.

46. Satoh T, Hatae M, Watanabe Y, et al. Outcomes of fertility-sparing surgery for stage I epithelial ovarian cancer: a proposal for patient selection. J Clin Oncol 2010;28(10):1727–32.

47. Gershenson DM. Treatment of ovarian cancer in young women. Clin Obstet Gynecol 2012;55(1): 65–74.

48. Expert Panel on Women's I, Atri M, Alabousi A, et al. ACR appropriateness Criteria((R)) clinically suspected adnexal mass, no acute symptoms. J Am Coll Radiol 2019;16(5S):S77–93.

49. Kinkel K, Lu Y, Mehdizade A, et al. Indeterminate ovarian mass at US: incremental value of second imaging test for characterization–meta-analysis and Bayesian analysis. Radiology 2005;236(1): 85–94.

50. Sohaib SA, Mills TD, Sahdev A, et al. The role of magnetic resonance imaging and ultrasound in patients with adnexal masses. Clin Radiol 2005;60(3): 340–8.

51. Timmerman D, Ameye L, Fischerova D, et al. Simple ultrasound rules to distinguish between benign and malignant adnexal masses before surgery: prospective validation by IOTA group. BMJ 2010;341:c6839.

52. Van Calster B, Timmerman D, Valentin L, et al. Triaging women with ovarian masses for surgery: observational diagnostic study to compare RCOG guidelines with an International Ovarian Tumour Analysis (IOTA) group protocol. BJOG 2012; 119(6):662–71.

53. Outwater EK, Siegelman ES, Talerman A, et al. Ovarian fibromas and cystadenofibromas: MRI features of the fibrous component. J Magn Reson Imaging 1997;7(3):465–71.

54. Siegelman ES, Outwater EK. Tissue characterization in the female pelvis by means of MR imaging. Radiology 1999;212(1):5–18.

55. Tang YZ, Liyanage S, Narayanan P, et al. The MRI features of histologically proven ovarian cystadenofibromas: an assessment of the morphological and enhancement patterns. Eur Radiol 2013;23(1): 48–56.

56. Rockall AG, Qureshi M, Papadopoulou I, et al. Role of imaging in fertility-sparing treatment of gynecologic malignancies. Radiographics 2016;36(7): 2214–33.

57. Bernardin L, Dilks P, Liyanage S, et al. Effectiveness of semi-quantitative multiphase dynamic contrast-enhanced MRI as a predictor of malignancy in complex adnexal masses: radiological and pathological correlation. Eur Radiol 2012;22(4):880–90.

58. Bent CL, Sahdev A, Rockall AG, et al. MRI appearances of borderline ovarian tumours. Clin Radiol 2009;64(4):430–8.

59. Ledermann JA, Raja FA, Fotopoulou C, et al. Newly diagnosed and relapsed epithelial ovarian carcinoma: ESMO Clinical Practice Guidelines for diagnosis, treatment and follow-up. Ann Oncol 2013; 24(Suppl 6):vi24–32.

60. Shaaban AM, Rezvani M, Elsayes KM, et al. Ovarian malignant germ cell tumors: cellular classification and clinical and imaging features. Radiographics 2014;34(3):777–801.

61. Mangili G, Sigismondi C, Gadducci A, et al. Outcome and risk factors for recurrence in malignant ovarian germ cell tumors: a MITO-9 retrospective study. Int J Gynecol Cancer 2011;21(8): 1414–21.

Imaging of Gynecologic Malignancy in a Reproductive Age Female
Cancer During Pregnancy

Charis Bourgioti, MD*, Marianna Konidari, MD,
Lia Angela Moulopoulos, MD

KEYWORDS

- Cancer • Pregnancy • Cervix • Ovaries • Cervical cancer • Ovarian cancer

KEY POINTS

- Cervical cancer is the most common gynecologic cancer during pregnancy. Magnetic resonance (MR) imaging is the preferred imaging modality for cervical cancer staging in the gravid population.
- Most ovarian tumors in pregnant patients are benign but they occasionally undergo pregnancy-related morphologic changes mimicking malignancy.
- Sonography is the initial imaging modality of choice for the evaluation of ovarian masses in the pregnant population. MR imaging is valuable when sonography is inconclusive, when the mass is too large, and for staging potentially malignant lesions.
- Uterine, vaginal, or vulvar cancers are extremely rare in the gravid population; imaging is used for determining the extent of the disease.

INTRODUCTION

Pregnancy-associated cancer includes any cancer diagnosed from the day of conception to 12 months after delivery to account for possible delays in diagnosis during the course of pregnancy and because postpartum cancer is considered a continuum of cancer in pregnancy (Box 1).[1,2]

Cancer in pregnancy is uncommon, with a reported incidence ranging from 0.02% to 0.1%.[3] Several epidemiologic studies suggest an increase in pregnancy-associated cancers in recent years.[4,5] Advanced maternal age is considered a strong predisposing factor, because the incidence of cancer increases with age[6]; however, the increased incidence of pregnancy-associated malignancies cannot be explained only by the delay in childbearing.[2,4]

Among cancers diagnosed during pregnancy, gynecologic malignancies are common, especially those of cervical and ovarian origin (Box 2).[3] Recently, in an international cohort of 1170 women with pregnancy-associated cancer, gynecologic tumors accounted for 20% of the cases (cervical cancer, 13%; ovarian cancer, 7%); breast cancer and hematological malignancies were diagnosed in 39% and 16% of the study patients, respectively.[7] A similar incidence of cervical (15%) and ovarian cancer (6%) was also reported in a recent study performed in the Swedish population.[8]

Note that pregnancy status does not seem to adversely affect maternal survival compared with

First Department of Radiology, School of Medicine, National and Kapodistrian University of Athens, Aretaieion Hospital, 76 Vassilisis Sofias Avenue, Athens 11528, Greece
* Corresponding author.
E-mail address: charisbourgioti@yahoo.com

Radiol Clin N Am 58 (2020) 413–430
https://doi.org/10.1016/j.rcl.2019.10.008

nonpregnant patients treated for cancer and, furthermore, outcomes concerning fetal safety are encouraging.[7] Early diagnosis of cancer is extremely important for successful treatment, regardless of gestational age, because advanced disease at the time of diagnosis is strongly associated with poorer prognosis. However, there is often a delay in the diagnosis of pregnancy-associated cancer for several reasons.[9] Common symptoms of malignancy, such as nausea, vomiting, pain, anemia, fatigue, or even vaginal spotting or bleeding, overlap with symptoms of pregnancy. Physical examination of breasts and abdomen is difficult because of hormonal changes and the enlarged gravid uterus. Commonly used tumor markers (eg, cancer antigen [CA] 15-3 for breast cancer, CA 125 for epithelial ovarian cancer, or alpha fetoprotein for germ cell tumors) are unreliable because they may be normally increased in pregnancy.[10] Moreover, physicians hesitate to use imaging studies other than sonography, particularly in the first trimester of pregnancy, to avoid any harmful effect on the fetus. For all these reasons and because cancer during pregnancy is a rare event, it may not be considered in the differential diagnosis of early symptoms.

IMAGING TECHNIQUES APPLIED IN PREGNANCY

Imaging of pregnant patients with cancer is challenging because conflict between maternal benefit and fetal risk needs to be addressed.[2] Before selecting the appropriate imaging modality for the diagnostic and staging work-up of pregnant patients with cancer, several issues need to be considered: fetal health (closely related to pregnancy trimester), maternal survival (closely related to tumor staging and possibility of metastases), and desire to continue the pregnancy.

It is generally suggested that imaging of the pregnant population is to be restricted to those methods that do not endanger fetal health and particularly, during the first trimester of pregnancy, only necessary radiological investigations are justified.[11] At present, sonography and magnetic resonance (MR) imaging are acceptable imaging modalities for assessing pregnant patients because they lack ionizing radiation.

Sonography is the modality of choice for the initial abdominal evaluation of gravid patients because it is widely available, low cost, and lacks adverse effects to mother and fetus. However, prolonged use of color Doppler imaging during the first trimester is better avoided, because there is a theoretic risk for tissue heating caused by acoustic energy deposition; appropriate settings for obstetric imaging minimize such risk.[12] However, as the pregnancy progresses, the enlarged gravid uterus obscures the pelvic organs and retroperitoneal space, rendering sonography less suitable for examination of the abdomen in patients with gynecologic malignancies.

Because of larger imaging fields of view, better reproducibility, and excellent soft tissue contrast, MR imaging is considered the imaging modality of choice for diagnosis and staging of gynecologic cancer during pregnancy. According to the American College of Radiology (ACR) guidelines, pregnant patients can be safely imaged with field strengths up to 3 T using a normal-level specific absorption rate (SAR) mode (<2 W/kg) with no adverse effects on organogenesis or fetal hearing documented.[13,14] Contrast-enhanced MR imaging may be used with caution and only when there is a significant benefit to the mother that outweighs the risk of fetal exposure to paramagnetic media, because gadolinium-based contrast agents cross the placenta-blood barrier.[15] Recently, whole-body diffusion-weighted imaging (DWI) has been proposed for oncologic staging of pregnant patients because it shows promising results and eliminates the need for intravenous contrast[16]; however, large prospective studies are needed to support its clinical implementation (Box 3).

The use of ionizing radiation is best avoided during pregnancy, especially in the first 2 trimesters because of potential risk of teratogenesis; although the absorbed doses for diagnostic imaging even for abdominal computed tomography (CT) are usually less than 50 mGy and considered safe for the fetus, cumulative radiation and stochastic effects should also be taken into consideration. CT in gravid patients should be performed

---

Box 3
Magnetic resonance imaging safety considerations during pregnancy

No special consideration for any trimester with field strengths up to 3 T

No known adverse effects on organogenesis or fetal auditory function

Gadolinium-based contrast agent may be used with caution

Imaging with DWI shows early promising results

Box 4
Prepare the pregnant patient for an magnetic resonance imaging study

Ask the patient to fast for 5 to 6 hours before imaging

May use antiperistaltic agents

Bladder should be moderately full (tip: ask the patient to void and then give her 1–2 cups of water, approximately 20–30 minutes before entering the scan room)

Use surface coil if possible

Apply ultrafast sequences as required

In late pregnancy, imaging may be performed in the left lateral decubitus position

---

only when the information required cannot be obtained with sonography or MR imaging and only after careful risk-benefit assessment, always keeping the radiation dose to the fetus as low as reasonably achievable (ALARA principle). In all cases, appropriate consultation for potential fetal risks and written informed consent from the patient is strongly advised.[17]

18F-fluorodeoxyglucose (FDG) PET/CT in pregnant patients is discouraged because of fetal exposure to radiation and potential toxicity of the radiopharmaceutical, even though reported total absorbed fetal doses are less than the threshold of 50 mGy. However, if it is medically indicated, PET/CT may be performed after careful risk-benefit assessment; PET/MR imaging can provide detailed imaging without the CT-related radiation, but its availability is still limited.[18]

More details regarding safety concerns of imaging pregnant women, and women of reproductive age in general, are provided in Michael A. Ohliger and Hailey H. Choi's article, "Imaging Safety and Technical Considerations in the Reproductive Age Female," elsewhere in this issue.

IMAGING PROTOCOLS TAILORED FOR CANCER IN PREGNANCY

Most investigators agree that it is difficult to advocate a single comprehensive protocol for maternal imaging in the setting of pregnancy, because several parameters must be considered, including clinical indications, gestational age, and technical issues. Imaging protocols should focus on answering a specific clinical question, taking into account fetal safety and maternal comfort and balancing short imaging times with acceptable image quality.[19]

Magnetic Resonance Imaging: Preparation

MR imaging of the abdomen and pelvis in pregnant patients is technically challenging (**Box 4**). It is not only maternal breathing and bowel peristalsis but also fetal motion that may degrade image quality. The effects of peristalsis and fetal motion may be reduced by asking the patient to fast for approximately 4 to 6 hours before the MR imaging study[19]; antiperistaltic agents (eg, 20 mg of hyoscine butyl bromide, intramuscularly) may be administered before the examination, because there is no contraindication for their use during pregnancy. The impact of fetal movement can be further minimized with the use of ultrafast sequences (single shot fast spin echo).[20] The urinary bladder should be moderately distended to allow adequate evaluation of its wall without causing maternal discomfort. Pregnant patients are typically imaged in the supine position. However, especially in the third trimester of the pregnancy, it may be difficult for the patient to suspend respiration and remain in the supine position for a long time. As the gravid uterus enlarges, it may cause pressure on abdominal organs and vessels, including the inferior vena cava. In such cases, imaging may be performed in the left lateral decubitus position to avoid impairing venous return from the pelvis and lower extremities, which may result in dizziness or even syncope.[19] Use of a surface phased-array coil is recommended because of superior signal/noise ratio and better contrast resolution. However, in larger patients with advanced pregnancy, imaging may be performed with the body coil.[21]

Magnetic Resonance Imaging: Sequences

There is insufficient data in the literature regarding MR imaging protocols in pregnant patients with gynecologic tumors. Therefore, oncologic protocols used in nonpregnant patients with suitable adjustments are mostly used. Overall scan time should not exceed 30 to 40 minutes because of concerns for tissue heating and maternal discomfort.

An example of an MR imaging protocol used to evaluate gynecologic malignancies in nonpregnant patients according to the European Society of Urogenital Radiology guidelines,[22,23] with modifications based on the needs of each pregnant patient, is presented in **Table 1**.

Computed Tomography

CT scan of the abdomen and the pelvis is justified in pregnant women with cancer if there is no other diagnostic alternative. Radiation dose-reduction techniques should be applied, including decreasing voltage (kilovolts) and current (milliamps), increasing pitch, widening beam collimation, limiting scanned areas, and performing a single-phase study. Automated settings may reduce dose by 40% to 50% while maintaining acceptable imaging quality.[24]

CT examinations with the fetus outside the field of view can be safely performed during any trimester of pregnancy, because fetal absorbed doses do not exceed 50 mGy; abdominal shielding may be used for protection from outside scatter radiation.

No teratogenic or mutagenic effects have been documented regarding the use of iodinated contrast media either in vivo or in vitro; however,

---

Table 1
Magnetic resonance imaging protocol for evaluation of pregnant patients with gynecologic malignancies

Sequence	Plane	Value
T2-W TSE (mandatory)	All 3 imaging planes • Axial (up to the level of renal hilum) • Sagittal • Coronal	Allows an overall view of the pelvic and abdominal organs and minimizes fetal motion artifacts
High-resolution T2-W TSE, with limited field of view in the pelvis (mandatory)	• Axial oblique plane (perpendicular to the cervical long axis), when cervical tumors are evaluated • True coronal plane (parallel to the uterine cavity), when adnexal masses are evaluated	Achieves optimal contrast difference between tumor and normal tissue. Fetal motion artifacts only rarely significantly compromise image interpretation
T1-W ±fat suppression (mandatory) TSE or Dixon	• Axial	Provides information on pelvic anatomy, hemorrhagic lesions, lymph nodes, and bone marrow. Fat suppression allows the diagnosis of hemorrhage vs fat and is particularly valuable in cases of ovarian tumors A Dixon technique reduces the number of sequences, but it is prone to artifacts from fetal movement
T2-W with fat suppression (optional)	• Axial	Detects fluid collections and bone marrow changes
DWI (0, 800, 1400 s/mm^2) (mandatory)	• Axial	Discriminates cancerous from normal tissue and detects lymph nodes
T1-W (2D or 3D GRE) DCE; not as routine	• Axial or Coronal	If contrast-enhanced imaging is required in case of ovarian tumors, use a macrocyclic gadolinium chelate at the lowest dose (0.1 mmol/kg) Use contrast media only if the information gained is critical for decision making

Abbreviations: 2D, two-dimensional; 3D, three-dimensional; DCE, dynamic contrast enhanced; GRE, gradient recalled echo; T1-W, T1 weighted; T2-W, T2 weighted; TSE, turbo spin echo.

their administration is recommended only under special circumstances and the exposed neonate should be checked for hypothyroidism soon after birth.

CERVICAL CANCER IN PREGNANCY
Epidemiology

Cervical carcinoma is the most common gynecologic malignancy in the gravid population, with an estimated incidence ranging from 0.05% to 0.1%. Cervical neoplasia (including intraepithelial lesions, in situ and invasive carcinomas) is expected to complicate 1.5 to 12 of 100,000 pregnancies, with invasive cancer affecting approximately 0.8 to 1.5 of 10,000 pregnancies.[25,26] About half of these cases are diagnosed during pregnancy, and the rest in the early postpartum period (within 12 months after delivery).[27] With the increased use of screening, most (up to 70%) cervical cancers of pregnancy are diagnosed at an early stage with small-volume disease (stage 1B)[3,28]; gravid patients with cervical cancer are 3 times more likely to have early disease (stage I) at diagnosis than nonpregnant patients.[2,3]

Relative to histology, there is no difference between cancer types of pregnant versus nonpregnant women, with most cases (90%) being of squamous cell origin, followed by adenocarcinomas.[29]

Diagnosis and Staging

The diagnostic approach for pregnancy-associated cervical cancer is similar to that in nonpregnant women.[30] Recommendations include routine performance of Pap smear at the first prenatal visit; in women with high-grade intraepithelial lesions, colposcopy and biopsies should follow, because endocervical curettage is contraindicated.[31] Colposcopy can be performed regardless of the pregnancy trimester; assessing the lesion's extent may be challenging because of pregnancy-related edema and increased vascularity of the vagina and cervix.[2]

The presence of symptoms is related to the clinical stage and tumor size.[25] Common symptoms of invasive cervical cancer include vaginal bleeding or discharge, and abdominal/pelvic pain,[2] which may be mistaken for threatened miscarriage or prepartum hemorrhage.

In cases of biopsy-confirmed invasive cervical cancer, staging work-up is indicated. The International Federation of Gynecology and Obstetrics (FIGO) classification system for staging cervical cancer may be applied to the pregnant population.[32] Clinical examination is the first step of staging patients with cervical cancer. However, in the pregnant population, bimanual physical examination may be technically difficult or painful and, therefore, less sensitive for determining the size and lateral extension of a cervical mass; also, it provides no information regarding nodal status, the most adverse prognostic factor for this disease (stage IIIC disease according to the revised FIGO staging system).[32]

New FIGO guidelines (2019) have incorporated imaging data into the staging system for cervical cancer; the use of imaging modalities, including sonography, CT, MR imaging, and PET (according to available resources), is permitted to provide information on tumor size, nodal status, or systemic tumor spread, and may influence the choice of treatment.[32] MR imaging is the preferred imaging technique for staging cervical cancer in gravid patients because it is safe for fetuses, reproducible, and non–operator dependent with excellent soft tissue contrast resolution and larger imaging field of view compared with sonography. It can accurately assess tumor size (all 3 dimensions); vaginal, parametrial, or adjacent organ invasion; hydronephrosis; and lymph node involvement.[28,30] Reported MR imaging accuracy values in the nonpregnant population for determining early (<IIB) versus advanced (≥IIB) disease are high, ranging from 75% to 96%. Clinical staging of early cervical cancer significantly improves when MR imaging information is added to the clinical data, enabling better selection of candidates for surgery.[33,34] Although, the clinical impact of pelvic MR imaging in cervical cancer of pregnancy has not been assessed in large cohorts, several investigators advocate its use for staging purposes in pregnant patients with pathologically confirmed cervical cancer and macroscopically visible disease (>IB1) or clinical signs suspicious for metastases.[26] Alternatively, if MR imaging is not feasible, because it is contraindicated or the patient has severe claustrophobia, CT or even PET-CT may be used to evaluate tumor local extent and nodal enlargement, after careful patient consultation.

Imaging Findings, Differences from Nonpregnant Patients, and Potential Pitfalls

MR imaging features of cervical cancer during pregnancy are similar to those observed in nonpregnant patients, although there are some differences that should be taken into account during interpretation. During pregnancy, the normal cervical stroma may be hyperintense because of pregnancy-related edema and, therefore, tumor may be difficult to detect on conventional T2-weighted images.[20] In such cases, DWI is valuable because typically only cancerous tissue shows restricted diffusivity (**Fig. 1**); because postbiopsy hemorrhage may be the cause of false-positive results on DWI, time interval between cone biopsy and MR imaging examination should be longer than 1 week.[35]

Small (<1 cm) cervical tumors may be easily overlooked on non–contrast-enhanced MR imaging and may appear only on early arterial dynamic contrast-enhanced MR imaging as small enhancing foci.[35] Although contrast enhancement may increase small lesion conspicuity, it is usually avoided in pregnant women because of fetal safety considerations; detection of cervical lesions less than 1 cm does not affect treatment decisions or maternal prognosis.[20]

When uterine-sparing surgery is planned, estimation of the distance between the tumor and the internal cervical os (ICO) is of utmost importance[36]; a tumor to ICO distance more than 1 cm is usually required for successful outcomes. Tumor extension to the ICO is a poor prognosticator for patient survival because it is associated with an increased incidence of nodal metastases. MR imaging is a noninvasive modality with high sensitivity (86%–91%) and specificity (94%–96%) values for evaluating tumor extension to the corpus uteri. However, in pregnant patients, ICO evaluation may be difficult because the gravid uterus distorts normal cervical anatomy and pregnancy-related edema may alter normal ICO T2 signal intensity; in such cases information derived from DWI may be helpful.[34]

Metastatic lymph nodes are strongly associated with poor clinical outcome in patients with cervical cancer. Surgical lymphadenectomy is considered the gold standard procedure for the diagnosis of nodal metastases; several investigators report no adverse fetal outcomes when the procedure is performed before 20 weeks of gestation.[31]

Recently, in 2019, imaging criteria for nodal assessment have been introduced in the new FIGO recommendations for staging cervical cancer. If imaging findings indicate pelvic nodal metastases, stage allocation is IIIC1r; with pathologic confirmation (via laparoscopic resection) it becomes IIIC1p. Accordingly, imaging diagnosis of para-aortic nodal involvement is classified as stage IIIC2r and pathologic confirmation as stage IIIC2p disease. In all cases, the type of imaging modality or pathology technique used should be documented.[32]

In pregnant women, care should be taken not to mistake dilated pelvic veins for enlarged pelvic lymph nodes in the axial plane; use of other planes (eg, coronal) is helpful to avoid misdiagnosis.[20]

Another potential pitfall in pregnant women is the prolonged use of vaginal progesterone gel to avoid premature birth. This prolonged use may result in the formation of a solid mass within the vagina, mimicking a cervical tumor; knowledge of the patient's history may raise suspicion of such a condition and the gel foam mass may be removed with colposcopy (**Fig. 2**).

Treatment Options and Prognosis

Management of invasive cervical cancer during pregnancy depends on the following criteria: tumor local extent (staging), nodal involvement, gestational age, and tumor histology (**Fig. 3**). Uterine-sparing surgery and pregnancy preservation may be considered under certain circumstances. Current treatment options for cervical cancer during pregnancy are summarized in **Box 5**.[7,36] Although there are no definitive conclusions about how overall prognosis differs between pregnant and nonpregnant patients with cervical cancer, it seems both groups have a similar

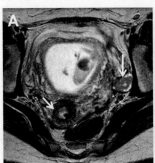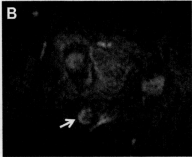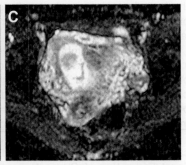

Fig. 1. FIGO IB2 cervical cancer of adenosquamous histology at gestational week 14. (*A*) Axial T2-weighted image shows a mildly hyperintense tumor confined to the cervix (*short arrow*). Note the presence of a corpus luteum at the left ovary (*long arrow*). (*B*) Corresponding axial high b value (1000) DWI shows a high signal intensity lesion (*arrow*) with restriction on the corresponding apparent diffusion coefficient (ADC) map. (*C*) The patient was treated with abdominal radical trachelectomy and successfully completed the pregnancy at gestational week 34.

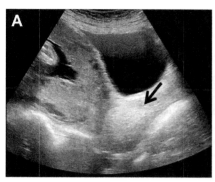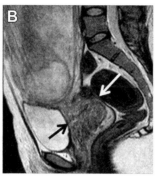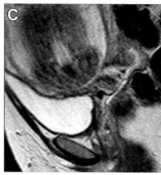

Fig. 2. An incidentally detected cervical mass at gestational week 36. (*A*) Transabdominal sonography shows a hyperechoic mass within the cervix (*black arrow*). (*B*) Corresponding T2-weighted sagittal image shows a low-signal-intensity mass within the cervical canal (*arrows*). Gelatinous material caused by prolonged use of a vaginal progesterone was removed at colposcopy. (*C*) Repeated sagittal T2-weighted image of the same patient 2 days after colposcopy shows no evidence of the mass.

survival profile. Recently, Cordeiro and colleagues[31] reported that the 30-year survival of pregnant women diagnosed with cervical cancer is similar to age-matched and disease-matched controls, concluding that pregnancy does not adversely affect survival. Therefore, most investigators agree that pregnancy in women with cervical cancer can be preserved in most cases.[3]

Follow-up

If management or conservative treatment until delivery is decided, close radiologic follow-up is recommended to choose between immediate intervention because of tumor progression or relapse and watchful waiting.[37]

MR imaging is the only examination that can reliably assess response to treatment (surgical or chemotherapy) during pregnancy[20]; it also best depicts the uterovaginal anastomosis and postoperative complications such as lymphocysts in cases of radical trachelectomy.[35] Some investigators propose an MR imaging examination every 4 weeks after diagnosis until the 30th week of pregnancy, to evaluate the course of disease and plan the cesarean section.[20]

OVARIAN CANCER IN PREGNANCY
Epidemiology

Ovarian cancer represents the fifth most common malignancy in the gravid population and the second most frequent gynecologic cancer in pregnancy. In general, adnexal masses are common in pregnancy, appearing in approximately 2.8 to 11 of 100,000 pregnancies.[38,39] However, most of these lesions are benign, with malignant tumors (including borderline tumors) accounting for only 1% to 5% of the cases.[2,39]

Corpus luteum of pregnancy and simple functional cysts are often observed during pregnancy, with a reported incidence ranging from 11% to 41%; because they are hormonally dependent,

Fig. 3. A biopsy-confirmed small cell cervical cancer at gestational week 12. Sagittal T2-weighted image shows a hypointense mass in the ectocervix (*arrow*). Also shown is contraction (*asterisk*) of the anterior myometrium. The patient was treated immediately with hysterectomy because of aggressive histology.

Box 5
Cervical cancer in pregnancy: treatment options

Pregnancy termination: first or early second trimester; undesirable pregnancy; advanced tumor stage

Immediate definitive treatment (regardless of gestational age): lymph node metastases (documented); disease progression during pregnancy; rare aggressive subtypes such as small cell carcinoma

Early cervical cancer

Gestational age greater than 22 weeks: may be treated after delivery with no known adverse oncologic effects

Gestational age less than 22 weeks: treatment during pregnancy; conization, simple trachelectomy or radical trachelectomy for fertility preservation only in early stages (FIGO IA, IB1); for tumors larger than 2 cm, abdominal radical trachelectomy may be considered, under strict eligibility criteria and careful consultation

For node-positive disease or tumors 4 cm or larger, radical hysterectomy and/or chemoradiation treatment to ensure effective oncologic outcome; if preservation of pregnancy is desired, platinum-based (±paclitaxel) neoadjuvant chemotherapy until fetal maturation (35–36 weeks)

Box 6
Adnexal masses in pregnancy

Asymptomatic

Benign (more common)

Functional (ie, corpus luteum): regress spontaneously, by 20 weeks

Persistent lesions: mature teratoma (most common), cystadenoma, endometrioma, paraovarian cyst, exophytic leiomyoma

Malignant (1%–5%)

Germ cell or stromal origin

Borderline tumor

Epithelial ovarian cancer (less common)

Symptomatic

Ectopic pregnancy (first trimester)

Ovarian torsion (check for underlying disorder)

Degenerated (red) leiomyoma

Tumor rupture (rare)

---

they tend to resolve spontaneously by 18 to 20 weeks.[39] In cases of persistent ovarian masses, mature cystic teratoma is the most common benign histopathologic diagnosis (7%–37%).[31,40] Other frequently observed benign adnexal lesions include serous (5%–28%) and mucinous (3%–24%) cystadenomas, endometriomas (0.8%–27%), paraovarian cysts (<5%), and leiomyomas (1%–2.5%)[31] (Box 6).

Germ cell tumors, sex cord (stromal) tumors, and borderline tumors are the most common malignancies among pregnancy-associated ovarian tumors,[2,41] possibly because of their increased prevalence in women of reproductive age; dysgerminoma and yolk sac tumor are the 2 most common malignant germ cell histologies.[41] Borderline ovarian tumors (BOTs) are neoplasms of low malignant potential, but in pregnant compared with nonpregnant women they have a higher incidence of more aggressive histologic features, such as microinvasion.[42] Epithelial ovarian cancer, the most aggressive and common histologic type of ovarian cancer outside pregnancy, is responsible for only 35%

of ovarian malignant tumors diagnosed during gestation.[31]

Most ovarian malignant tumors are associated with a good prognosis because they usually present as stage I disease.[2]

Diagnosis and Staging

The number of asymptomatic ovarian masses during pregnancy has increased because of the routine use of prenatal fetal sonography.[39] However, it is common for adnexal masses in the gravid population to present as an acute abdominal event caused by torsion, rupture, or even intraperitoneal hemorrhage.[3]

Diagnosis of ovarian malignancy in gravid patients may be challenging, because levels of common tumor markers are usually increased in pregnancy. In particular, CA125 is typically increased during the first trimester, whereas in the second and third trimesters its levels are low in the maternal serum but high in the amniotic fluid.[39] Levels of other more specific tumor markers, including inhibin B, antimüllerian hormone, Human Epididymis protein 4 (HE4), CA 19-9, and lactate dehydrogenase, are not expected to increase in pregnancy and can be used for the diagnosis of pregnancy-related ovarian cancer.[2]

Transvaginal and/or abdominal sonography is the initial imaging modality for evaluating pelvic masses in pregnancy. International Ovarian Tumor

Analysis (IOTA) simple rules[43] is a commonly used model to characterize ovarian disorders outside pregnancy, using specific tumor features such as size, morphologic characteristics, color Doppler flow, and evidence of extraovarian disease; several different algorithms have also been developed over recent years to stratify the risk of malignancy in adnexal masses.[44] However, the usefulness of scoring systems in the pregnant population has not yet been established.[3] When sonographic diagnosis is inconclusive even when performed by an experienced sonographer, the mass is too large to be accurately assessed, or there is a high risk of malignancy, further imaging is required (Fig. 4).[44]

Pelvic MR imaging is the optimal second-line imaging technique to characterize complex or indeterminate adnexal masses discovered incidentally on ultrasonography during pregnancy [45] MR imaging is highly accurate in the characterization of complex adnexal masses; applying the ADNEX MR imaging score seems to further improve the characterization of ovarian lesions and, particularly, the detection of cancer with an overall accuracy higher than 80%.[46] Functional imaging such as DWI may reduce the need for gadolinium chelate administration, the use of which is discouraged in the pregnant population (Fig. 5). If imaging characteristics remain equivocal, there may be a role for endovaginal ultrasonography–guided biopsy to obtain definitive tissue diagnosis to guide management.

Ovarian cancer is surgically staged according to the updated, revised FIGO classification system (2018) for ovarian, fallopian tube, and peritoneal cancer and it is the same for both epithelial and nonepithelial ovarian tumors.[47] Imaging is helpful for presurgical evaluation of the extent of disease and particularly for determining peritoneal dissemination and nodal metastases (Fig. 6). Even though CT is recommended for initial staging, MR imaging is preferable for pregnant patients because of the lack of ionizing radiation. Whole-body DWI MR imaging has shown good accuracy values, regardless of lesion size, compared with contrast-enhanced MR imaging or CT and FDG-PET/CT.[44] CT may be used in pregnant patients when MR imaging is not feasible, mainly to map the extraovarian spread of the disease; however, fetal exposure to radiation should be carefully taken into consideration.[39]

Imaging Findings

Size and morphology of ovarian lesions are the key sonographic features used to decide between surveillance or intervention. The ultrasonography criteria for suspected malignancy are similar to those applied in nonpregnant women. IOTA simple rules for sonographic characterization of ovarian tumors show 78% specificity and 87% sensitivity.[43] A lesion is characterized as benign when only B features are observed or malignant, when only M features are observed; when no features or both B and M features apply, the mass is considered indeterminate (Box 7).[48] Note that Doppler indices may change rapidly in pregnancy and, therefore, this M criterion should be applied with caution.[40]

Tumors of low malignant potential or BOTs may show the ovarian crescent sign on ultrasonography examination; that is, a rim of normal ovarian tissue seen adjacent to the tumor. This sign practically excludes invasion of tumor into the ovary. In the absence of this sign, it may not be possible to discriminate between BOTs and invasive ovarian epithelial neoplasms, a

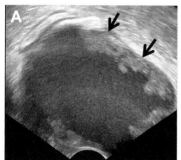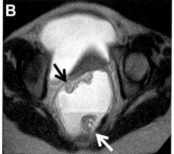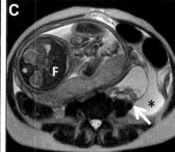

Fig. 4. High-grade serous ovarian cancer at gestational week 30. (A) Transvaginal sonography shows a cystic mass in the posterior cul-de-sac with multiple internal papillary projections (black arrows). Corresponding T2 weighted images in the axial plane (B, C) clearly show intratumoral solid foci (arrows in B) and fluid-fluid level as well as tumor extension beyond the pelvis (arrow in C). Ascites is also present (asterisk); malignant cells were detected on cytology. F, fetus.

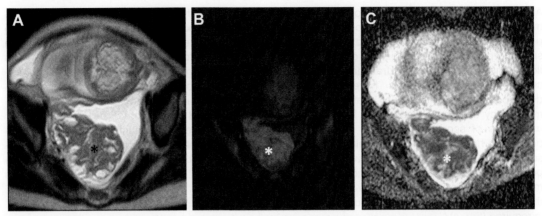

Fig. 5. High-grade serous cystadenocarcinoma at gestational week 28. (*A*) Axial T2-weighted image shows complex mass with large solid components (*asterisk*) showing restricted diffusion on the corresponding high b value (1000) (*B*) and ADC map (*C*) images.

crucial differential diagnosis particularly for the pregnant population.

It is reported that, even with experienced readers, 5% to 25% of adnexal masses are indeterminate on ultrasonography. MR imaging can assist sonographic diagnosis of adnexal masses in pregnancy by assessing specific morphologic features and signal intensity characteristics. The ADNEX MR scoring system developed by Thomassin-Naggara and colleagues[46,49] is a well-established classification system that can be used to stratify the risk of malignancy for ovarian masses (**Box 8**).

An important limitation of this classification system in the gravid population is that the use of dynamic contrast-enhanced MR imaging is mandatory for the characterization of the lesion's solid component, unless it displays both low signal intensity on T2 and high b value DWI[46];

furthermore, there is lack of data regarding tumor enhancement characteristics in pregnant patients and it is not clear whether differences exist between pregnant and nonpregnant patients[41] (see **Box 7**).

Differential Diagnosis and Pitfalls

Evaluation of adnexal masses during pregnancy is challenging because they may undergo pregnancy-related morphologic changes mimicking malignancy (**Box 9**). The most common pregnancy-related adnexal masses are the corpus luteum of pregnancy and the theca lutein cyst, both of which resolve after 18 weeks of pregnancy, although sometimes they can persist until after delivery.[44]

Corpus luteum persisting into the second trimester accounts for 13% to 17% of all cystic

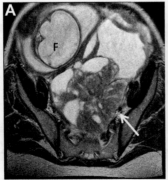
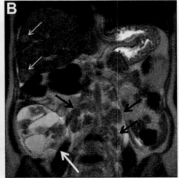

Fig. 6. FIGO IV bilateral high-grade epithelial ovarian cancer complicating an in vitro fertilization twin pregnancy at gestational week 24. (*A*) Axial T2-weighted image shows a large cystic/solid mass located in the left adnexa (*arrow*) displacing the gravid uterus. (*B*) Coronal T2-weighted image shows a second tumor with similar characteristics on the right side of the pelvis (*thick white arrow*). Also shown are liver metastases (*thin white arrows*) and multiple enlarged para-aortic lymph nodes (*black arrows*). F, fetus.

Box 7
Adnexal masses in pregnancy: benign versus malignant features

Sonography (initial modality of choice)

B rules: unilocular or smooth multilocular lesions less than 10 cm, presence of solid internal component less than 7 mm, presence of acoustic shadowing and no color Doppler flow

M rules: irregular solid tumor, ascites, at least 4 internal papillary projections, presence of an irregular multilocular solid tumor greater than 10 cm, and strong blood flow on color Doppler

Only B, benign; only M, malignant; no features or both B and M, indeterminate

Tips: ovarian crescent sign (excludes invasion), color Doppler indices may change during pregnancy, direct probe pressure to determine paraovarian origin

MR imaging (use with indeterminate ultrasonography findings, large masses, high-risk lesions, staging purposes)

ADNEX MR score

Score 1 to 3, benign or probably benign; score 4, indeterminate; score 5, probably malignant

Tips: use specific morphologic features; ie, no solid tissue or solid tissue with low signal on T2 and high b value DWI (benign), blood products (endometrioma, functional cyst), fat (teratoma), very low T2 signal (fibrous tissue), solid with multiple low-T2 enhancing septa (dysgerminoma), evidence of extraovarian disease (ie, peritoneal deposits), ascites, or lymph node enlargement (invasive carcinoma)

Limitations: usefulness of the above scoring systems in the pregnant population has not yet been tested in large cohorts; use of gadolinium chelate is discouraged in pregnancy (reserve for cases in which maternal benefit outweighs potential fetal risks)

Box 8
ADNEX magnetic resonance score

Score 1: mass detected by ultrasonography, not visible at MR imaging

Score 2: purely cystic mass (ie, high-T2, low-T1 signal; no enhancement); purely endometriotic mass (ie, T2 shading, high-T1 signal, no solid components); purely fatty mass (ie, high T2, high T1, signal decrease on fat-saturated images); mass without wall enhancement; solid tissue with low T2 and low signal on high b value DWI

Score 3: mass without solid tissue that cannot be rated as score 2 or mass with solid tissue that enhances with a type 1 time intensity curve (TIC) (ie, gradual enhancement)

Score 4: mass with solid tissue that enhances with a type 2 TIC (ie, early enhancement, but later than myometrium, followed by plateau) or unfeasible dynamic contrast-enhanced MR analysis

Score 5: mass with solid tissue that enhances with type 3 TIC (ie, rapid contrast uptake, faster than myometrium, early washout) and any lesion with peritoneal implants

The imaging characteristics of hemorrhagic cysts vary depending on the stages of clot evolution; a reticular pattern consisting of fibrin septa and blood products (fishnet appearance) is a characteristic ultrasonography feature. As hemorrhagic cysts evolve, solid and cystic components may be evident, with the avascular solid component corresponding to a retracting clot. The MR imaging appearance of hemorrhagic cysts also varies. Typically, they manifest with homogeneous or layering high T1 and low T2 signal; subtracted postcontrast images show no contrast uptake.[41]

Hyperreactio luteinalis is a rare, benign pregnancy-related entity that presents with bilateral, functional, multicystic ovarian enlargement caused by increased levels of human chorionic gonadotropin (hCG) and is typically seen in the third trimester. This entity is often associated with gestational trophoblastic disease, triplet pregnancies, or polycystic ovarian disease and it is similar to the ovarian hyperstimulation syndrome, although the latter is iatrogenic and usually occurs in the first trimester. Imaging features of hyperreactio luteinalis include the presence of massively enlarged ovaries with multiple thin-walled small theca lutein cysts rendering a spoke-wheel appearance; ascites may be present. This entity may be misdiagnosed as a mucinous borderline ovarian tumor, although these tumors

adnexal masses. On sonography, corpus luteum cysts manifest as simple or complex cysts (because of hemorrhagic components), 3 to 6 cm in size, with thick walls. Typically, on Doppler imaging, a peripheral vascular rim is seen, the so-called ring of fire. The MR imaging appearance of corpus luteum cysts is also variable; typically, a cystic mass with components of variable signal intensity, ragged internal walls, and avid peripheral enhancement is seen (**Fig. 7**).[41]

Box 9
Adnexal masses in pregnancy mimicking malignancy

Hyperreactio luteinalis (rare): bilateral, multicystic ovarian masses (spoke-wheel appearance), increased human chorionic gonadotropin (hCG) level, third trimester. Mimics ovarian hyperstimulation syndrome (dd: iatrogenic, first trimester) or mucinous BOT (smaller cysts, less rounded, less solid tissue).

Luteoma of pregnancy (rare): solid mass, strong association with virilization. Mimics ovarian stromal tumor (spontaneously regresses after delivery).

Decidualized endometrioma (uncommon): cystic with hemorrhagic content and mural solid components, papillary projections, or internal septa. Mimics mucinous BOT (decidualization nodules are smaller, show higher T2 signal, no restriction on DWI, and may regress during the course of the pregnancy).

Degenerated leiomyoma (common): rapidly growing leiomyoma with areas of infarction, necrosis, and hemorrhage (red degeneration). If it is subserosal or pedunculated, it may mimic an ovarian lesion (leiomyomas show beak-shaped or claw-shaped interface with the uterus, vascular pedicle, or bridging vessels, and they are often painful).

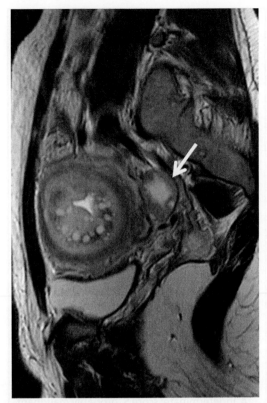

Fig. 7. Pregnancy-related corpus luteum. Sagittal T2-weighted image shows a cystic ovarian mass with ragged wall, typical of corpus luteum (*arrow*). The patient was diagnosed with gestational trophoblastic disease (partial mole).

---

usually have smaller, less rounded locules, and less solid tissue compared with the hyperreactio luteinalis lesions.[50]

Luteoma of pregnancy is a rare, nonneoplastic ovarian lesion that develops during pregnancy when proliferating luteinized stromal cells under the influence of hCG replace normal ovarian parenchyma. These tumors may produce androgens, which may cause maternal as well as female fetus virilization. On sonography, luteomas appear as heterogeneous, predominantly hypoechoic masses with increased vascularity on Doppler imaging.[41] Because of the solid nature of these masses, it is virtually impossible even on MR imaging to differentiate luteomas from other solid ovarian neoplasms, particularly those of stromal origin; when there is clinical suspicion of luteoma, conservative management is advocated because these lesions tend to spontaneously regress in the early postpartum period.[51]

Most of the endometriotic cysts spontaneously decrease in size during the course of pregnancy, possibly because of high progesterone levels and interruption of menstruation. However, 12% of ovarian endometriomas may undergo ectopic

decidualization of their walls, mimicking a borderline ovarian tumor. Sonography may show smooth solid nodules within the wall of an endometrioma with a similar echotexture to the placenta and blood flow on Doppler imaging. This appearance may raise suspicion for malignancy, and MR imaging is usually required for further investigation. MR imaging features of decidualized endometriomas include high T1 signal and solid mural components, papillary projections, or internal septa. These specific features may explain the more frequent ADNEX MR score misclassification (benign lesions classified as potentially malignant, score 4) in the gravid population compared with the nonpregnant population.[46] However, MR imaging diagnosis of this benign entity is feasible because decidualized nodules are usually smaller than those of ovarian carcinomas and they follow the signal intensity of normal placenta (higher signal intensity on T2-weighted images, no restriction on high b value DWI).[52] Most decidualized endometriomas are surgically removed because they resemble ovarian malignancies; however,

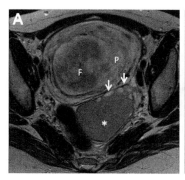
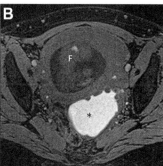

Fig. 8. Decidualized endometrioma incidentally found at gestational week 18. (*A*) Axial T2-weighted image shows a low-T2-signal mass (*asterisk*, T2 shading sign) with multiple mural nodules (*arrows*). (*B*) Corresponding T1-weighted fat-suppressed image (*asterisk*) confirms the hemorrhagic content of the lesion. Note the high T2 signal intensity of the nodules (*arrows in A*), similar to that of the placenta (P). On follow-up examination at gestational week 34, the mass had significantly decreased in size, confirming the diagnosis. F, fetus. (*Courtesy of* Diomidis Botsikas M.D., University Hospital of Geneva, Geneva, Switzerland.)

when the diagnosis is clinically suspected, conservative management may be decided, because decidualized endometriomas tend to regress rapidly during follow-up studies, unlike ovarian malignancies (**Fig. 8**).

When a painful unilateral adnexal mass is diagnosed in early pregnancy and the intrauterine gestational sac is absent, then an extrauterine (ectopic) pregnancy must be ruled out. Painful ovarian lesions in the correct clinical setting may also indicate an ovarian abscess or even ovarian torsion. When sonography is inconclusive, MR imaging can be helpful. Tubo-ovarian abscesses appear as tubular or multiseptated adnexal cystic structures with thick walls, variable T1, and high or heterogeneous T2 signal intensity; pus content typically shows strongly restricted diffusivity.[41]

Discrimination between ovarian versus paraovarian origin of lesions is important, because the latter are almost always of benign cause. Both sonography and MR imaging have the potential to accurately identify the origin of adnexal lesions. During transvaginal ultrasonography, direct probe pressure may be adequate to separate the lesion

from the ovary, confirming a paraovarian origin. In large lesions, MR imaging may identify the borders of normal ovarian tissue and, thus, define a possible extraovarian origin.[41] Pedunculated leiomyomas, which may grow under the hormonal effects of pregnancy, are the most common solid adnexal masses found in pregnancy. MR imaging is superior to sonography for the diagnosis of a large degenerated leiomyoma, which can simulate an ovarian neoplasm on sonography. Typical leiomyoma features include a well-circumscribed solid lesion with low T2 signal and a beak-shaped or claw-shaped interface with the uterus. The presence of a vascular pedicle (bridging vessels) extending from the uterus to the adnexal mass is also a useful sign for discriminating between an exophytic leiomyoma and an ovarian fibroma. Rapid growth of a leiomyoma may result in impairment of its blood supply, infarction, and hemorrhage (red degeneration), causing acute pain in gravid patients (**Fig. 9**). In this case, MR imaging features show a leiomyoma with uniform or peripheral high T1 signal intensity, whereas sonographic findings may be less specific.[41]

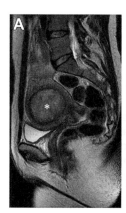
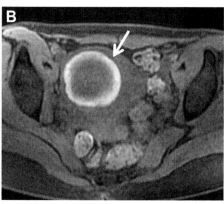

Fig. 9. Degenerated (red) leiomyoma at gestational week 8 presenting with acute abdominal pain. (*A*) Sagittal T2-weighted image shows a right-sided intramural leiomyoma (*asterisk*) in the uterine corpus. (*B*) T1-weighted image with fat suppression shows a hemorrhagic rim at the periphery of the leiomyoma (*arrow*), typical of red degeneration.

Treatment

Treatment approach depends on tumor size, imaging morphology, histologic subtype, presence of extraovarian disease, gestational age, and the patient's desire to keep the pregnancy or to preserve fertility potential.[3,30,38] Current guidelines for treatment of ovarian tumors are summarized in **Box 10**.

RARE GYNECOLOGIC CANCERS IN PREGNANCY
Endometrial Cancer and Uterine Sarcomas

Coexistence of pregnancy with endometrial cancer is very rare, with only 35 cases reported so far in the literature. The presence of endometrial tumor makes fertilization extremely difficult and pregnancy has a protective effect against endometrial cancer growth, because of the increased progesterone levels. Pregnancy and endometrial cancer is a paradox, and it may be attributed to the presence of focally immature endometrium with impaired receptivity that is sensitive to estrogen and resistant to progesterone.[53] Information on this condition is based only on individual case reports, most of which were diagnosed at the time of curettage for spontaneous first-trimester abortion, whereas some were identified because of postpartum uterine bleeding. Most tumors were well differentiated with no or minimal myometrial invasion (FIGO stage 1) with excellent overall survival.[53]

Because the reported cases are so few, there is lack of evidence regarding imaging diagnosis and work-up in these patients. When endometrial cancer is diagnosed, staging according to FIGO guidelines is recommended[37]; however, although the standard of care for endometrial cancer is total abdominal hysterectomy and bilateral salpingo-oophorectomy, fertility-sparing options in young women may be considered after careful consultation.

Female genital sarcomas diagnosed during pregnancy are also extremely rare. A review by Matsuo and colleagues[54] reported a total of 40 cases within a 50-year interval (1955–2007). Uterine sarcomas accounted for 37.5% of cases, followed by retroperitoneal (27.5%), vulvar (22.5%), and vaginal (12.5%) sarcomas. Most of the cases were diagnosed in the third trimester because of the presence of a large growing mass; abdominal pain and abnormal vaginal bleeding were also common symptoms. Diagnosis was incidental in approximately 22.5% of the cases. Diagnosis is frequently delayed because these masses are misdiagnosed for leiomyomas because of low suspicion rate; even histopathologic evaluation may be confusing and requires expertise because of pregnancy-induced histologic alterations (hemorrhage, necrosis, degeneration), which also occur in benign leiomyomas. In large tumors, MR imaging may help to determine the extent of disease (**Fig. 10**). Five-year survival is similar to that of advanced-stage sarcoma in nonpregnant women.

Vaginal Cancer

Vaginal cancer is often observed secondary to other primaries, including cervical, vulvar, and adjacent pelvic organ cancer. Primary carcinoma of the vagina is also rare in the nonpregnant population, with most (>90%) of the tumors being of squamous cell origin. Coexistence of vaginal cancer and pregnancy is extremely rare and described only in individual case reports.[53] Vaginal malignancies are associated with discharge and irregular bleeding. Diagnosis is made by assessment of smears and biopsies taken under colposcopy. Because of the rarity of the disease, there are no

---

Box 10
Adnexal masses in pregnancy: treatment options

Case-by-case approach

Operate when the mass is too large (>6 cm) because of high risk for acute events (ie, torsion, rupture, or infarction) or when the mass is already symptomatic or suspicious for malignancy (perform surgery after gestational week 16, to avoid luteal function or fetal loss)

Check histologic type, gestational age, and cancer stage

Germ cell: consider pregnancy preservation plus or minus chemotherapy.

Borderline: up-front salpingo-oophorectomy and planned restaging surgery postpartum

Invasive epithelial cancer: depends on the stage

Early stage (I–II): surgery (consider pregnancy preservation) plus or minus chemotherapy

Advanced stage (III–IV):

Before gestational week 20: terminate pregnancy; neoadjuvant chemotherapy; cytoreduction

After gestational week 20: may preserve pregnancy, neoadjuvant chemotherapy (carboplatinum plus paclitaxel); complete cytoreduction after delivery

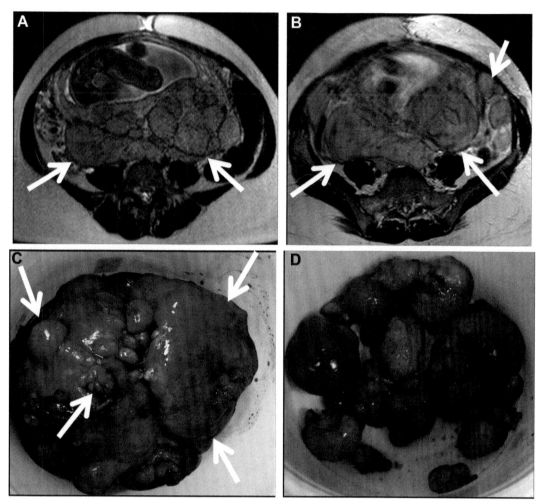

Fig. 10. Low-grade endometrial stromal sarcoma and multiple peritoneal deposits at gestational week 34. Axial T2-weighted images (*A, B*) show several soft tissue masses (*long arrows*) involving the posterior myometrium and within the peritoneal cavity (*short arrow in B*). Multiple soft tissue nodules along the posterior uterine surface are shown on the corresponding surgicopathologic specimen (*arrows in C*) along with numerous resected peritoneal nodules (*D*).

radiologic or clinical guidelines considering the pregnant patients and management should be tailored to each patient, depending on the extent of disease, tumor histology, gestational age, and desire to maintain pregnancy; regardless of the coexistence of pregnancy, advanced disease has a poor prognosis with low 5-year survival rates.[53]

Vulvar Cancer

Vulvar cancer is very rare in the premenopausal population, and therefore in pregnant women, although the incidence of invasive squamous cell carcinoma of the vulva in women less than 40 years of age has increased because of human papilloma virus and human immunodeficiency virus infections.[53]

Diagnosis of vulvar cancer is clinical, and biopsies should be taken from the suspicious lesion to establish diagnosis. The treatment of vulvar cancer in pregnant women is not different from that performed in nonpregnant women; however, gestational age should be taken into account in treatment decisions.[53] In patients with clinically negative nodal disease, radical local surgery with unilateral or bilateral lymph node dissection is advocated. The role of preoperative imaging (sonography, MR imaging) is to better evaluate the inguinal lymph nodes, because in cases of involvement the prognosis is less favorable and local radiotherapy should be applied to prevent groin recurrence. Termination of pregnancy in the first and second trimesters and immediate radiotherapy treatment is recommended. In the third

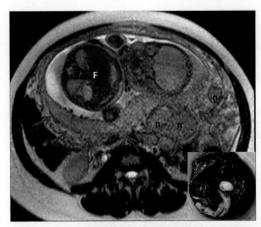

Fig. 11. T2-weighted image of the same patient as in **Fig. 10** shows several soft tissue nodules (n) abutting the placenta (*red arrows*). Intrauterine growth retardation fetus was diagnosed. The placenta was easily removed at cesarean section and it was intact on surgicopathologic examination (*inset*).

trimester, a delay of radiotherapy by 6 to 8 weeks until fetal delivery is within the accepted safety limits.[30]

Cancer Transfer via Placenta

It is reported that the only natural route available for transfer of cancer cells between humans is via the placenta. Therefore, it may be assumed that maternal cancer during pregnancy may be transmitted to the fetus. However, transplacental transmission of a maternal cancer to a fetus is exceedingly rare, with approximately 26 cases reported in the literature. In all recorded cases of maternal-fetal transmission, cancer in the neonate was of the same type as in the mother. Melanoma and leukemia/lymphoma accounted for most of such cases.[55] The role of imaging in identifying placental cancerous involvement remains unknown (**Fig. 11**).

SUMMARY

Management of malignant tumors during pregnancy is challenging because clinicians need to consider maternal and fetal safety and the potential loss of the patient's reproductive potential caused by cancer therapy. Pregnancy and cancer evoke strong opposite emotions and careful counseling is advised to reduce the psychological distress of the patients and their families. According to FIGO recommendations, such patients should be handled by a dedicated multidisciplinary team and imaging is an important part of the diagnosis, staging, and follow-up of pregnancy-associated malignancies.

DISCLOSURE

The authors have nothing to disclose.

REFERENCES

1. Zagouri F, Dimitrakakis C, Marinopoulos S, et al. Cancer in pregnancy: disentangling treatment modalities. ESMO Open 2016;1:e000016.
2. Botha M, Rajaram S, Karunaratne K. FIGO CANCER REPORT 2018. Cancer in pregnancy. Int J Gynecol Obstet 2018;143(Suppl. 2):137–42.
3. Morice P, Uzan C, Gouy S, et al. Gynaecological cancers in pregnancy. Lancet 2012;379:558–69.
4. Lee YY, Roberts CL, Dobbins T, et al. Incidence and outcomes of pregnancy-associated cancer in Australia, 1994–2008: A population-based linkage study. BJOG 2012;119:1572–82.
5. Parazzini F, Franchi M, Tavani A, et al. Frequency of pregnancy related cancer: a population based linkage study in Lombardy, Italy. Int J Gynecol Cancer 2017;27:613–9.
6. Peccatori FA, Azim HA Jr, Orecchia R, et al. Cancer, pregnancy and fertility: ESMO Clinical Practice Guidelines for diagnosis, treatment and follow-up. Ann Oncol 2013;24(Suppl 6):vi160–70.
7. de Haan J, Verheecke M, Van Calsteren K, et al. Oncological management and obstetric and neonatal outcomes for women diagnosed with cancer during pregnancy: A 20-year international cohort study of 1170 patients. Lancet Oncol 2018;19: 337–46.
8. Andersson TM, Johansson AL, Fredriksson I, et al. Cancer during pregnancy and the postpartum period: A population-based study. Cancer 2015; 121:2072–7.
9. Salani R, Billingsley C, Crafton S. Cancer and pregnancy: an overview for obstetricians and gynecologists. Am J Obstet Gynecol 2014;211(1):7–14.
10. Sarandakou A, Protonotariou E, Rizos D. Tumor markers in biological fluids associated with pregnancy. Crit Rev Clin Lab Sci 2007;44:151–78.
11. Surbone A, Peccatori F, Pavlidis N. Why is the topic of cancer and pregnancy so important? why and how to read this book. In: Surbone A, Peccatori F, Pavlidis N, editors. Cancer and Pregnancy. Recent Results in Cancer Research, vol 178. Springer-Verlag, Berlin, Heidelberg; 2008. p. 1–2.
12. American College of Radiology Guidelines and Standards Committee. AIUM-ACR-ACOG-SMFM-SRU practice parameter for the performance of obstetrical ultrasound. J Ultrasound Med 2018;37: E13–24.
13. Kanal E, Barkovich J, Bell C. Expert Panel on MR safety. ACR guidance document on MR safe practices. J Magn Reson Imaging 2013;37: 501–30.

14. Weisstanner C, Gruber GM, Brugger PC, et al. Fetal MRI at 3T-ready for routine use? Br J Radiol 2017; 90(1069):20160362.

15. ACR Committee on Drugs and Contrast Media. ACR manual on contrast media. Version 10.3 2018. Available at: https://www.acr.org/-/media/ACR/Files/Clinical-Resources/Contrast_Media.pdf.

16. Han SN, Amant F, Michielsen K, et al. Feasibility of whole-body diffusion-weighted MRI for detection of primary tumour, nodal and distant metastases in women with cancer during pregnancy: a pilot study. Eur Radiol 2018;28(5):1862–74.

17. ACR–SPR practice parameter for imaging pregnant or potentially pregnant adolescents and women with ionizing radiation. Available at: https://www.acr.org/-/media/ACR/Files/Practice-Parameters/pregnant-pts.pdf.

18. Zanotti-Fregonara P, Laforest R, Wallis JW. Fetal radiation dose from 18F-FDG in pregnant patients imaged with PET, PET/CT, and PET/MR. J Nucl Med 2015;56:1218–22.

19. Leyendecker JR, Gorengaut V, Brown JJ. MR imaging of maternal diseases of the abdomen and pelvis during pregnancy and the immediate postpartum period. Radiographics 2004;24(5):1301–16.

20. Balleyguier C, Fournet C, Ben Hassen W. Management of cervical cancer detected during pregnancy: role of magnetic resonance imaging. Clin Imaging 2013;37(1):70–6.

21. Masselli G, Derchi L, McHugo J, et al. Acute abdominal and pelvic pain in pregnancy: ESUR recommendations. Eur Radiol 2013;23(12):3485–500.

22. Balleyguier C, Sala E, Cunha TM, et al. Staging of uterine cervical cancer with MRI: guidelines of the European Society of Urogenital Radiology. Eur Radiol 2011;21(5):1102–10.

23. Forstner R, Sala E, Kinkel K, et al. ESUR guidelines: ovarian cancer staging and follow-up. Eur Radiol 2010;20(12):2773–80.

24. Raman SP, Johnson PT, Deshmukh S. CT dose reduction applications: available tools on the latest generation of CT scanners. J Am Coll Radiol 2013; 10(1):37–41.

25. Hunter MI, Monk BJ, Tewari KS. Cervical neoplasia in pregnancy. Part 1: Screening and management of preinvasive disease. Am J Obstet Gynecol 2008;199:3–9.

26. Hunter MI1, Tewari K, Monk BJ. Cervical neoplasia in pregnancy. Part 2: current treatment of invasive disease. Am J Obstet Gynecol 2008;199(1):10–8.

27. Smith LH, Dalrymple JL, Leiserowitz GS, et al. Obstetrical deliveries associated with maternal malignancy in California, 1992 through 1997. Am J Obstet Gynecol 2001;184:1504–12.

28. La Russa M, Jeyarajah AR. Invasive cervical cancer in pregnancy. Best Pract Res Clin Obstet Gynaecol 2016;33:44–57.

29. Doyle S, Messiou C, Rutherford JM. Cancer presenting during pregnancy: radiological perspectives. Clin Radiol 2009;64(9):857–71.

30. Amant F, Halaska MJ, Fumagalli M, et al. Gynecologic cancers in pregnancy: Guidelines of a second international consensus meeting. Int J Gynecol Cancer 2014;24:394–403.

31. Cordeiro CN, Gemignani ML. Gynecologic malignancies in pregnancy: Balancing fetal risks with oncologic safety. Obstet Gynecol Surv 2017;72: 184–93.

32. Bhatla N, Berek JS, Cuello Fredes M, et al. Revised FIGO staging for carcinoma of the cervix uteri. Int J Gynaecol Obstet 2019;145(1):129–35.

33. Bourgioti C, Chatoupis K, Rodolakis A, et al. Incremental prognostic value of MRI in the staging of early cervical cancer: a prospective study and review of the literature. Clin Imaging 2016;40(1):72–8.

34. Bourgioti C, Chatoupis K, Moulopoulos LA. Current imaging strategies for the evaluation of uterine cervical cancer. World J Radiol 2016;8(4):342–54.

35. Bourgioti C, Koutoulidis V, Chatoupis K, et al. MRI findings before and after abdominal radical trachelectomy (ART) for cervical cancer: a prospective study and review of the literature. Clin Radiol 2014; 69(7):678–86.

36. Rodolakis A, Thomakos N, Sotiropoulou M, et al. Abdominal radical trachelectomy for early-stage cervical cancer during pregnancy. A provocative surgical approach. Overview of the literature and a single-institute experience. Int J Gynecol Cancer 2018;28:1743–50.

37. Kehoe S. Cervical and endometrial cancer during pregnancy. Recent Results Cancer Res 2008;178: 69–74.

38. Ledermann JA, Raja FA, Fotopoulou C, et al. ESMO Guidelines Working Group. Newly diagnosed and relapsed epithelial ovarian carcinoma: ESMO Clinical Practice Guidelines for diagnosis, treatment and follow-up. Ann Oncol 2013;24(Suppl 6):vi24–32.

39. Boussios S, Moschetta M, Tatsi K, et al. A review on pregnancy complicated by ovarian epithelial and non-epithelial malignant tumors: Diagnostic and therapeutic perspectives. J Adv Res 2018;12:1–9.

40. Mukhopadhyay A, Shinde A, Naik R. Ovarian cysts and cancer in pregnancy. Best Pract Res Clin Obstet Gynaecol 2016;33:58–72.

41. Yacobozzi M, Nguyen D, Rakita D. Adnexal masses in pregnancy. Semin Ultrasound CT MR 2012;33(1): 55–64.

42. Fauvet R, Brzakowski M, Morice P, et al. Borderline ovarian tumors diagnosed during pregnancy exhibit a high incidence of aggressive features: results of a French multicenter study. Ann Oncol 2012;23(6): 1481–7.

43. Timmerman D, Ameye L, Fischerova D, et al. Simple ultrasound rules to distinguish between benign and

malignant adnexal masses before surgery: prospective validation by IOTA group. BMJ 2010;341:c6839.

44. Fruscio R, de Haan J, Van Calsteren K, et al. Ovarian cancer in pregnancy. Best Pract Res Clin Obstet Gynaecol 2017;41:108–17.

45. Forstner R, Thomassin-Naggara I, Cunha TM, et al. ESUR recommendations for MR imaging of the sonographically indeterminate adnexal mass: an update. Eur Radiol 2017; 27(6):2248–57.

46. Thomassin-Naggara I, Fedida B, Sadowski E, et al. Complex US adnexal masses during pregnancy: Is pelvic MR imaging accurate for characterization? Eur J Radiol 2017;93:200–8.

47. Berek JS, Kehoe ST, Kumar L, et al. Cancer of the ovary, fallopian tube, and peritoneum. Int J Gynecol Obstet 2018;143(Suppl. 2):59–78.

48. Garg S, Kaur A, Mohi JK, et al. Evaluation of IOTA simple ultrasound rules to distinguish benign and malignant ovarian tumours. J Clin Diagn Res 2017; 11(8):TC06–9.

49. Thomassin-Naggara I, Aubert E, Rockall A, et al. Adnexal masses: development and preliminary validation of an MR imaging scoring system. Radiology 2013;267(2):432–43.

50. Van Holsbeke C, Amant F, Veldman J, et al. Hyperreactio luteinalis in a spontaneously conceived singleton pregnancy. Ultrasound Obstet Gynecol 2009;33(3):371–3.

51. Verma V, Paul S, Chahal KS, et al. Pregnancy luteoma: a rare case report. Int J Appl Basic Med Res 2016;6(4):282–3.

52. Bourgioti C, Preza O, Panourgias E, et al. MR imaging of endometriosis: spectrum of disease. Diagn Interv Imaging 2017;98(11):751–67.

53. Skrzypczyk-Ostaszewicz A, Rubach M. Gynaecological cancers coexisting with pregnancy - a literature review. Contemp Oncol (pozn) 2016;20(3): 193–8.

54. Matsuo K, Eno ML, Im DD, et al. Pregnancy and genital sarcoma: a systematic review of the literature. Am J Perinatol 2009;26(7):507–18.

55. Greaves M, Hughes W. Cancer cell transmission via the placenta. Evol Med Public Health 2018;1: 106–15.

Imaging of Postpartum/ Peripartum Complications

Sherry S. Wang, MBBS[a],*, Dorothy Shum, MD[b], Anne Kennedy, MB BCh BAO[a,c]

KEYWORDS

- Cesarean section complications • Retained products of conception • Postpartum complications
- Endometritis • Uterine artery pseudoaneurysm • Uterine torsion • Uterine dehiscence
- Bladder injury

KEY POINTS

- There is significant overlap between normal postpartum findings and complications.
- Hematoma management is based on location.
- Endometritis is a clinical diagnosis and negative imaging does not exclude it.
- The immediate postpartum period has high risk for adnexal torsion when a mass is present.
- Enhanced myometrial vascularity can be seen with normal placental implantation site involution or associated with retained products of conception.

INTRODUCTION

The postpartum period extends from delivery of the placenta to the completion of uterine involution, which may take as long as 8 weeks. Maternal mortality in the United States rose from 12 per 100 000 births in 1990 to 28 per 100,000 in 2013. Postpartum hemorrhage (PPH) is the most frequent cause of severe maternal morbidity.[1]

Diagnosis of postpartum complications requires a team approach with careful imaging, laboratory studies, and clinical surveillance. There is considerable overlap between the normal appearance during involution and pathologic states; gas within the uterine cavity may be seen for several weeks after delivery, increased myometrial blood flow and echogenic material in the endometrial cavity (Fig. 1) are not necessarily abnormal and do not always predict the need for intervention.[2]

The imaging findings in postpartum complication can be grouped anatomically or in relationship to mode of delivery. Cesarean delivery (CD) carries higher risk of complications, which are reviewed specifically followed by an overview of the findings associated with PPH, retained products of conception (RPOCs), placental site subinvolution, fibroid infection/infarction, and adnexal or uterine torsion.

COMPLICATIONS RELATED TO CESAREAN SECTION

Cesarean section (CS) accounts for one-third of deliveries in the United States.[3] The overall complication rate of CD is 14.5%, with infection (eg, endometritis, ovarian vein thrombophlebitis, and wound infection) the most common.[4] Risk factors for complications include prolonged rupture of membranes, long duration of labor prior to surgery, anemia, and obesity. Other perioperative complications include hematoma, uterine artery pseudoaneurysm formation, bladder injury, and fistula development.

[a] Department of Radiology and Imaging Sciences, University of Utah, 30 North 1900 East # 1A71, Salt Lake City, UT 84132, USA; [b] Department of Radiology, University of California San Francisco, 505 Parnassus Avenue, 3rd Floor Box #0628, San Francisco, CA 94143, USA; [c] Maternal Fetal Diagnostic Center, University of Utah, 30 North 1900 East # 1A71, Salt Lake City, UT 84132, USA
* Corresponding author.
E-mail address: SHERRY.WANG@UTAH.EDU
Twitter: @DRSHERRYWANG (S.S.W.)

Radiol Clin N Am 58 (2020) 431–443
https://doi.org/10.1016/j.rcl.2019.10.007

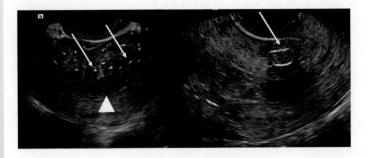

Fig. 1. Normal findings post-CS. Endovaginal US on gray scale (*left*) demonstrates clot within the endometrial cavity (*arrowhead*) and (*right*) suture material post-CS (*arrows*).

Scar endometriosis tends to present later when menses resume. Scar dehiscence and/or rupture, cesarean scar ectopic pregnancy, and placenta accreta spectrum occur in future pregnancies.

Endometritis

Endometritis is the most common cause for persistent low-grade postpartum fever; it is a clinical diagnosis[5] and the imaging findings are nonspecific, overlapping with expected postpartum changes. It is approximately 30 times more common with CS than with vaginal birth.[6]

Ultrasound (US) and computed tomography (CT) show nonspecific uterine enlargement and endometrial fluid and/or gas. US is superior for the detection of RPOCs; CT is superior for identification of parametrial inflammation and pelvic abscess. The treatment is antibiotic administration with appropriate management of any associated RPOC-infected hematoma or pelvic abscess.

Ovarian Vein Thrombophlebitis

Pelvic septic thrombophlebitis occurs in 0.05% to 0.18%[7] of all deliveries and 1% to 2% of those with endometritis[6]; thus, it is more common after CD. The right ovarian vein is involved in 80% to 90% but both veins may be involved.[8]

CT or MR imaging is preferred over US due to limited acoustic access. The vein is enlarged; luminal enhancement is absent or diminished due to central thrombus but the vein walls may enhance and the ovary may be enlarged.[7]

Postoperative Hematomas

Bladder flap hematoma is extraperitoneal, between the bladder and the lower uterine segment (LUS) secondary to bleeding[9] after low transverse CS. It is common, occurring in 50% of women[9] and should be less than or equal to 4 cm in greatest thickness. Hematomas greater than 5 cm increase concern for scar dehiscence.[10] Bladder flap hematomas tend to have thicker edges compared with hematomas at the incision defect, which are thickest at the center (**Fig. 2**A).

US shows a hypoechoic mass between the bladder and the intact LUS. Echogenicity decreases over time as clot liquefies. On CT, look for the typical location and lack of enhancement. Bleeding may spread to the broad ligaments and retroperitoneum with resultant hydronephrosis due to mass effect on the distal ureters. Superimposed infection may manifest as echogenic foci with dirty posterior shadowing on US or as rim-enhancing collections with or without septations and gas locules.

A subfascial hematoma also is extraperitoneal, arising from the inferior epigastric vessels. Hemorrhage is posterior to the rectus and transversalis muscles, anterior to the peritoneum, and contiguous with the space of Retzius (**Fig. 2**B, C), with the potential for large-volume blood loss (up to 2.5 L[11]) and hemodynamic instability; thus, recognition is critical. On US, there is a complex, solid, or cystic heterogeneous mass anterior to the bladder.[12] Contrast-enhanced CT may identify active bleeding, which can be treated with embolization.

Subcutaneous hematomas are anterior to the rectus muscle.

Uterine Artery Pseudoaneurysm

Uterine artery pseudoaneurysm is a rare but important complication of CS because rupture can lead to life-threatening hemorrhage. The sonographic diagnosis is made when color Doppler demonstrates turbulent, bidirectional flow, increased velocity, and the pathognomonic yin-yang sign in a hypoechoic lesion adjacent to the scar (**Fig. 3**A). CT and MR imaging show an enhancing mass in the myometrium or parametrium (**Fig. 3**B). Definitive diagnosis is made at angiography. Treatment by embolization has a 97% success rate.[13]

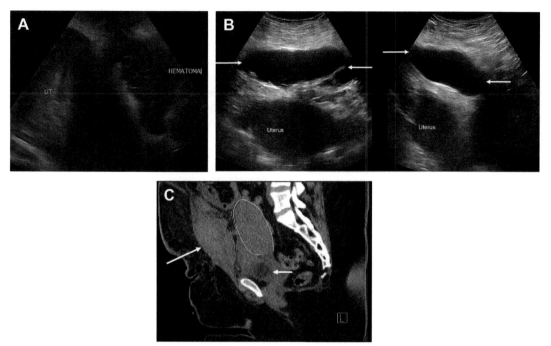

Fig. 2. Hematomas of different locations. (*A*) Transabdominal US demonstrates a heterogeneous hematoma just anterior to the uterus and posterior to a collapsed urinary bladder in keeping with a bladder flap hematoma. (*B*) Axial (*left*) and sagittal (*right*) US of a subfascial hematoma show large hypoechoic hematoma (*arrows*) deep to the rectus abdominis and subcutaneous fat, anterior to the uterus. The bladder was decompressed by a Foley catheter in this patient who also sustained a bladder injury at the time of CS. (*C*) Sagittal noncontrast CT demonstrates slightly hyperdense clot in the rectus sheath (*longarrow*). Foley catheter balloon (*short arrow*) marks bladder location. The uterus is outlined in white; the space of Retzius (the location of a subfascial hematoma) is outlined in red.

Bladder Injury

Urogenital fistulas are more likely to follow CD than obstructed labor.[14] The incidence of bladder injury during CS is 0.28%,[15] with the greatest risk during creation of the bladder flap (43%), especially with adhesive disease from previous CS; 95% occur at the bladder dome, the rest at the trigone.[15] Diagnosis usually is made intraoperatively with prompt repair. Imaging is used to confirm healing before catheter removal and to evaluate later complications, such as vesicovaginal, vesicouterine, or ureterovaginal fistula. Surgery is the definitive treatment. Post-CS fistulae repair is delayed by 3 months to wait for involution of the uterus and tissue healing.[16]

Scar Endometriosis Implant

Endometriosis can occur in abdominal incisions with an average 3.6-year delay between surgery

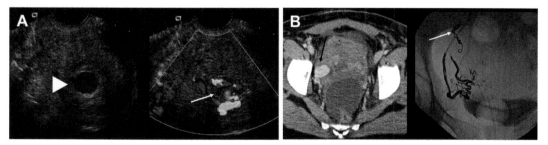

Fig. 3. Uterine artery pseudoaneurysm. (*A*) Endovaginal US on gray scale (*left*) demonstrates an anechoic well circumscribed structure within the uterus (*white arrowhead*). On Doppler US (*right*), there is a typical yin-yang sign (*arrow*), in keeping with a uterine artery pseudoaneurysm. (*B*) Axial image of a contrast-enhanced CT (*left*) demonstrates a right uterine artery pseudoaneurysm characterized by pooling of intravenous contrast (*black arrow*). (*Right*) Coils (*white arrow*) placed selectively in the right uterine artery obliterated flow to the pseudoaneurysm.

and the development of symptoms.[17] The incidence is 0.03% to 1.5% with prior CD.[18] The ectopic endometrium is functional, which causes cyclic pain due to recurrent soft tissue bleeding. Sonographic evaluation of abdominal wall pain or mass is best performed with a linear high-frequency transducer. Routine pelvic US employs 4 MHz to 6 MHz transducers for transabdominal views and 4 MHz to 9 MHz transducers for transvaginal imaging, neither of which is optimal for assessment of the anterior abdominal wall.

On US, the implants usually are solid, hypoechoic, and heterogeneous with irregular margins. Increased echogenicity adjacent to the implant reflects inflammatory/reactive changes secondary to bleeding, which creates small cystic space within the mass. Internal blood flow may be present.

On CT, abdominal wall endometriosis manifests as an enhancing mass with adjacent inflammatory change (Fig. 4). On MR imaging, the key finding is areas of T1 hyperintensity due to subacute blood, which distinguishes endometriotic implant from other abdominal wall masses. Biopsy is definitive for diagnosis. Treatment is

wide local excision; there is a recurrence rate of 4.3%.[17]

Uterine Dehiscence

Uterine dehiscence is defined as separation of the endometrium and myometrium with intact serosa. The imaging diagnosis is difficult due to normal physiologic thinning of the LUS myometrium but should be considered in a pregnant patient with pain and LUS myometrial thickness of less than 2 mm[19] or with a bladder flap hematoma greater than 5 cm in thickness in a postpartum patient.[10] CT is the modality of choice postpartum, and reformatted images perpendicular to the incision scar may be useful. Treatment usually is conservative with antibiotics, with surgery reserved for complete ruptures (Fig. 5).

Uterine Rupture

Uterine rupture is defined as separation of all layers of the uterine wall, including the serosa, creating a connection between the uterine cavity and the peritoneal space.[7] Intrapartum rupture is a surgical emergency and imaging is not performed. Rupture may occur in association with

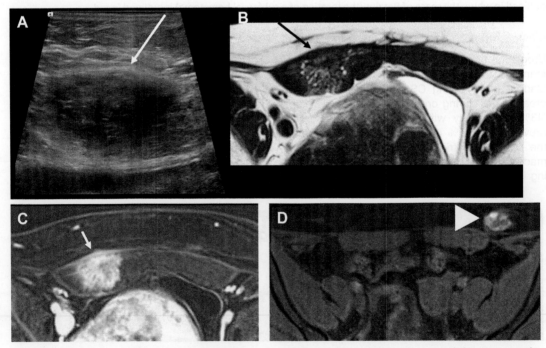

Fig. 4. CS endometriosis. (A) Transabdominal US on gray-scale images demonstrates a rectus abdominus mass (arrow). (B) Axial T2-weighted image of the same patient demonstrates T2 hyperintense foci within the lesion (arrow). (C) Axial T1 fat saturation postcontrast image of the same patient demonstrates avid enhancement (arrow), in keeping with CS scar endometriosis. (D) Axial T1 fat saturation image of a different patient demonstrates T1 hyperintense foci (arrowhead), in keeping with CS scar endometriosis.

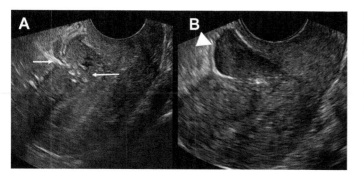

Fig. 5. Cesarean scar dehiscence. (*A*) Sagittal endovaginal US 2 days after this patient's fourth CS shows hematoma (*arrows*) at the myometrial incision as well as intracavitary blood. (*B*) Follow-up 1 year later shows an organized hematoma (*arrowhead*) in the dehiscence.

prior uterine surgery or maternal trauma and should be suspected when there is focal discontinuity of the myometrium, hemoperitoneum, gas extending into the uterine cavity, or abnormal location of the fetus.[20,21]

Cesarean Scar Ectopic Pregnancy and Placenta Accreta Spectrum

Both entities, cesarean scar ectopic pregnancy and placenta accrete spectrum, are manifestations of abnormal pregnancy implantation and

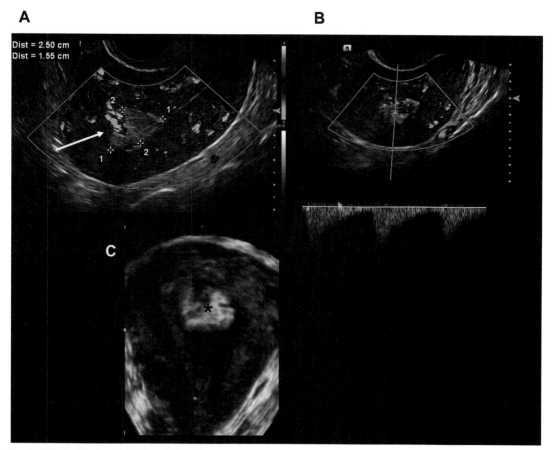

Fig. 6. RPOCs. Vaginal bleeding 5.5 weeks post–spontaneous vaginal delivery. (*A*) Endovaginal US of the uterus demonstrates focal echogenic endometrial mass (*arrow*), measuring approximately 16 mm in thickness. (*B*) Spectral waveform demonstrates arterial flow. (*C*) Three-dimensional reformat of endometrial abnormality (*asterisk*). β-hCG was 50. Pathology after hysteroscopic removal compatible with RPOCs.

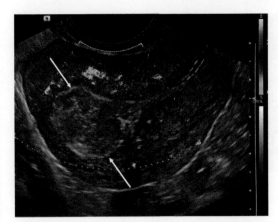

Fig. 7. Type 0 vascularity RPOCs. Fetal demise at 26 weeks, followed by D&C for endometritis and RPOCs with 2 months of spotting after D&C. Endovaginal US of the uterus demonstrates focal echogenic thickening measuring up to 30 mm (measurement not shown). Note lack of demonstrable internal flow despite low-flow settings (between *arrows*). β-hCG was less than 5. Follow-up D&C confirmed RPOCs.

placenta adherence to the cesarean scar. Early recognition and management is of the utmost importance, with some investigators suggesting that a 5-week to 7-week scan is mandatory in women with a prior CD.[22] These topics are discussed in detail elsewhere in this issue.

POSTPARTUM HEMORRHAGE

PPH is the leading cause of maternal morbidity worldwide. Primary (immediate) PPH occurs within 24 hours of delivery whereas secondary (delayed or late) PPH occurs between 24 hours and 12 weeks after delivery. In the United States, PPH complicates 3% of all deliveries[23] and 77% are due to uterine atony.[23] Atony commonly presents in the immediate phase and is diagnosed and managed clinically with little role for imaging. Other causes of primary PPH include delivery-related trauma or coagulopathy.

Secondary PPH complicates approximately 0.2% to 1% of pregnancies,[24,25] with RPOCs accounting for at least 30% of cases.[25] Other causes of secondary PPH include subinvolution of the placental implantation site, endometritis, uterine artery pseudoaneurysm, and benign or malignant uterine masses.

Retained Products of Conception

RPOCs are postpregnancy intrauterine remnants of placental and/or fetal tissue. The all-inclusive term of postpregnancy includes after spontaneous abortion, medical and surgical termination, and vaginal delivery or CD. RPOCs are more common after terminations, miscarriages, and second-trimester demises than term deliveries[26] and after vaginal deliveries than CDs.[25] Presentation is nonspecific, with bleeding, pelvic pain, fever, and/or uterine tenderness. Beta human chorionic gonadotrophin (β-hCG) may not be clinically useful because it can be positive or negative[27] in the setting of retained products. It is beneficial, however, to obtain a baseline to exclude markedly

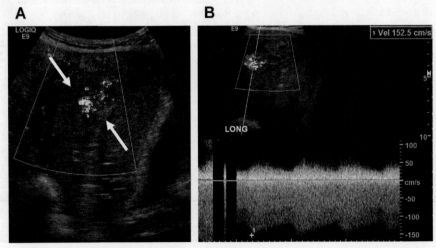

Fig. 8. Type 3 RPOCs. Vaginal bleeding 2 weeks post-CS complicated by intraoperative retained placenta. (*A*) Transabdominal US with heterogeneous vascular endometrial mass measuring greater than 20 mm (between *arrows*) (measurement not shown). (*B*) Color doppler shows greater vascularity within the endometrium than myometrium. β-hCG was 2. Pathology confirmed necrotic RPOCs.

elevated or rising levels seen with gestational trophoblastic disease.

US is the primary imaging modality for evaluation of PPH. The greatest diagnostic strength of US lies in its negative predictive value. Durfee and colleagues[28] showed no intervention was required for patients who lacked an endometrial mass or had an endometrial thickness less than 10 mm.

Sonographic findings of RPOCs include a focal endometrial mass and/or endometrial thickness greater than 10 mm[28–31] (**Fig. 6**). Rarely, retained placenta can present as a calcified mass. Gray-scale findings alone have a false-positive rate up to 34%,[32] which is understandable given the significant overlap in imaging features between RPOCs and expected postpartum lochia.[33]

Identification of color Doppler flow within the endometrium increases the positive predictive value[29,31] with greater vascularity associated with higher likelihood for surgical management.[34] Kamaya and colleagues[29] proposed a vascular grading system based on comparison of endometrial versus myometrial color Doppler flow. Type 0 is no endometrial vascularity (**Fig. 7**), which can be seen with intracavitary clot or avascular RPOCs. Type 1 is minimal endometrial vascularity on color

Doppler and less than in the myometrium; type 2 is moderate endometrial vascularity equal to the myometrium; and type 3 is marked endometrial vascularity greater than the myometrium (**Fig. 8**).

If endometrial evaluation is limited on US by technical factors, such as body habitus, postoperative gas, or intracavitary blood clot, contrast-enhanced MR imaging can be an adjunctive tool to detect enhancing retained products (see **Fig. 6**).

Subinvolution of the Placental Site and Enhanced Myometrial Vascularity

Normal placental development requires trophoblast differentiation into villous trophoblasts, which form the chorionic villi, and extravillous trophoblasts (EVTs), which replace the musculoelastic component of the endothelial lining of maternal spiral arteries. This vascular remodeling extends into the inner third of the myometrium (endomyometrium or junctional zone); results in dilated uteroplacental vessels, which facilitate maternal blood flow for maximal oxygen and nutrient exchange; and exhibits high-flow, low-resistance waveforms. This vascular pattern corresponds with the peritrophoblastic flow seen sonographically at intrauterine implantation sites.[35]

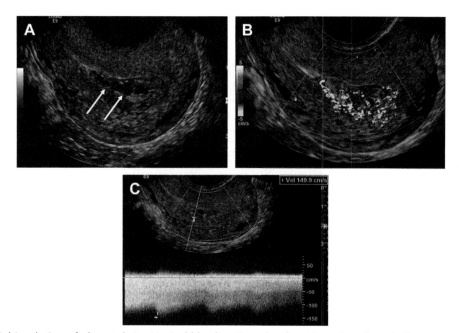

Fig. 9. Subinvolution of placental site. Vaginal bleeding 3 weeks after 10-week embryonic demise treated with misoprostol. (*A*) Endovaginal US demonstrates prominent subendometrial vessels on gray scale (*arrows*) and myometrial vascularity as seen on color Doppler (*B*). (*C*) Spectral Doppler demonstrates high-velocity low-resistance arterial flow. Subsequent manual uterine aspiration with dilated decidual vessels containing trophoblasts within vessel walls compatible with placental subinvolution. No chorionic villi or membranes to suggest RPOCs.

Involution of the placental site initiates in the third trimester and accelerates postpartum with resumption of the pregravid small-caliber arterial size and complete disappearance of the EVTs with replacement by maternal endothelial cells. Subinvolution at the placental site (SIPS) is a histologic diagnosis of delayed or inadequate conversion of the maternal spiral arteries back to baseline with persistence of the EVTs within vessels.[36] Subinvolution commonly occurs in the setting of RPOCs and gestational trophoblastic disease to maintain vascular demand but also can be seen postpregnancy without retained products as a transient (Fig. 9) or even prolonged finding several years after delivery.[37]

Postpregnancy-detected low-resistance waveforms of variable velocities spanning the full thickness of the myometrium to the uterine cavity has been referred to as enhanced myometrial vascularity (EMV)[38] and is postulated to be the sonographic representation of SIPS. EMV is a common early postpartum finding seen in 50% of asymptomatic patients on postpartum day 3, reducing to 4% by week 6 with concomitant decrease in velocity and increase in resistance. Typically EMV recedes by week 10[39] but has been reported up to 15 weeks[40] postpregnancy. Similar to SIPS, EMV also can be seen in asymptomatic and symptomatic bleeding patients with or without RPOCs38–41 (see Fig. 9), gestational trophoblastic disease,[41] and even cesarean scar pregnancies.[40] If EMV is associated with RPOCs,

this can be managed conservatively (Fig. 10) or with surgical resection (Fig. 11), which can immediately resolve the vascular finding. Currently, there are no definitive imaging features that distinguish between EMV that spontaneously resolve versus those that necessitate surgical or percutaneous embolic therapy.

The high flow, low-resistance waveforms of EMV also have been confusingly reported as uterine arteriovenous malformations (AVMs), acquired AVMs, and uterine vascular malformation in the literature because of their shared spectral pattern. Most areas of EMV without excessive bleeding, molar pregnancy, or abnormal implantation site resolve spontaneously.[40,41] These cases are unlikely to be true AVMs because they are evident only after pregnancy; can spontaneously resolve, which is in contradistinction to the classic congenital AVM description by Mulliken and Glowacki[42]; and do not consistently demonstrate an early draining vein on angiography, the gold standard for diagnosis of a true AVM. True congenital AVMs and their treatment re discussed in detail elsewhere in this issue.

There is significant overlap in clinical and imaging features of normal and pathologic conditions, which can present with PPH (Table 1). Ultimately, the decision on how best to treat should be predicated on clinical presentation and hemodynamic status. EMV should not be misconstrued as a true vascular malformation

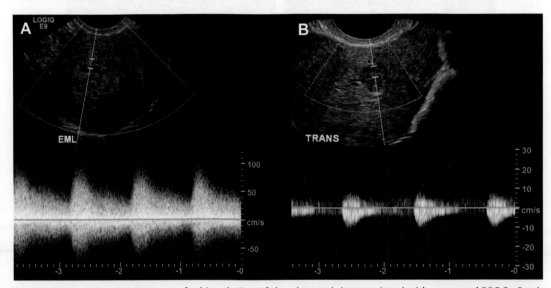

Fig. 10. Conservative management of subinvolution of the placental site associated with presumed RPOCs. Persistent vaginal spotting after manual uterine aspiration for 10-week pregnancy failure. (A) Initial imaging with small focus of endometrial thickening and adjacent elevated myometrial velocity up to 100 cm/s. Patient opted for conservative management and was hemodynamically stable with decreasing β-hCG. (B) After 2.5 weeks, 10-fold decrease in systolic velocity to less than 10 cm/s.

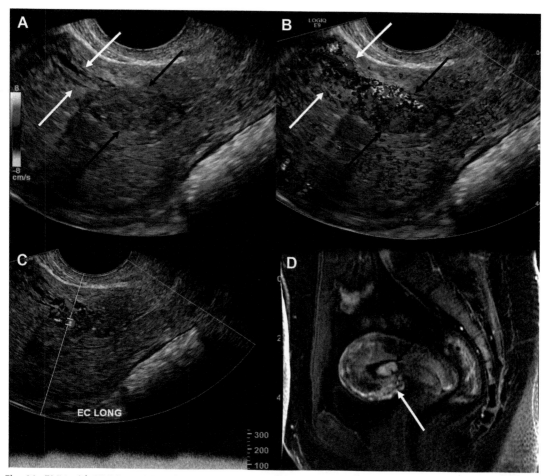

Fig. 11. EMV with RPOCs on US and MR imaging. Vaginal bleeding 5 days after D&C found RPOCs post 18-week pregnancy loss. (*A*) Endovaginal US on gray-scale and (*B*) color Doppler images demonstrate dilated vascular tubular structures (*white arrows*) extending from myometrium to endometrial mass (*black arrows*). Subsequent D&C of proved RPOCs (*black arrows*) at implantation site. (*C*) Spectral Doppler of high-velocity low-resistance arterial waveform. (*D*) Postcontrast MR imaging with enhancing RPOCs along anterior endometrium (*black arrow*) and adjacent full-thickness increased myometrial vascularity extending to RPOCs (*white arrow*).

because it can be a normal part of uterine involution. Even if EMV is associated with suspected RPOCs, it can be conservatively managed,[40,41] particularly within the first 6 weeks to 10 weeks postpregnancy, and monitored with serial US. Other treatment options for stable patients include dilation and curettage (D&C) regardless of peak systolic velocity within areas of EMV[43] or a staged approach with uterotonic agents followed by surgical evacuation if needed. Unstable patients may require UAE and/or hysterectomy.

Vaginal Wall Hematoma

Lacerations to the lower portion of the genital tract account for 2% to 4% of PPH.[10] Paravaginal hematoma can be divided into infralevator and supralevator. Infralevator hematomas are clinically visible as they extend to the vulva, perineum, and ischiorectal fossa and are managed with transvaginal drainage (**Fig. 12**).

Supralevator hematomas extend upward through the broad ligament into the retroperitoneum and are difficult to diagnose clinically, presenting as vague abdominal pain and hypovolemic shock. This entity should be considered in all patients with blood loss without uterine atony.[44] Contrast-enhanced CT is the modality of choice for location of hematoma and identification of the culprit vessel, which may require embolization. Surgical excision and drainage improves pelvic pain and prevent secondary infection.

POSTPARTUM FIBROID COMPLICATIONS

Uterine fibroids are associated with many gynecologic and obstetric complications but in the

Table 1
Overlap of imaging and clinical features between intracavitary blood clot, retained products of conception, enhanced myometrial vascularity/subinvolution of the placental site, and true congenital arteriovenous malformation

	Blood Clot	Retained Products of Conception	Enhanced Myometrial Vascularity/ Subinvolution of the Placental Site	True Arteriovenous Malformation
Endometrial mass or thickening >10 mm	+	+	± (+ if RPOCs)	−
Endometrial vascularity	−	±	± (+ if RPOCs)	−
Myometrial vascularity	± (+ if SIPS)	+	+	+
β-hCG	±	±	±	± (+if concurrent pregnancy)

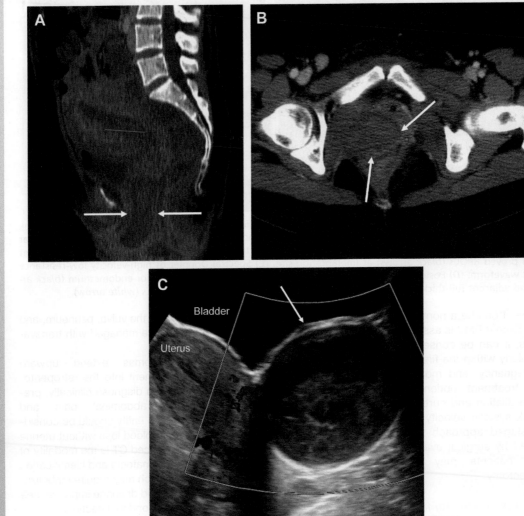

Fig. 12. Vaginal wall hematoma. Post–forceps-assisted delivery. (*A*) Sagittal and (*B*) axial non contrast CT demonstrates a heterogeneous mass in the right vaginal wall in keeping with an infralevator hematoma (*arrows*). This was drained vaginally. (*C*) Transabdominal color Doppler US of a different patient demonstrates a heterogeneous, avascular mass (*arrow*) in the vaginal wall in keeping with an infralevator hematoma.

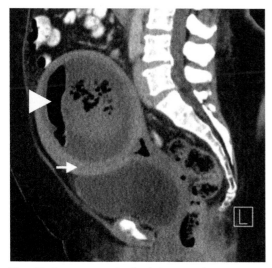

Fig. 13. Pyomyoma. Sagittal image of a contrast-enhanced CT demonstrates a large heterogeneous hypodense structure within the myometrium with a thick enhancing rim (*arrow*) and gas (*arrowhead*), in keeping with a pyomyoma.

postpartum setting the 2 most important are bleeding[45] and infection.[46] Fibroids that degenerate during pregnancy are particularly at risk for secondary infection if endometritis develops. In this setting, a pyomyoma may develop and can cause severe sepsis despite antibiotic therapy. CT is the most helpful modality because gas in the pyomyoma may compromise US image quality (**Fig. 13**). CT also allows detection of other complications, such as associated ovarian vein thrombophlebitis and deep pelvic abscess formation.

POSTPARTUM TORSION

The risk of adnexal torsion in pregnancy is highest at the end of the first trimester when the uterus expands out of the pelvis and postpartum with sudden decrease in uterine size after delivery. Any patient with an adnexal mass (eg, mature cystic teratoma) should be forewarned of the risk and cautioned to report any postpartum pain (**Fig. 14**).

Clinical symptoms of adnexal torsion include severe, sharp, sudden-onset pelvic pain with a palpable pelvic mass and nausea and vomiting. US is the imaging modality of choice to evaluate morphology and size of the ovary, to detect any mass, and for Doppler interrogation but grayscale findings are more sensitive and specific for torsion that Doppler findings. In 1 study, 60% of surgically confirmed cases of ovarian torsion had normal Doppler flow.[47] If peripheral blood flow is seen around a corpus luteum in an enlarged edematous ovary, however, that is a strong negative predictor for torsion on both US and CT.[48] Laparoscopy provides definitive diagnosis and allows treatment, the goal of which is ovarian preservation if possible. In the absence of infarction, the ovary is untwisted and oophoropexy is performed whereby the utero-ovarian ligament is fixed to the lateral pelvic wall or posterior to the uterus to prevent recurrent torsion.[49]

Another rare postpartum complication is uterine torsion defined as a twist of greater than 45° between the uterus and the cervix.[50] Clinical presentation is usually nonspecific as are the US findings.[51] Change in position of a previously documented fibroid should raise suspicion torsion of a myomatous uterus. MR imaging is particularly helpful because the upper vaginal configuration changes from the usual H shape to an X shape.[52,53] Confirmation is surgical and treatment is hysterectomy for irreversible and bilateral plication of the round ligaments[54] or

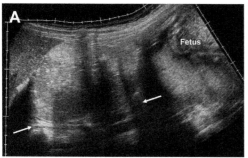
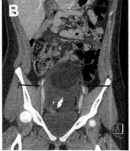
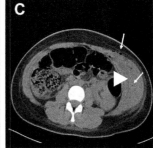

Fig. 14. Postpartum torsion of dermoid. (*A*) Transabdominal US demonstrates a 17-cm dermoid on the right (*arrows*) between the liver and the gravid uterus. (*B*) Coronal contrast-enhanced CT demonstrates the dermoid has now moved to the midline (*arrows*). The patient had acute severe pain immediately postpartum. Findings are in keeping with torsion of the right ovary, given the acute change in dermoid position. (*C*) Axial image of a nonenhanced CT of the same patient post-oophorectomy demonstrates a large left abdominal wall hematoma (*arrowhead*) with gas locules (*arrows*), which are most likely postsurgical in etiology rather than due to infection.

uterosacral ligaments[55] to prevent recurrence when the uterus is salvageable.

SUMMARY

Radiologists should be aware of the various complications that can occur in the postpartum patient with pain, bleeding, or signs of infection. Many can be assessed with US but judicious use of CT and MR imaging can be helpful. The specific postpartum complications of pelvic floor dysfunction and placenta accreta spectrum are covered in detail in other articles in this issue.

DISCLOSURE

Royalties from Elsevier (A. Kennedy). Nothing to disclose (S.S. Wang and D. Shum).

REFERENCES

1. Troiano NH, Witcher PM. Maternal mortality and morbidity in the United States: classification, causes, preventability, and critical care obstetric implications. J Perinat Neonatal Nurs 2018;32(3): 222–31.
2. Plunk M, Lee JH, Kani K, et al. Imaging of postpartum complications: a multimodality review. AJR Am J Roentgenol 2013;200(2):W143–54.
3. Martin J, Hamilton B, Osterman M, et al. National vital statistics reports. Births: final data for 2016, vol. 67. Hyattsville (MD): National Center for Health Statistics; 2018.
4. Nielsen T, Hökegård K. Postoperative cesarean section morbidity: a prospective study. Gynecol 1983; 146(8):911–6.
5. Twickler D, Setiawan A, Harrell R, et al. CT appearance of the pelvis after cesarean section. Am J Roentgenol 1991;156(3):523–6.
6. Maharaj D. Puerperal pyrexia: a review. Part I. Obstet Gynecol Surv 2007;62:393–9.
7. Di Salvo D. Sonographic imaging of maternal complications of pregnancy. J Ultrasound Med 2003; 22(1):69–89.
8. Bennett G, Slywotzky C, Giovanniello G. Gynecologic causes of acute pelvic pain: spectrum of CT findings. Radiographics 2002;22(4):785–801.
9. diFlorio-Alexander R, Harris R. Gynecologic imaging. Philadelphia: Elsevier; 2011.
10. Sierra A, Burrel M, Sebastia C, et al. Utility of multidetector CT in severe postpartum hemorrhage. Radiographics 2012;32(5):1463–81.
11. Auh Y, Rubenstine W, Schneider M, et al. Extraperitoneal paravesical spaces: CT delinieation with US correlation. Radiology 1986;159(2):319–28.
12. Wiener M, Bowie J, Baker M, et al. Sonography of subfascial hematoma after cesarean delivery. Am J Roentgenol 1987;148(5):907–10.
13. Chitra T, Panicker S. Pseudoaneurysm of uterine artery: a rare cause of secondary postpartum hemorrhage. J Obstet Gynaecol India 2011;61(6): 641–4.
14. Osman SA, Al-Badr AH, Malabarey OT, et al. Causes and management of urogenital fistulas. A retrospective cohort study from a tertiary referral center in Saudi Arabia. Saudi Med J 2018;39(4):373–8.
15. Phipps M, Watabe B, Clemons J, et al. Risk factors for bladder injury during cesarean delivery. Obstet Gynecol 2005;105(1):156–60.
16. Wong M, Wong K, Rezvan A, et al. Urogenital fistula. Female Pelvic Med Reconstr Surg 2012;18:71–8.
17. Horton J, Dezee K, Ahnfeldt E, et al. Abdominal wall endometriosis: a surgeon's perspective and review of 445 cases. Am J Surg 2008;196(2):207–12.
18. Francica G, Scarano F, Scotti L, et al. Endometriomas in the region of a scar from cesarean section: sonographic appearance and clinical presentation vary with the size of the lesion. J Clin Ultrasound 2009;37:215–20.
19. Suzuki S, Sawa R, Yoneyama Y, et al. Preoperative diagnosis of dehiscence of the lower uterine segment in patients with a single previous caesarean section. Aust N Z J Obstet Gynaecol 2000;40(4):402–4.
20. Antonelli E, Morales M, Dumps P, et al. Sonographic detection of fluid collections and postoperative morbidity following cesarean section and hysterectomy. Ultrasound Obstet Gynecol 2004;23(4): 388–92.
21. Maldjian C, Milestone B, Schnall M, et al. MR appearance of uterine dehiscence in the postcesarean section patient. J Comput Assist Tomogr 1998;22(5):738–41.
22. Timor-Tritsch IE, D'Antonio F, Cali G, et al. Early first trimester transvaginal ultrasound is indicated in pregnancies after a previous cesarean delivery: should it be mandated? Ultrasound Obstet Gynecol 2019;54(2):156–63.
23. Marshall AL, Durani U, Bartley A, et al. The impact of postpartum hemorrhage on hospital length of stay and inpatient mortality: a National Inpatient Sample-based analysis. Am J Obstet Gynecol 2017;217(3):344.e1-6.
24. Hoveyda F, MacKenzie IZ. Secondary postpartum haemorrhage: incidence, morbidity and current management. BJOG 2001;108(9):927–30.
25. Dossou M, Debost-Legrand A, Dechelotte P, et al. Severe secondary postpartum hemorrhage: a historical cohort. Birth 2015;42(2):149–55.
26. Van den Bosch T, Daemen A, Van Schoubroeck D, et al. Occurrence and outcome of residual trophoblastic tissue: a prospective study. J Ultrasound Med 2008;27(3):357–61.
27. Achiron R, Goldenberg M, Lipitz S, et al. Transvaginal duplex doppler ultrasonography in bleeding

patients suspected of having residual trophoblastic tissue. Obstet Gynecol 1993;81(4):507–11.

28. Durfee SM, Frates MC, Luong A, et al. The sonographic and color Doppler features of retained products of conception. J Ultrasound Med 2005;24(9):1181–6.

29. Kamaya A, Petrovitch I, Chen B, et al. Retained products of conception spectrum of color doppler findings. J Ultrasound Med 2009;28(8):1031–41.

30. Sellmyer MA, Desser TS, Maturen KE, et al. Physiologic, histologic, and imaging features of retained products of conception. Radiographics 2013;33(3): 781–96.

31. Esmaeillou H, Jamal A, Eslamian L, et al. Accurate detection of retained products of conception after first-and second-trimester abortion by color doppler sonography. J Med Ultrasound 2015; 23(1):34–8.

32. Sadan O, Golan A, Girtler O, et al. Role of Sonography in the diagnosis of retained products of conception. J Ultrasound Med 2004;23(3):371–4.

33. Mulic-Lutvica A, Bekuretsion M, Bakos O, et al. Ultrasonic evaluation of the uterus and uterine cavity after normal, vaginal delivery. Ultrasound Obstet Gynecol 2001;18(5):491–8.

34. Kamaya A, Krishnarao PM, Nayak N, et al. Clinical and imaging predictors of management in retained products of conception. Abdom Radiol (NY) 2016; 41(12):2429–34.

35. Dillon EH, Feyock AL, Taylor KJW. Pseudogestational sacs - doppler us differentiation from normal or abnormal intrauterine pregnancies. Radiology 1990;176(2):359–64.

36. Weydert JA, Benda JA. Subinvolution of the placental site as an anatomic cause of postpartum uterine bleeding - A review. Arch Pathol Lab Med 2006;130(10):1538–42.

37. Wachter DL, Thiel F, Agaimy A. Subinvolution of the placental site 6 years after last delivery. Int J Gynecol Pathol 2011;30(6):581–2.

38. Van den Bosch T, Van Schoubroeck D, Lu C, et al. Color Doppler and gray-scale ultrasound evaluation of the postpartum uterus. Ultrasound Obstet Gynecol 2002;20(6):586–91.

39. van Schoubroeck D, van den Bosch T, Scharpe K, et al. Prospective evaluation of blood flow in the myometrium and uterine arteries in the puerperium. Ultrasound Obstet Gynecol 2004;23(4):378–81.

40. Timor-Tritsch IE, Haynes MC, Monteagudo A, et al. Ultrasound diagnosis and management of acquired uterine enhanced myometrial vascularity/arteriovenous malformations. Am J Obstet Gynecol 2016; 214(6):731.e1–10.

41. Timmerman D, Wauters J, Van Calenbergh S, et al. Color Doppler imaging is a valuable tool for the diagnosis and management of uterine vascular malformations. Ultrasound Obstet Gynecol 2003;21(6): 570–7.

42. Mulliken JB, Glowacki J. Hemangiomas and vascular malformations in infants and children - a classification based on endothelial characteristics. Plast Reconstr Surg 1982;69(3):412–20.

43. Groszmann YS, Murphy ALH, Benacerraf BR. Diagnosis and management of patients with enhanced myometrial vascularity associated with retained products of conception. Ultrasound Obstet Gynecol 2018;52(3):396–9.

44. Yamashita Y, Torashima M, Harada M, et al. Postpartum extraperitoneal pelvic hematoma: imaging findings. Am J Roentgenol 1993;161(4):805–8.

45. Akrivis C, Varras M, Bellou A, et al. Primary postpartum haemorrhage due to a large submucosal nonpedunculated uterine leiomyoma: a case report and review of the literature. Clin Exp Obstet Gynecol 2003;30(2–3):156–8.

46. Nguyen QH, Gruenewald SM. Sonographic appearance of a postpartum pyomyoma with gas production. J Clin Ultrasound 2008;36(3):186–8.

47. Pena J, Ufberg D, Cooney N, et al. Usefulness of Doppler sonography in the diagnosis of ovarian torsion. Fertil Steril 2000;73:1047–50.

48. Rogers D, Al-Dulaimi R, Rezvani M, et al. Peripheral hypervascularity of the corpus luteum with ovarian edema (CLOE) may decrease false positive diagnoses of ovarian torsion. Abdom Radiol (NY) 2019; 44(9):3158–65.

49. Abeş M, Sarihan HEJPS. Oophoropexy in children with ovarian torsion. Eur J Pediatr Surg 2004;14: 168.

50. Cipullo LMA, Milosavljevic S, van Oudgaarden ED. Uterus didelphys: report of a puerperal torsion and a review of the literature. Case Rep Obstet Gynecol 2012;2012:190167.

51. Nesbitt R, Corner G. Torsion of the human pregnant uterus. Obstet Gynecol Surv 1956;11(3):311–32.

52. Luk S, Leung J, Cheung M, et al. Torsion of a nongravid myomatous uterus: radiological features and literature review. Hong Kong Med J 2010; 16(4):304–6.

53. Nicholson W, Coulson C, McCoy M, et al. Pelvic magnetic resonance imaging in the evaluation of uterine torsion. Obstet Gynecol 1995;85(5): 888–90.

54. Pelosi M, Pelosi M. Managing extreme uterine torsion at term: a case report. J Reprod Med 1998; 43(2):153–7.

55. Mustafa M, Shakeel F, Sporrong B. Extreme torsion of the pregnant uterus. Aust N Z J Obstet Gynaecol 1999;39(3):360–3.

Role of Interventional Procedures in Obstetrics and Gynecology

Michael Weston, MB ChB, MRCP, FRCR[a],*, Philippe Soyer, MD, PhD[b],
Matthias Barral, MD, PhD[b], Anthony Dohan, MD, PhD[b],
Sacha Pierre, BSc, MBBS, MRCS, FRCR[a], Rana Rabei, MD[c],
Kirema Garcia-Reyes, MD[c], Maureen P. Kohi, MD, FSIR[c]

KEYWORDS

- Interventional radiology • Postpartum hemorrhage • Invasive placenta
- Ultrasonography-guided drainage • Ultrasonography-guided adnexal/ovarian/ pelvic mass biopsy
- Ultrasonography-guided omental biopsy • Ultrasonography-guided ascites drainage
- Ultrasonography-guided diagnosis of gynecologic disorder

KEY POINTS

- Uterine artery embolization is an effective means for the treatment of postpartum hemorrhage of several causes, including atony and invasive placenta.
- Ultrasonography-guided intervention can be used in daily practice in the diagnosis and treatment of benign and malignant gynecologic conditions.
- Clinicians should be familiar with the clinical presentations, procedural steps, and outcomes of high-intensity focused ultrasonography, fallopian tube recanalization, and pelvic congestion.
- Interventional radiology can be used for the treatment of pelvic congestion syndrome, uterine fistula, and uterine leiomyomas, and for fallopian tube recanalization.

INTRODUCTION

This article introduces some of the many techniques of imaging-guided intervention that are available in the pelvis. Many facets of obstetric and gynecologic disorders from assisted fertility, through biopsy or aspiration of adnexal masses to embolization of postpartum bleeding, are considered. The techniques are often common to nongynecologic applications but this article provides an aide memoire to how they can be used in the female pelvis.

Fallopian Tube Recanalization

Infertility is a common problem that affects many couples. According to the Centers for Disease Control and Prevention, infertility affects 6.1 million or 10% of women of reproductive age in the United States.[1] Fallopian tube obstruction contributes to one-third of cases of infertility, with 10% to 25% of these cases attributed to proximal fallopian tube obstruction.[2,3] The unique anatomy of the proximal fallopian tube, with its muscular wall, small diameter, and tortuosity, makes this segment prone to spasm, mucus plugging, and scarring from inflammation leading to obstruction and infertility.[4] The American Society for Reproductive Medicine recommends fallopian tube recanalization (FTR) as a treatment of infertility in women with proximal tubal occlusion.[5]

FTR is a minimally invasive and cost-effective alternative to in vitro fertilization (IVF) with the

[a] Department of Radiology, St James's University Hospital, Leeds LS9 7TF, UK; [b] Department of Radiology, Service de Radiologie A, Hopital Cochin, APHP & Université de Paris-Descartes Paris 5, 27 rue du Faubourg Saint-Jacques, Paris 75014, France; [c] Department of Radiology and Biomedical Imaging, University of California, San Francisco, 505 Parnassus Avenue, M-361, San Francisco, CA 94143, USA
* Corresponding author.
E-mail address: Michael.weston2@nhs.net

Radiol Clin N Am 58 (2020) 445–462
https://doi.org/10.1016/j.rcl.2019.11.006

added advantage of allowing women the ability to conceive naturally, at their own pace and without hormonal intervention. FTR is a well-established and well-tolerated procedure with similar outcomes to IVF.[6]

Preprocedural planning

This minimally invasive procedure is performed in an ambulatory setting, during the follicular phase of the menstrual cycle, before ovulation. Preprocedural prophylactic antibiotics such as doxycycline 100 mg twice a day is recommended 2 days before FTR. The procedure is routinely performed with moderate sedation. Postprocedural pain and cramping are predominately managed with nonsteroidal antiinflammatory drugs (NSAIDs). Following FTR, patients can attempt to conceive soon after the procedure.[7]

Fallopian tube recanalization procedure

FTR is performed using a sterile technique with the patient in the lithotomy position. The procedure is composed of 3 components: uterine access, hysterosalpingogram (HSG), and tubal recanalization. Uterine access is performed using a balloon occluding sheath or catheter. Next, the HSG is performed with slow injection of a dilute nonionic contrast agent to localize the uterine cornua (**Fig. 1**). Once proximal fallopian tubal obstruction is confirmed, selective catheterization of the blocked tube is performed using a 5-French or 3-French coaxial catheter system (**Fig. 2**). A hydrophilic guidewire is used to cross the obstruction, followed by selective tubal injection (salpingogram) to confirm patency (**Fig. 3**). A postrecanalization HSG can also then be performed (**Fig. 4**).

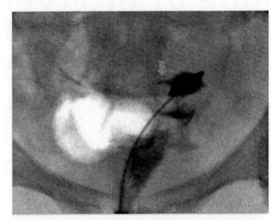

Fig. 2. Selective catheterization of the blocked tube confirms right proximal tubal blockage with no opacification of right fallopian tube (*arrow*).

In light of recent evidence showing higher rates of pregnancy and live births following HSG with oil-based contrast, a small amount of oil-based contrast can be injected following confirmation of tubal recanalization.[8]

Clinical outcomes

The technical success rate of this procedure is in the range of 70% to 90%, and patency rates are reported to be over 60% for up to 1 year after recanalization, and reocclusion of the fallopian tube can be treated with repeat recanalization.[6] The pregnancy rates following the procedure are in the range of 30% to 60%.

Adverse events

The minor complications of FTR include mild uterine cramping and vaginal bleeding 1 to

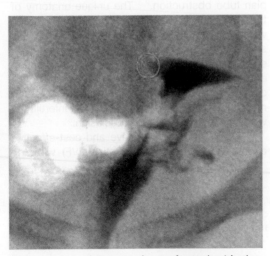

Fig. 1. Hysterosalpingography performed with slow injection of a dilute nonionic iodinated contrast agent shows right proximal tubal occlusion (*circle*).

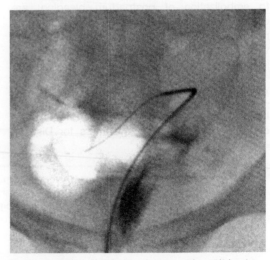

Fig. 3. Crossing of tubal occlusion with a Glidewire.

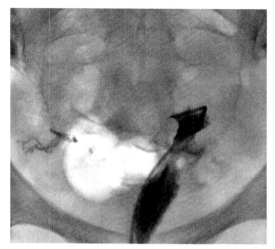

Fig. 4. Selective salpingogram confirms patency of the recanalized tube.

3 days following recanalization. Complications of tubal perforation, ectopic pregnancy, and adnexal infections have been reported but are rare. Radiation doses to the ovaries from this procedure are less than 1 rad (10 mGy), with a mean dose of 2.7 mGy and patient effective dose of 1.2 mSV.[5,9,10]

POSTPARTUM HEMORRHAGE

Postpartum hemorrhage (PPH) occurs in 6% of all deliveries. PPH is defined as a blood loss greater than 500 mL within 24 hours after vaginal or cesarean delivery that requires specific administration of oxytocin, which is a first-line uterotonic drug.[11] Severe PPH is a life-threatening condition with hemodynamic instability that requires the use of prostaglandins; uterine tamponade; and, in case of failure, uterine artery embolization (UAE) or surgery. Severe PPH represents 1.86% of all deliveries.[12] PPH that occurs less than 24 hours after delivery is also called primary or early PPH.[12] When PPH occurs more than 24 hours but less than 6 to 12 weeks after delivery it is called secondary or late PPH.[13]

Uterine atony and trauma or laceration of the lower portion of the genital tract are the main causes of primary PPH, occurring in approximately 80% and 5% of PPH, respectively.[14] Other less frequent causes of primary PPH consist of abnormally invasive placentation, congenital or acquired coagulation disorders, uterine rupture or inversion, bladder flap hematoma, retention of blood clots or placental fragments, and leiomyomas. Retained placenta, abnormally invasive placentation, uterine subinvolution, coagulopathies, and ruptured pseudoaneurysm represent

the main causes of secondary PPH.[15,16] Usually, pseudoaneurysms occur on uterine arteries after cesarean section and on cervicovaginal arteries after vaginal delivery.[17]

The overall success rate of UAE in women with PPH approaches 91%.[12,13,18–20] Predictive factors of failed UAE include disseminated intravascular coagulation,[21,22] transfusion of 5 to 10 packed red cells, blood loss greater than 1.5 L,[21,22] severe arterial vasoconstriction on angiography,[23] and abnormally invasive placentation.[8,14] Repeat UAE when the first uterine embolization session has failed has a success rate of 67% to 80%.[12,18,19] Of note, active bleeding during angiography has been suggested as a predictive factor of repeat UAE.[24]

Complications of UAE occur in 3% of women with PPH. They include hematoma at the puncture site, dissection of the uterine artery dissection, transient sciatic nerve palsy, and synechiae, without need of surgical intervention, which are all benign complications.[19,21,25] Major complications such as uterine necrosis[26] or nontarget embolization[27] are rare events. Endometritis and infected pelvic hematoma have been reported and usually resolve with antibiotic therapy and sometime drainage.[28] Consequently, in women with unexplained fever after UAE, computed tomography (CT) examination should be performed to exclude abscess, pelvic thrombosis, or infected hematoma.

Uterine Atony

Uterine atony mainly occurs in women without prior obstetric history. However, multiple pregnancies, polyhydramnios or fetal macrosomia, prolonged labor, and general anesthesia are predisposing factors of uterine atony. Uterine atony represents 70% to 80% of all causes of PHH.[16] On angiogram, uterine atony is associated with dilated uterine and arcuate arteries and there is no contrast extravasation.[16]

Most interventional radiologists use gelatin sponge torpedoes because they are temporary occluding agents and provide proximal arterial occlusion.[29] Nontarget embolization is the main complication, especially in the posterior trunk and external iliac artery, which can be responsible for sciatic nerve and distal leg ischemia, respectively.

The increase of arterial blood pressure after UAE is a strong indicator of clinical success. External bleeding should promptly stop and the uterus should quickly become well retracted soon after UAE.[16] In women with persisting hypotension and hemorrhage, second-look angiography should be performed to exclude reperfusion of the bleeding site by spontaneous anastomosis.[30] Aortogram with delayed images is needed to search for distal recanalization of uterine arteries through patent collaterals.[30]

Placenta Accreta Spectrum Disorder

Several approaches are now available for the management of placenta accreta spectrum (PAS) disorders. They include an aggressive approach (ie, extirpative approach with placental removal, yielding high morbidity), cesarean hysterectomy (in which the placenta is removed along with the uterus, resulting in no future fertility), and full conservative management (ie, the placenta is left in place).[31,32]

Regarding UAE, PPH caused by PAS disorder is a complex and challenging situation for several reasons. First, it is performed in an emergency setting, often with hemodynamically unstable women.[33] Second, angiographic findings are often unpredictable, resulting in variable procedure time.[16] Third, PAS disorder remains a main cause of failed embolization, with repeat embolization needed in a subset of patients.[16,27,33]

To date, UAE in women with PPH caused by PAS disorder is the treatment option for which the highest degrees of evidence are available.[16,18,34] However, other options have been tested, including prophylactic catheter placement, balloon occlusion of the iliac arteries, and abdominal aorta balloon occlusion.[35,36]

Uterine artery embolization

PAS disorder is a complex situation. The angiographic findings in women with PAS disorder depend on several variables. The patient may have undergone arterial ligations that result in further recruitment of extrauterine arteries.[37] In addition, the degree of aggressiveness of PAS disorder (accreta or percreta) correlates with the technical difficulty. For these reasons, full pelvic angiogram is needed to understand the complex vascularization of the remaining placenta and pelvis. The goals of arterial embolization in women with PPH caused by PAS disorder are to stop the bleeding to avoid surgical morbidity and induce thrombosis of intervillous space, reduce the risk of further bleeding, and improve the speed of placental resorption.[16]

The success rate of UAE in women with PPH caused by PAS disorder ranges between 76% and 92.5%.[25,33,34] A systematic review including 177 women with AIP reported a success rate of 90% for UAE.[38] Repeat embolization is feasible, resulting in an increased

success rate.[34] The need for further hysterectomy because of failed embolization is reported in 7.5% to 18% of women, with a mean rate of 11.3%.[16,33,34,38]

The overall complication rate of UAE rate reaches 11%, consisting of minor complications such as pelvic pain, nausea, urticaria, and fever, or more severe complications such as deep venous thrombosis, uterine necrosis, endometritis, and synechiae.[16,19,22,34,38,39] Besides the well-acknowledged hemostatic effect of UAE, another useful role of UAE is to shorten the resorption delay of the placenta in women with PAS disorder treated conservatively with the invasive placenta left in place.[40]

Prophylactic catheter placement and/or balloon occlusion

The use of prophylactic catheter placement and embolization in women with PAS disorder has gained recent interest because in many institutions interventional radiologists are not permanently available for emergency UAE. Several studies have investigated the potential of this approach in women with PAS disorder.[41–43] The embolic agents are mainly gelatin pledgets, alone or used in combination with metallic coils.[42,43]

Clinical success rates of up to 86% have been reported.[41] However, hysterectomy following this approach because of ineffectiveness is needed in 8% to 30% of women.[43–45] Complications include transient paresthesia of lower limb,[41] peritonitis, and endometritis.[45] Large blood transfusion requirement was reported in 14% of women,[41,46] with mean blood loss ranging from 1200 mL[43] to 2279 mL[45] and up to 9000 mL in 1 study.[47]

Of interest, in 1 study, 2 women with prophylactic placement of catheters had severe PPH that was treated with immediate peripartum hysterectomy and UAE was not attempted, thus seriously questioning the value of prophylactic placement.[44] In addition, 43% of women (6 out of 14) underwent hysterectomy.[44] In addition, PPH occurred in 7 out of 14 women (50%) only, indicating that UAE may be needed in 50% of women with PAS disorder.[44]

Balloon catheters in iliac arteries

The value of prophylactic placement of balloon catheters in the iliac arteries in women with PAS disorder is controversial, mainly owing to the higher risks of complications compared with UAE, and the lack of direct comparison with UAE.[36,48] The impact of this approach on the amount of blood loss is not fully established.[36] One randomized controlled trial found no differences in the number of women with blood loss greater than 2500 mL, number of plasma products transfused, duration of surgery, peripartum complications, and hospitalization length using prophylactic placement of balloon catheters in the iliac arteries compared with a conventional approach.[49] However, other studies found some benefits in terms of reduced blood loss.[48,50] In addition, only 50% of women who undergo prophylactic placement of balloon catheters in the internal iliac arteries for PAS disorder have balloon inflation during delivery when excessive bleeding occurs.[51]

Several complications caused by the use of balloon catheters in the internal iliac arteries have been reported, with a rate of up to 16%.[52] Balloon-related complications include left iliac artery rupture, internal iliac artery dissection, leg ischemia, and permanent claudication.[52]

Despite using low-radiation-dose techniques, fetal radiation exposure is a major concern when considering internal iliac artery balloon occlusion. Although variable, mean fetal radiation exposure is 4.4 mGy.[53]

Uterine Vascular Malformations

Uterine vascular malformations (UVMs) are categorized according their content and flow characteristics.[54,55] UVMs can be congenital or acquired, but congenital UVMs are less frequent than acquired UVMs. Congenital UVMs are caused by the abnormal development of a vessel resulting in multiple vascular connections invading surrounding structures. Acquired UVMs usually occur after uterine trauma such as curettage (Fig. 5) or cesarean section.

Because treatment strategy depends on the type of UVM, correct classification is essential. Slow-flow vascular malformations (venous and lymphatic malformations) are often treated by sclerotherapy, whereas fast-flow lesions (arteriovenous malformations [AVMs]) are generally managed with embolization.[54] Fast-flow AVMs are classified and treated according to their angioarchitecture (ie, caliber and multiplicity of shuntings and draining veins). Pretherapeutic evaluation is based on transvaginal color Doppler ultrasonography and magnetic resonance (MR) imaging. Transvaginal color Doppler ultrasonography has a main role for deciding on the best treatment option. Some investigators suggest that AVMs with peak systolic velocity (PSV) less than 40 cm/s and nonsignificant bleeding should be treated expectantly, whereas those with high PSV (>80 cm/s) or significant blood flow should undergo embolization.[55] However, the treatment should be individualized based on the clinical evaluation. MR imaging with MR angiography sequences provides useful information regarding the size and extent of AVMs. When embolization of AVMs is considered, liquid embolic agents have been reported to be useful for fast-flow AVM treatment, and seem more appropriated because they are able to progress distally through the smallest capillaries to reach the nidus,[56] but n-butyl-2-cyanoacrylate also showed excellent results.[57]

BENIGN GYNECOLOGIC DISEASE
Benign Uterine Disease

Uterine artery embolization for uterine leiomyoma

UAE is now a well-established uterine-sparing treatment of women with uterine leiomyoma.[58] Treatment of uterine leiomyoma is restricted to symptomatic leiomyomas (ie, menorrhagia, dysmenorrhea, pain, infertility). UAE of leiomyomas allows uterus preservation and short recovery time compared with surgery.[58,59] In addition, UAE can be used in conjunction with minimally invasive surgery for the resection of multiple uterine

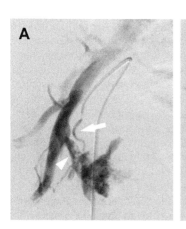
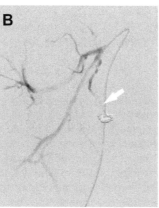

Fig. 5. A 44-year-old woman presenting with acute vaginal bleeding and hemodynamic instability after uterine curettage. (*A*) Angiogram of right internal iliac artery shows direct communication between right uterine vein (*arrow*) and right uterine artery (*arrowhead*). (*B*) Control angiogram after uterine artery embolization using metallic coils (*arrow*) and gelatin sponge shows complete exclusion of anterior trunk of right internal iliac artery. After a follow-up of 12 months, no repeat bleeding was observed.

leiomyomas.[60] The clinical success rate for menorrhagia symptoms and bulk-related symptoms has been reported as 81% to 94% and 64% to 96% of women, respectively, along with a reduction of the uterine and leiomyoma volume of 35% to 52% and 37% to 69% respectively.[61] Contraindications include uterine infection, pregnancy, and gynecologic malignancies. Future fertility is now considered a relative contraindication, because successful pregnancies have been reported after UAE for leiomyomas, as well as for postpartum hemorrhage and ectopic pregnancies.[61]

MR imaging is the best imaging modality for mapping, characterization, and follow-up of uterine leiomyomas after UAE.[62,63] During the follow-up, MR imaging shows devascularization of uterine leiomyomas, which correlates with long-term success.[62,64,65] The technique is similar to the general protocol of UAE in female pelvis with a few specificities: (1) microparticles 500 μm or larger are used to prevent nontargeted embolization of ovarian arteries through the utero-ovarian anastomosis[66]; (2) embolization should be performed distal to the cervicovaginal branch to prevent vaginal ischemia and sexual dysfunction; (3) a good result is achieved when angiogram shows a pruned-tree appearance with sluggish forward flow in the main uterine artery. Interventional radiologists should keep in mind that pseudo-occlusion caused by arterial spasm or embolic material clumping is followed by delayed restoration of flow. In addition, arterial blood supply to leiomyomas from ovarian arteries should be thoroughly investigated to prevent embolization failure. When using UAE, knowledge of the potential ovarian-uterine anastomoses is important because they provide collateral blood flow that may result in failed embolization or ovarian nontargeted embolization.[5] Complications of arterial embolization include uterine ischemia and necrosis, unwanted embolization of cervicovaginal branches, amenorrhea, and ovarian failure.[65]

High-intensity focused ultrasonography

High-intensity focused ultrasonography is a noninvasive, outpatient, novel treatment of uterine leiomyomas that uses tightly focused, high-energy ultrasound waves to destroy tissue, a process known as sonication. This high-energy targeted beam heats tissue to a temperature ranging between 55°C and 85°C (131°–185° Fahrenheit) resulting in coagulative necrosis and cell death.[67] This technology can be used under MR imaging guidance (MR-guided focused ultrasonography [MRgFUS]). MR imaging provides increased image contrast and spatial resolution resulting in improved tissue targeting, and MR thermometry offers real-time thermal imaging of the treated region[68]

Preprocedure assessment Preprocedure contrast-enhanced MR imaging of the pelvis should be obtained to determine whether the patient is a good candidate for MRgFUS. The goal is to evaluate for size, number, location, and imaging characteristics of leiomyomas and review surrounding anatomy for treatment planning. Studies have shown that patients with fewer than 4 leiomyomas that are each less than 10 cm across or less than 500 cm^3 in volume tend to have better response.[68] Uterine leiomyomas with homogeneous hypointense signal on T2-weighted imaging and homogeneous enhancement on fat-saturated T1-weighted postcontrast imaging have better treatment response than those with heterogeneous signal characteristics.[67,69]

Preprocedure assessment should also include evaluation for standard contraindications to MR imaging. In addition, if the patient has an intrauterine device, it should be removed before treatment to prevent heating.[68] The skin overlying the lower abdomen and pelvis should be evaluated for scars or tattoos along the projected beam path, which may result in skin injury or burns during the procedure.

High-intensity focused ultrasonography procedure This noninvasive procedure is routinely performed in an outpatient setting with moderate sedation. The patient is positioned prone on the MR imaging table with the pelvis over the ultrasound transducer and the feet in the MR imaging bore (Fig. 6A). Multiplanar rapid gradient echo localizer sequences are performed to ensure appropriate positioning with the patient's uterus in line with the transducer (Fig. 6B). If bowel loops are seen along the projected ultrasound beam, they can be moved by distending the bladder or filling the rectum with gel (Fig. 7). Ideally the posterior aspect of the uterine leiomyoma is no more than 12 cm from the skin, and the rectum can be filled to mobilize the uterus anteriorly, if needed.

Once the patient is appropriately positioned, multiplanar T2-weighted MR imaging sequences are obtained and transferred to the workstation for treatment planning. The leiomyoma region of interest is marked and landmarks including skin, uterus, bowel, and bone are outlined to avoid injury. Multiple sonications are then performed, each lasting approximately 20 to 30 seconds, followed by a cooling period of 80 to 100 seconds.[67] Real-time temperature measurements are also plotted throughout the sonication, and the parameters can be adjusted to ensure areas with

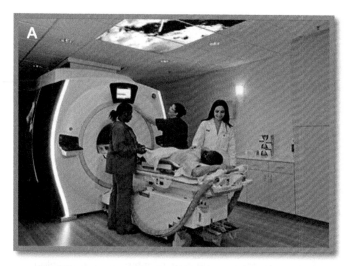

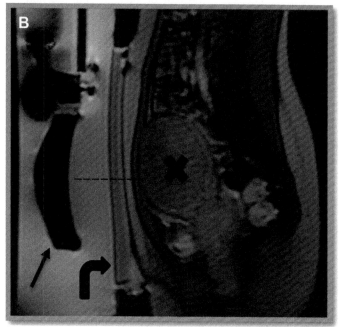

Fig. 6. Patient positioning for high-intensity focused ultrasonography ablation of uterine leiomyoma. The patient is positioned prone with the pelvis over the transducer and (A) feet in the MR imaging bore. (B) An MR imaging rapid gradient echo localizer sequence is then obtained showing the transducer (arrow), targeted uterine leiomyoma (X), gel pad (curved arrow), and expected trajectory of the ultrasonography beam (dashed line).

suboptimal heating can be retreated. A typical treatment lasts approximately 3 hours. Throughout the procedure, the patient holds a panic button and can stop the sonication in case of pain or skin warmth/burning.

After treatment is complete, multiplanar, fat-saturated, T1-weighted noncontrast and contrast-enhanced images are obtained to evaluate procedural outcomes potential adverse events. Using the postcontrast imaging, the non-perfused volume (NPV) can be calculated. The NPV is the area of the leiomyoma that no longer enhances and does not have any blood flow (Fig. 8).[67] Technical and clinical success can be evaluated via the NPV because values greater than 50% to 60% have been correlated to improved symptoms.[70]

Following a brief period of recovery, the patient can be discharged home. Most patients do not require any medications in the postprocedural setting. Patients are instructed to take over-the-counter acetaminophen or ibuprofen for any postprocedural pain.

Outcomes Patients report improvement in bulk symptoms and heavy menstrual bleeding after approximately 3 menstrual cycles.[71] Approximately 92.9% of women who undergo MRgFUS report

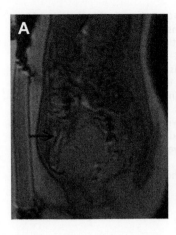
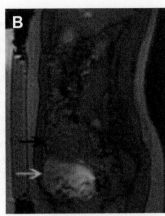

Fig. 7. Treatment planning. Rapid gradient echo localizer sequence images reveal (*A*) bowel anterior to the uterus (*black arrow*), which (*B*) was displaced superiorly (*black arrow*) by distending the urinary bladder (*white arrow*). (*From* Devulapalli K, Kohi MP, Rieke V, Ozhinsky E, Jacoby VL, Westphalen A, Weinstein S. Expected Imaging Findings and Potential Complications after MR Guided Focused Ultrasound Surgery (MRgFUS) of Symptomatic Fibroids. Imaging in Medicine 2016; 8.3; with permission.)

symptom improvement at 6 months and 87.6% at 12 months. However, younger women, women with heterogeneous uterine leiomyomas on imaging, and those with NPV of less than 50% are more likely to require additional treatment.[71,72]

A prospective randomized controlled trial that compared the efficacy of UAE versus MRgFUS in the treatment of symptomatic uterine leiomyomas found that women undergoing MRgFUS had a higher reintervention rate than those undergoing UAE. Both treatment groups experienced significant improvement in symptoms, but women undergoing UAE had greater improvement in overall quality of life and symptom scores[73]

Adverse events The most common side effects of the procedure are cramping and nausea/vomiting. Postprocedural pain and cramping are predominantly managed with NSAIDs, and most patients return to their normal routines after 1 to 3 days.[67] Uncommon complications include skin burns, nerve injury, injury to adjacent organs such as bowel or ovaries, and deep venous thrombosis.

Gynecologic Infections

Pelvic inflammatory disease may be related to iatrogenic, gynecologic, or nongynecologic causes.[74] The role of interventional radiology is to obtain a sample for diagnosis, to provide drainage, or both.

Actinomycosis is a pelvic infection that is related to long-term use of an intrauterine device. It has a characteristic feature of the infection sweeping through tissue planes and may be mistaken for malignancy. The diagnosis is often achieved by culture of the removed intrauterine device. However, sometimes biopsy of the abnormal tissue is needed. This biopsy can be performed via a transvaginal route or, if present, percutaneous biopsy of omental disease. Tuberculosis is another disease that may present as peritoneal and omental abnormal soft tissue, in which radiologically guided biopsy may be the only way to confirm the diagnosis.

Most gynecologic-related infections involve the development of a tubo-ovarian abscess. A typical scenario is someone with preexisting abnormal fallopian tubes, such as hematosalpinges, who has undergone an intrauterine intervention (coil placement, HSG, or hysteroscopy) and who then presents a few days later with pelvic sepsis (**Fig. 9**). Management with a course of intensive antibiotics is only successful in 37% to 88% of patients.[75] Gynecologic infections are also seen in

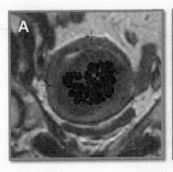
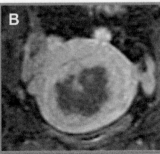

Fig. 8. Nonperfused volume. (*A*) Posttreatment fat-saturated, T1-weighted noncontrast MR image in the axial plane with blue overlay representing the targeted region. (*B*) Posttreatment gadolinium chelate–enhanced fat-saturated, T1-weighted axial image shows no residual enhancement in the treated region.

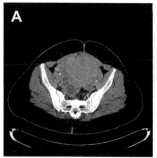
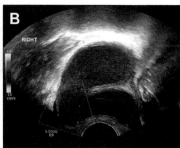

Fig. 9. (A) CT image in the axial plane shows a right pyosalpinx. (B) Transvaginal ultrasonography shows the pyosalpinx. The dotted line indicates the intended needle path. Color Doppler is used to check the needle path and avoid large blood vessel injury. Note the short distance the needle has to travel from the vaginal wall to the pyosalpinx.

the postoperative setting (eg, for benign/malignant gynecologic or colorectal surgery). Drainage of the resulting abscess is used to speed the recovery (**Fig. 10**). Many of these abscesses lie deep in the pelvis and are not accessible to traditional percutaneous routes of access. Alternative routes of access are transgluteal, transvaginal, or transrectal.[76] In general, the transrectal route should

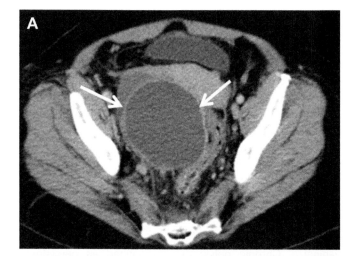

Fig. 10. (A) CT image in the axial plane shows a postappendicectomy pelvic abscess (*arrows*). (B) Transvaginal ultrasonography shows a needle (*arrows*) having been passed into the abscess via the transvaginal route.

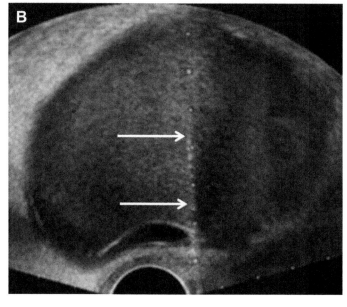

be avoided in gynecologic infections for fear of introducing bowel pathogens into the abscess.[74] The transgluteal route has been well described. However, this can be a painful and poorly tolerated route of access, particularly if a drain is left in place.

Our preference is to offer transvaginal aspiration of the tubal abscess, because of its proximity to vaginal fornix, allowing easy, safe, and quick assess. All patients with an abscess should be established on antibiotic therapy before any aspiration is attempted. Otherwise, there is a risk of causing septic shock. Clotting abnormalities should be corrected before the intervention.

Transvaginal aspiration/drainage

The patient lies in the usual supine position for a transvaginal scan. Stirrups are not needed. A wedge or pillow under the bottom can be helpful. Some authorities advocate vaginal cleansing with povidone-iodine because the vaginal route of access is only semisterile. However, in our practice, the authors have found that use of an antiseptic cream as the probe lubricant is sufficient.[76]

Sedation is not essential and in our practice we have found it is rarely needed. Careful discussion with the woman beforehand and an appropriate reassuring environment usually allow the procedure to take place without undue discomfort.

A transvaginal probe with a needle guide is essential. It should be possible to identify the abscess and to position the probe such that the needle path is only a few millimeters from the vagina to the target. Care needs to be taken to keep intervening structures such as bladder or blood vessels out of the way.[74,77] A long black spinal needle is used to infiltrate local anesthetic into the vaginal wall. Gentle pressure with the transvaginal probe helps to keep the vaginal wall taut and facilitate passage of the needle. Our preference for an aspiration needle is a sheathed 19-gauge needle, in which the sheath has side holes as well as the end hole. Once this needle is placed in the abscess and the inner stylet withdrawn, an assistant can drain the lesion by connecting a syringe via some tubing to the hub of the sheath. If there is more than 1 abscess collection (commonly there are bilateral pyosalpinges), it is reasonable to do a second puncture to the second collection at the same sitting.

On occasion, if the abscess is very large or the material too thick to aspirate down the 19-gauge needle sheath, it may be necessary to upsize to a drain. A wire is passed through the sheath into the collection under ultrasonography vision. Once the wire is in place, the whole transducer, guide, and sheathed needle have to be withdrawn

back over the wire, taking care not to displace it. The rest of the procedure is done by feel. Dilators and then the required drain (usually 8 French is enough) are passed over the wire, taking care to push along the line of the initial needle puncture. This method ensures that the wire does not buckle back out of the abscess.

It is always good practice to try to empty the abscess collection as completely as possible rather than relying on spontaneous drainage through the catheter.

Complications are, theoretically, septic shock, hematoma, hemorrhage, and damage to adjacent organs. However, the literature does not report any of these events in the absence of blood dyscrasias and if antibiotics have been given. The woman will see some blood per vagina after the procedure, which typically spontaneously ceases within 24 hours.[74]

Other pelvic collections Posthysterectomy pelvic hematoma can be substantial and can be managed conservatively, by surgical evacuation or by transvaginal drainage. The latter depends on whether the surgeon has oversewn the vault of the vagina. If not, then the surgeon can reopen the vault at speculum examination. Failing this, the transvaginal ultrasonography-guided drain insertion can be used as described earlier. If a larger drain is required, an alternative technique is to dilate over the wire until a peel-away sheath can be introduced. A Foley balloon catheter can then be placed through the sheath to provide longer-term drainage.

Pelvic Congestion Syndrome

Chronic pelvic pain is defined as persistent, noncyclic pain in the pelvis that lasts longer than 6 months. In the United States there is a 15% prevalence of chronic pelvic pain in women, which accounts for 10% of all outpatient gynecologic visits. The differential diagnosis for pelvic pain is broad and includes gynecologic, genitourinary, gastrointestinal, and musculoskeletal abnormalities.[78] Common causes of pelvic pain include endometriosis, adhesions, adenomyosis, uterine leiomyoma, and inflammatory bowel syndrome. Pelvic congestion syndrome (PCS) is a commonly overlooked condition characterized by pelvic venous congestion that can cause chronic pelvic pain. Typically, patients with PCS are multiparous women of childbearing age with dull and chronic pelvic pain that is exacerbated by menses, heavy activity, and prolonged standing and is associated with dyspareunia. The diagnostic criteria for PCS include pelvic venous distension on imaging coupled with pelvic pain for longer than 6 months. Pelvic venous congestion can be caused by venous insufficiency from valvular incompetence or venous outflow obstruction, as in the case of left renal vein compression by the superior mesenteric artery (ie, Nutcracker syndrome) or left common iliac vein compression by the right common iliac artery (May-Thurner syndrome).[79] It can also be a hormonally mediated process, so treatment options include ovarian-suppression therapy, surgical venous ligation, and endovascular therapy with gonadal vein embolization and/or venous stenting.[80]

Imaging work-up

Although venography remains the gold standard for the diagnosis of PCS, ultrasonography and MR imaging are critical for work-up and procedural planning. Transvaginal gray-scale and Doppler ultrasonography is a dynamic and radiation-free modality with the added advantage that patients can be in the semiupright position and perform Valsalva during imaging to accentuate venous reflux. Ultrasonography finding of dilated tortuous parauterine veins with enlarged diameter more than 4 mm with slow flow (<3 cm/s) is diagnostic (**Fig. 11**). MR imaging is an excellent modality for evaluation of pelvic congestion and ruling out other pelvic causes, and time-resolved MR angiography can show gonadal vein reflux. The diagnostic criteria for MR imaging and CT consist of at least 4 ipsilateral parauterine veins of varying caliber, at least 1 measuring more than 4 mm in diameter, or an ovarian vein diameter greater than 8 mm.[81] CT has a limited role in work-up of PCS because, unlike ultrasonography, MR imaging, and venography, it allows limited assessment of flow rates and reflux.[82]

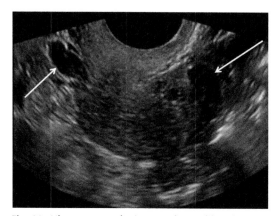

Fig. 11. Ultrasonography images shows dilated parauterine veins (*arrows*) in a woman with PCS.

Gonadal vein embolization

Gonadal vein embolization is performed in an ambulatory setting under moderate sedation or with anesthesia support. Prophylactic antibiotics are administered. The procedure can be performed via an internal jugular vein or common femoral vein approach. The key technical steps of this procedure include venography of gonadal veins and iliac veins to assess for reflux and/or obstruction. Commonly, intravenous ultrasonography is used in addition to venography to evaluate for compression of the renal vein or the left common iliac vein (**Fig. 12**). Once reflux is diagnosed, the incompetent pelvic veins can be sclerosed and the gonadal veins can be embolized with a combination of sclerosant and coils (**Fig. 13**). If obstruction is diagnosed via venography and/or intravenous ultrasonography, a self-expanding stent can be deployed to restore luminal caliber and improve blood flow.

Clinical outcomes The reported clinical success rates of gonadal vein embolization are 60% to 90% in reducing pelvic pain. Although most patients experience improvement in intensity and frequency of symptoms, a few have complete resolution of pelvic pain.[83] Therefore, it is critical to counsel patients in the clinic before the procedure and set realistic expectations with regard to the goal of therapy.

Adverse events Complications from this procedure are rare, occurring at a rate of 0% to 4%, and include thrombophlebitis, nontarget embolization, and coil migration. Postprocedural pain is managed with NSAIDs and a short course of narcotics for break-through relief. Patients should be reevaluated at 3 months in clinic to assess their response to treatment. Patients with severe pain at presentation may take longer to experience benefit from the procedure, and repeat venography and intervention can be considered in patients without improvement after 6 months.[80]

Nonsurgical Management of Pelvic Cysts: Drainage and Sclerosis

Aspiration of simple pelvic cysts is, in general, neither advised nor needed. It is known that the rate of resolution of simple cysts is the same whether treated with watchful waiting or with aspiration. Cysts often recur after aspiration. Endometriomas often recur after drainage and are painful to drain. Malignant cysts should be managed surgically.

There are exceptions to these rules:

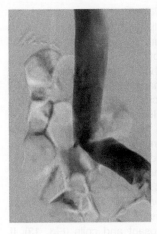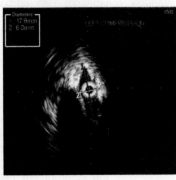

Fig. 12. Venography (*A*) and intravenous ultrasonography (*B*) show external compression of the left common iliac vein by the right common iliac artery in a woman with pelvic congestion syndrome.

1. Symptomatic cysts in women who are too high risk to undergo surgical removal (either because of their comorbidities or because there is a hostile pelvis caused by adhesions)
2. Women in whom it is uncertain whether the cyst is the cause of their symptoms and do not wish to accept surgery until it is proved
3. Women undergoing palliative care looking for respite from the pressure effects of a malignant cyst in the pelvis

The technique of transvaginal aspiration of a cyst is the same as described for drainage of a pelvic collection earlier. Ideally the cyst is emptied as completely as possible. Our experience is that these procedures can be done as an outpatient. The women are warned to expect vaginal bleeding, similar to menstrual loss, and can usually leave the department after half an hour provided they have a companion.

Some authorities recommend the injection of a sclerosant agent into the cyst after it has been aspirated. Agents such as tetracycline or alcohol have been used, with some short-term preliminary results in drainage of endometriomas showing a recurrence rate of only 12%.[84] The technique is to try to replace the aspirated volume with a similar volume of sclerosant, leave it in place for a short period of time, and then reaspirate to dryness. Clearly this is more practical with smaller cysts. The literature reports good results with low levels of recurrence. Our experience has been that the cysts still recur but do so in a complex multiloculated fashion that precludes any further aspiration attempts.

MALIGNANT GYNECOLOGIC DISEASES
Adnexal Masses

Percutaneous biopsy
The management of women with ovarian or peritoneal carcinoma has traditionally been by primary cytoreductive surgery followed by chemotherapy. However, there has been a

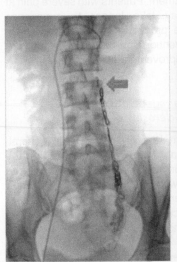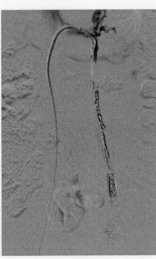

Fig. 13. Left pelvic venous sclerotherapy with coil embolization of the left gonadal vein. Arrows indicate metallic coils in left gonadal vein.

paradigm shift to management with primary chemotherapy followed by interval debulking surgery, which shows the same survival rates but much lower morbidity.[85] In order to give the appropriate primary chemotherapy, it becomes necessary to obtain a biopsy to confirm the tumor type.[86] Peritoneal carcinomatosis may be caused by ovary, breast, colon, appendix, pancreas, and stomach cancers, among others. The treatment of these tumors varies and surgery is contraindicated in some patients. Modern histology techniques, including immunohistochemistry, enable a site-specific diagnosis in more than 93% of biopsies taken.[87]

Seeding of a tumor along the biopsy track or into the peritoneum is a potential risk. However, it is not one that has been quantified despite anecdotal case reports.[88] This perceived risk influences practice. Percutaneous biopsy should not be done in pelvic malignancy unless there is already evidence of spread from the primary tumor.

Omental infiltration or lymph nodes are the commonest targets. The choice of imaging guidance is a matter of the operator's preference. Some radiologists use CT guidance. Our view is that ultrasonography guidance is quicker and more reliable, provided that ultrasonography is able to identify the target.[89] The staging CT or MR imaging scan is invaluable in planning any biopsy. These scans help identify the target with ultrasonography. Time spent in preparation is never wasted when planning a biopsy. The presence of ascites is a benefit when using ultrasonography to biopsy an omental cake. It makes the target and the needle readily visible (Fig. 14).

Studies have shown that needle core biopsy techniques outperform fine-needle aspiration cytology in diagnostic rates without changing the risk of complications.[87] The technique of percutaneous biopsy is common to any other radiological percutaneous biopsy.

Transvaginal biopsy

Transvaginal biopsy is appropriate when there is no percutaneous route of biopsy available.[90] It provides the ability to reach pelvic sidewall masses, vaginal vault masses (Fig. 15), or pelvic peritoneal deposits.

The technique is the same as for transvaginal aspiration described earlier except that, instead of an aspiration needle, a core biopsy needle is used.

Image-guided Endometrial Biopsy

Endometrial biopsy is typically done by gynecologists either with the Pipelle suction technique or at hysteroscopy. However, there are occasions when the gynecologist is unable to access the endometrial cavity; for example, because of a prior trachelectomy, cervical stenosis,[91] or a Manchester repair. Ordinarily, the next step might be to discuss the merits of a diagnostic hysterectomy with the woman. An alternative is to undertake transvaginal ultrasonography-guided access to the endometrial cavity. There are 3 techniques:

1. The indirect guidance method. The radiologist does a transabdominal scan while the gynecologist probes the cervix at speculum examination. This technique can facilitate the gynecologist negotiating a stenosed cervical canal without causing a false track.
2. The direct guidance method. The radiologist does a transvaginal ultrasonography needle-guided puncture to the endocervix that enables passage of a wire through the needle into the endometrial cavity. Once the wire is in place, the track can be dilated and a suction catheter positioned to take a sample (Fig. 16).

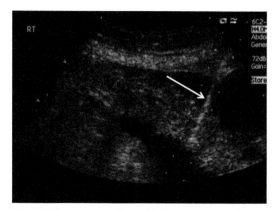

Fig. 14. Ultrasonography-guided percutaneous biopsy of a large omental cake surrounded by ascites in a woman with peritoneal carcinomatosis. Arrow indicates the biopsy needle.

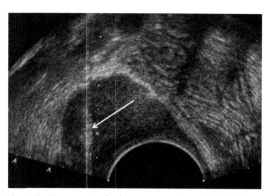

Fig. 15. Transvaginal ultrasonography-guided biopsy of a vaginal vault mass. The needle (arrow) can be seen in the mass.

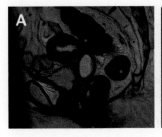
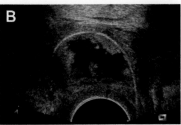

Fig. 16. (A) T2-weighted MR image in the sagittal plane shows distended endometrial cavity with suspected endometrial cancer and distended endocervix. (B) Transvaginal ultrasonography scan shows how a wire has been guided via a transcervical needle into the endometrial cavity to allow subsequent catheter aspiration.

3. The most direct method of obtaining a biopsy of the endometrium is to do a transvaginal guided-needle core biopsy across the myometrium into the endometrium. This technique inevitably runs the risk of contaminating the needle path with tumor and upstaging a tumor that might otherwise be confined to the endometrial cavity.

Brachytherapy Placement in Cervical Cancer

Oncologists are usually able to access the endocervical canal and endometrial cavity to position the applicator without the need for any radiological guidance. Sometimes, the cervical tumor is such that the site and course of the endocervical canal is hidden and it is possible to push the applicator through the tumor and make a false channel. In these instances, transabdominal ultrasonography through a filled bladder can be used to guide the oncologist while sounding the cervix to ensure the applicator is passed into the endometrial canal (**Fig. 17**).

Symptom Control in Gynecologic Malignancy

Intermittent drainage of symptomatic ascites with a fine-bore tube is a well-recognized procedure. An alternative, palliative procedure that allows the patients to manage their ascites themselves at home is to place a tunneled long-term drainage catheter. The concept is similar to the placement of continuous ambulatory peritoneal dialysis catheters. The advantage is that the patients can take control of their own symptoms and quality of life by connecting a drainage bottle to the tubing as and when they wish; the disadvantage is having the

drainage tube present at all times. The long-term tunneled drain can also be placed into a large pelvic cyst when that is the main cause of the recurrent abdominal distension during the palliative care.

The technique is to identify the target for drainage and site of percutaneous access with ultrasonography. This target marks the entry point. An exit point for the tubing from the skin is then identified about 10 cm from the entry point. Usually the exit point from the skin is positioned above (more cephalad to) the entry point. Care is taken to avoid any superficial vessels in this path.

An aseptic technique is used. The procedure is done under local anesthesia. Skin incisions are made at both the entry and exit sites. The long-term tubing is tunneled subcutaneously from the exit to the entry incision. The fibrous cuff on the tubing is positioned under the skin. A needle puncture is made through the entry incision down to the target fluid. A wire is passed through the needle and the track dilated to take a peel-away sheath. The free end of the tubing (currently coming out of the entry skin incision) is passed down the peel-away sheath and the sheath peeled away such that the free end of the tubing no longer protrudes from the entry skin incision but is entirely within the patient and the target fluid. The entry skin incision is then closed with a couple of stitches. A purse-string suture can be placed around the tubing as it comes out through the exit wound.

The risks of placing a long-term drainage tube are the same as for placing a temporary ascitic drain (bleeding and damage to bowel) but also include the added risks of ascitic leakage,

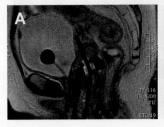
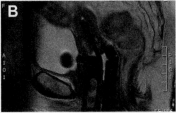

Fig. 17. (A) T2-weighted MR image in the sagittal plane shows a brachytherapy applicator that does not lie within the endometrial cavity. (B) T2-weighted MR image in the sagittal plane following ultrasonography-assisted repositioning of the brachytherapy applicator shows it is now correctly located.

peritoneal infection, and the tubing ceasing to be effective if it becomes blocked or walled off from the rest of the fluid.[92,93]

SUMMARY

There are many ways in which radiology can help in the diagnosis and management of female pelvic conditions. Applying well-known general techniques to specific gynecologic problems or remembering the endoluminal route of access to the pelvis is of the essence.

DISCLOSURE

M. Weston, S. Pierre, P. Soyer, M. Barral, and A. Dohan have nothing to disclose in relation to this article. M.P. Kohli disclosures: advisory committee for Boston Scientific, Medtronic, Philips; consulting for Medtronic, Cook, Boston Scientific, Philips, and Penumbra.

REFERENCES

1. Centers for Disease Control and Prevention. Infertility: key statistics from the national survey of family growth 2011-2015. Available at: https://www.cdc.gov/nchs/fastats/infertility.htm.
2. Steinkeler JA, Woodfield CA, Lazarus E, et al. Female infertility: a systematic approach to radiologic imaging and diagnosis. Radiographics 2009;29(5):1353–70.
3. Al-Omari MH, Obeidat N, Elheis M, et al. Factors affecting pregnancy rate following fallopian tube recanalization in women with proximal fallopian tube obstruction. J Clin Med 2018;7(5) [pii:E110].
4. Papaioannou S. A hypothesis for the pathogenesis and natural history of proximal tubal blockage. Hum Reprod 2004;19:481–5.
5. Lopera J, Suri R, Kroma GM, et al. Role of interventional procedures in obstetrics/gynecology. Radiol Clin North Am 2013;51:1049–66.
6. Thurmond AS. Fallopian tube catheterization. Semin Intervent Radiol 2008;25(4):425–31.
7. Thurmond AS. Fallopian tube catheterization. Semin Intervent Radiol 2013;30(4):381–7.
8. Dreyer K, Van Rijswijk J, Mijatovic V, et al. Oil-based or water-based contrast for hysterosalpingography in infertile women. N Engl J Med 2017;376(21):2043–52.
9. Hedgpeth PL, Thurmond AS, Fry R, et al. Radiographic fallopian tube recanalization: absorbed ovarian radiation dose. Radiology 1991;180(1):121–2.
10. Perisinakis K, Damilakis J, Grammatikakis J, et al. Radiogenic risks from hysterosalpingography. Eur Radiol 2003;13(7):1522–8.
11. Pelage JP, Le Dref O, Jacob D, et al. Selective arterial embolization of the uterine arteries in the management of intractable post-partum hemorrhage. Acta Obstet Gynecol Scand 1999;78(8):698–703.
12. Pelage JP, Le Dref O, Mateo J, et al. Life-threatening primary postpartum hemorrhage: treatment with emergency selective arterial embolization. Radiology 1998;208(2):359–62.
13. Pelage JP, Soyer P, Repiquet D, et al. Secondary postpartum hemorrhage: treatment with selective arterial embolization. Radiology 1999;212(2):385–9.
14. Sierra A, Burrel M, Sebastia C, et al. Utility of multidetector CT in severe postpartum hemorrhage. Radiographics 2012;32(5):1463–81.
15. Soyer P, Fargeaudou Y, Morel O, et al. Severe postpartum haemorrhage from ruptured pseudoaneurysm: successful treatment with transcatheter arterial embolization. Eur Radiol 2008;18(6):1181–7.
16. Soyer P, Dohan A, Dautry R, et al. Transcatheter arterial embolization for postpartum hemorrhage: indications, technique, results, and complications. Cardiovasc Intervent Radiol 2015;38(5):1068–81.
17. Dohan A, Soyer P, Subhani A, et al. Postpartum hemorrhage resulting from pelvic pseudoaneurysm: a retrospective analysis of 588 consecutive cases treated by arterial embolization. Cardiovasc Intervent Radiol 2013;36(5):1247–55.
18. Poujade O, Zappa M, Letendre I, et al. Predictive factors for failure of pelvic arterial embolization for postpartum hemorrhage. Int J Gynaecol Obstet 2012;117(2):119–23.
19. Doumouchtsis SK, Papageorghiou AT, Arulkumaran S. Systematic review of conservative management of postpartum hemorrhage: what to do when medical treatment fails. Obstet Gynecol Surv 2007;62(8):540–7.
20. Kim YJ, Yoon CJ, Seong NJ, et al. Failed pelvic arterial embolization for postpartum hemorrhage: clinical outcomes and predictive factors. J Vasc Interv Radiol 2013;24(5):703–9.
21. Lee HY, Shin JH, Kim J, et al. Primary postpartum hemorrhage: outcome of pelvic arterial embolization in 251 patients at a single institution. Radiology 2012;264(3):903–9.
22. Cheong JY, Kong TW, Son JH, et al. Outcome of pelvic arterial embolization for postpartum hemorrhage: a retrospective review of 117 cases. Obstet Gynecol Sci 2014;57(1):17–27.
23. Park JK, Shin TB, Baek JC, et al. Failure of uterine artery embolization for controlling postpartum hemorrhage. J Obstet Gynaecol Res 2011;37(8):971–8.
24. Kirby JM, Kachura JR, Rajan DK, et al. Arterial embolization for primary postpartum hemorrhage. J Vasc Interv Radiol 2009;20(8):1036–45.
25. Sentilhes L, Gromez A, Clavier E, et al. Predictors of failed pelvic arterial embolization for severe postpartum hemorrhage. Obstet Gynecol 2009;113(5):992–9.

26. Poujade O, Ceccaldi PF, Davitian C, et al. Uterine necrosis following pelvic arterial embolization for post-partum hemorrhage: review of the literature. Eur J Obstet Gynecol Reprod Biol 2013;170(2): 309–14.

27. La Folie T, Vidal V, Mehanna M, et al. Results of endovascular treatment in cases of abnormal placentation with post-partum hemorrhage. J Obstet Gynaecol Res 2007;33(5):624–30.

28. Gilbert WM, Moore TR, Resnik R, et al. Angiographic embolization in the management of hemorrhagic complications of pregnancy. Am J Obstet Gynecol 1992;166(2):493–7.

29. Dohan A, Pelage JP, Soyer P. How to avoid uterine necrosis after arterial embolization for post-partum hemorrhage: a proposal based on a single center experience of 600 cases. Eur J Obstet Gynecol Reprod Biol 2013;171(2):392–3.

30. Leleup G, Fohlen A, Dohan A, et al. Value of round ligament artery embolization in the management of postpartum hemorrhage. J Vasc Interv Radiol 2017;28(5):696–701.

31. Allen L, Jauniaux E, Hobson S, et al, for the FIGO Placenta Accreta Diagnosis and Management Expert Consensus Panel. FIGO consensus guidelines on placenta accreta spectrum disorders: nonconservative surgical management. Int J Gynaecol Obstet 2018;140(3):281–90.

32. Sentilhes L, Kayem G, Chandraharan E, et al, for the FIGO Placenta Accreta Diagnosis and Management Expert Consensus Panel. FIGO consensus guidelines on placenta accreta spectrum disorders: conservative management. Int J Gynaecol Obstet 2018;140(3):291–8.

33. Soyer P, Morel O, Fargeaudou Y, et al. Value of pelvic embolization in the management of severe postpartum hemorrhage due to placenta accreta, increta or percreta. Eur J Radiol 2011;80(3):729–35.

34. Hwang SM, Jeon GS, Kim MD, et al. Transcatheter arterial embolisation for the management of obstetric haemorrhage associated with placental abnormality in 40 cases. Eur Radiol 2013;23(3):766–73.

35. Petrov DA, Karlberg B, Singh K, et al. Perioperative internal iliac artery balloon occlusion, in the setting of placenta accreta and its variants: the role of the interventional radiologist. Curr Probl Diagn Radiol 2018;47(6):445–51.

36. Dilauro MD, Dason S, Athreya S. Prophylactic balloon occlusion of internal iliac arteries in women with placenta accreta: literature review and analysis. Clin Radiol 2012;67(6):515–20.

37. Morel O, Malartic C, Muhlstein J, et al. Pelvic arterial ligations for severe post-partum hemorrhage: indications and techniques. J Visc Surg 2011;148(2): e95–102.

38. Mei J, Wang Y, Zou B, et al. Systematic review of uterus-preserving treatment modalities for abnormally invasive placenta. J Obstet Gynaecol 2015;35(8): 777–82.

39. Hequet D, Morel O, Soyer P, et al. Delayed hysteroscopic resection of retained tissues and uterine conservation after conservative treatment for placenta accreta. Aust N Z J Obstet Gynaecol 2013;53(6): 580–3.

40. Soyer P, Sirol M, Fargeaudou Y, et al. Placental vascularity and resorption delay after conservative management of invasive placenta: MR imaging evaluation. Eur Radiol 2013;23(1):262–71.

41. Izbizky, Meller C, Grasso M, et al. Feasibility and safety of prophylactic uterine artery catheterization and embolization in the management of placenta accreta. J Vasc Interv Radiol 2015;26(2):162–9.

42. Chou MM, Hwang JI, Tseng JJ, et al. Internal iliac artery embolization before hysterectomy for placenta accreta. J Vasc Interv Radiol 2003;14(9 Pt 1): 1195–9.

43. D'Souza DL, Kingdom JC, Amsalem H, et al. Conservative management of invasive placenta using combined prophylactic internal iliac artery balloon occlusion and immediate postoperative uterine artery embolization. Can Assoc Radiol J 2015;66(2): 179–84.

44. Bouvier A, Sentilhes L, Thouveny F, et al. Planned caesarean in the interventional radiology cath lab to enable immediate uterine artery embolization for the conservative treatment of placenta accreta. Clin Radiol 2012;67(11):1089–94.

45. Yu PC, Ou HY, Tsang LL, et al. Prophylactic intraoperative uterine artery embolization to control hemorrhage in abnormal placentation during late gestation. Fertil Steril 2009;91(5):1951–5.

46. Meller C, Grasso M, Velazco A, et al. Feasibility and safety of prophylactic uterine artery catheterization and embolization in the management of placenta accreta. J Vasc Interv Radiol 2015;26(2):162–9.

47. Sivan E, Spira M, Achiron R, et al. Prophylactic pelvic artery catheterization and embolization in women with placenta accreta: can it prevent cesarean hysterectomy? Am J Perinatol 2010;27(6):455–61.

48. Tan CH, Tay KH, Sheah K, et al. Perioperative endovascular internal iliac artery occlusion balloon placement in management of placenta accreta. AJR Am J Roentgenol 2007;189(5):1158–63.

49. Salim R, Chulski A, Romano S, et al. Precesarean prophylactic balloon catheters for suspected placenta accreta: a randomized controlled trial. Obstet Gynecol 2015;126(5):1022–8.

50. Angstmann T, Gard G, Harrington T, et al. Surgical management of placenta accreta: a cohort series and suggested approach. Am J Obstet Gynecol 2010;202(1):38.e1-9.

51. Ballas J, Hull AD, Saenz C, et al. Preoperative intravascular balloon catheters and surgical outcomes in pregnancies complicated by placenta accreta: a

management paradox. Am J Obstet Gynecol 2012; 207(3):216.e1-5.

52. Shrivastava V, Nageotte M, Major C, et al. Case-control comparison of cesarean hysterectomy with and without prophylactic placement of intravascular balloon catheters for placenta accreta. Am J Obstet Gynecol 2007;197(4):402.e1-5.

53. Patel SJ, Reede DL, Katz DS, et al. Imaging the pregnant patient for nonobstetric conditions: algorithms and radiation dose considerations. Radiographics 2007;27(6):1705–22.

54. Barral M, Dautry R, Foucher R, et al. Combined transarterial and transvenous embolization of a ruptured utero-ovarian arteriovenous malformation with ethylene vinyl alcohol copolymer (Onyx®). Diagn Interv Imaging 2018;99(6):417–9.

55. Timor-Tritsch IE, Haynes MC, Monteagudo A, et al. Ultrasound diagnosis and management of acquired uterine enhanced myometrial vascularity/arteriovenous malformations. Am J Obstet Gynecol 2016; 214(6):731.e1-10.

56. Hugues C, Le Bras Y, Coatleven F, et al. Vascular uterine abnormalities: comparison of imaging findings and clinical outcomes. Eur J Radiol 2015; 84(12):2485–91.

57. Picel AC, Koo SJ, Roberts AC. Transcatheter arterial embolization with n-butyl cyanoacrylate for the treatment of acquired uterine vascular malformations. Cardiovasc Intervent Radiol 2016;39(8):1170–6.

58. Pinto I, Chimeno P, Romo A, et al. Uterine fibroids: uterine artery embolization versus abdominal hysterectomy for treatment–a prospective, randomized, and controlled clinical trial. Radiology 2003;226(2): 425–31.

59. Hehenkamp WJ, Volkers NA, Donderwinkel PF, et al. Uterine artery embolization versus hysterectomy in the treatment of symptomatic uterine fibroids (EMMY trial): peri- and postprocedural results from a randomized controlled trial. Am J Obstet Gynecol 2005;193(5):1618–29.

60. Malartic C, Morel O, Fargeaudou Y, et al. Conservative two-step procedure including uterine artery embolization with embosphere and surgical myomectomy for the treatment of multiple fibroids: preliminary experience. Eur J Radiol 2012;81(1):1–5.

61. Morris CS. Update on uterine artery embolization for symptomatic fibroid disease (uterine artery embolization). Abdom Imaging 2008;33(1):104–11.

62. Deshmukh SP, Gonsalves CF, Guglielmo FF, et al. Role of MR imaging of uterine leiomyomas before and after embolization. Radiographics 2012;32(6):E251–81.

63. Malartic C, Morel O, Rivain AL, et al. Evaluation of symptomatic uterine fibroids in candidates for uterine artery embolization: comparison between ultrasonographic and MR imaging findings in 68 consecutive patients. Clin Imaging 2013;37(1): 83–90.

64. Sutter O, Soyer P, Shotar E, et al. Diffusion-weighted MR imaging of uterine leiomyomas following uterine artery embolization. Eur Radiol 2016;26(10): 3558–70.

65. Pelage JP, Cazejust J, Pluot E, et al. Uterine fibroid vascularization and clinical relevance to uterine fibroid embolization. Radiographics 2005;25(Suppl 1):S99–117.

66. Pelage JP, Le Dref O, Beregi JP, et al. Limited uterine artery embolization with tris-acryl gelatin microspheres for uterine fibroids. J Vasc Interv Radiol 2003;14(1):15–20.

67. Sridhar D, Kohi MP. Updates on MR-guided focused ultrasound for symptomatic uterine fibroids. Semin Intervent Radiol 2018;35(1):17–22.

68. Roberts A. Magnetic resonance-guided focused ultrasound for uterine fibroids. Semin Intervent Radiol 2008;25(4):394–405.

69. Funaki K, Fukunishi H, Funaki T, et al. Magnetic resonance-guided focused ultrasound surgery for uterine fibroids: relationship between the therapeutic effects and signal intensity of preexisting T2-weighted magnetic resonance images. Am J Obstet Gynecol 2007;196(2):184.e1-6.

70. Coakley FV, Foster BR, Farsad K, et al. Pelvic applications of MR-guided high intensity focused ultrasound. Abdom Imaging 2013;38(5):1120–9.

71. Silberzweig JE, Powell DK, Matsumoto AH, et al. Management of uterine fibroids: a focus on uterine-sparing interventional techniques. Radiology 2016; 280(3):675–92.

72. Gorny KR, Borah BJ, Brown DL, et al. Incidence of additional treatments in women treated with MR-guided focused US for symptomatic uterine fibroids: review of 138 patients with an average follow-up of 2.8 years. J Vasc Interv Radiol 2014;25(10): 1506–12.

73. Laughlin-Tommaso S, Barnard EP, AbdElmagied AM, et al. FIRSTT study: randomized controlled trial of uterine artery embolization vs focused ultrasound surgery. Am J Obstet Gynecol 2019;220(2):174.e1-13.

74. Weston MJ. Gynaecological intervention techniques. In: Allan PL, Baxter GM, Weston MJ, editors. Clinical ultrasound. Chapter 37. 3rd edition. London: Churchill Livingstone; 2011. p. 720–8.

75. McNeeley SG, Hendrix SL, Mazzoni MM, et al. Medically sound, cost-effective treatment for pelvic inflammatory disease and tuboovarian abscess. Am J Obstet Gynecol 1998;178(6):1272–8.

76. Ryan RS, McGrath F, Haslam PJ, et al. Ultrasound-guided endocavitary drainage of pelvic abscesses: technique, results and complications. Clin Radiol 2003;58(1):75–9.

77. O'Neill MJ, Rafferty EA, Lee SI, et al. Transvaginal interventional procedures: aspiration, biopsy, and catheter drainage. Radiographics 2001;21(3): 657–72.

78. Carter JE. A systematic history for the patient with chronic pelvic pain. JSLS 1999;3(4):245–52.

79. Molière S, Rotaru-Hincu N. Pelvic hematoma due to spontaneous left iliac vein rupture in May-Thurner syndrome. Diagn Interv Imaging 2020;101(1):55–6.

80. Durham JD, Machan L. Pelvic congestion syndrome. Semin Intervent Radiol 2013;30(4):372–80.

81. Coakley FV, Varghese SL, Hricak H. CT and MRI of pelvic varices in women. J Comput Assist Tomogr 1999;23(3):429–43.

82. Knuttinen MG, Xie K, Jani A, et al. Pelvic venous insufficiency: imaging diagnosis, treatment approaches, and therapeutic issues. AJR Am J Roentgenol 2015;204(2):448–58.

83. Lopez AJ. Female pelvic vein embolization: indications, techniques, and outcomes. Cardiovasc Intervent Radiol 2015;38(4):804–20.

84. García-Tejedor A, Castellarnau M, Ponce J, et al. Ethanol sclerotherapy of ovarian endometrioma: a safe and effective minimal invasive procedure. preliminary results. Eur J Obstet Gynecol Reprod Biol 2015;187:25–9.

85. Kobal B, Noventa M, Cvjeticanin B, et al. Primary debulking surgery versus primary neoadjuvant chemotherapy for high grade advanced stage ovarian cancer: comparison of survivals. Radiol Oncol 2018;52(3):307–19.

86. Hewitt M, Anderson K, Hall G, et al. Women with peritoneal carcinomatosis of unknown origin: efficacy of image-guided biopsy to determine site-specific diagnosis. BJOG 2006;114(1):46–50.

87. Spencer JA, Swift SE, Wilkinson N, et al. Peritoneal carcinomatosis: image-guided peritoneal core biopsy for tumor type and patient care. Radiology 2001;221(1):173–7.

88. Morris J, Weston MJ. Ultrasound guided intervention in gynaecology: a review. BMUS Bulletin 1998;6(1):26–9.

89. Yarram SG, Nghiem HV, Higgins E, et al. Evaluation of imaging-guided core biopsy of pelvic masses. AJR Am J Roentgenol 2007;188(5):1208–11.

90. Dadayal G, Weston M, Young A, et al. Transvaginal ultrasound (TVUS)-guided biopsy is safe and effective in diagnosing peritoneal carcinomatosis and recurrent pelvic malignancy. Clin Radiol 2016;71(11):1184–92.

91. Hammoud AO, Deppe G, Elkhechen SS, et al. Ultrasonography-guided transvaginal endometrial biopsy: a useful technique in patients with cervical stenosis. Obstet Gynecol 2006;107(2 Pt 2):518–20.

92. Stukan M. Drainage of malignant ascites: patient selection and perspectives. Cancer Manag Res 2017;12(9):115–30.

93. Fleming ND, Alvarez-Secord A, Von Gruenigen V, et al. Indwelling catheters for the management of refractory malignant ascites: a systematic literature overview and retrospective chart review. J Pain Symptom Manage 2009;38(3):341–9.

Printed and bound by CPI Group (UK) Ltd, Croydon, CR0 4YY

08/05/2025

01864745-0014